THE KIDNEY

THE KIDNEY

*An Outline of Normal and Abnormal
Structure and Function*

By

H. E. de WARDENER

M.B.E., M.D., F.R.C.P.

*Professor of Medicine in the University of London
(Charing Cross Hospital Medical School)*

FOURTH EDITION

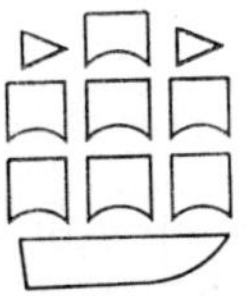

CHURCHILL LIVINGSTONE

EDINBURGH AND LONDON

1973

To

B. E. MILES

P. J. LITTLE

E. M. CLARKSON

and

R. W. SCHRIER

First Edition	.	.	.	.	*1958*
Reprinted .	.	.	.	.	*1960*
Translated into Spanish		.	.	.	*1960*
Translated into Portuguese		.	.	.	*1961*
Second Edition	.	.	.	.	*1961*
Translated into Greek .		.	.	.	*1962*
Reprinted .	.	.	.	.	*1963*
Third Edition	.	.	.	.	*1967*
Reprinted .	.	.	.	.	*1969*
Translated into Japanese		.	.	.	*1969*
Fourth Edition	.	.	.	.	*1973*

PREFACE TO THE FOURTH EDITION

SINCE the third edition there have been many important developments in nephrology. Among those that have made me make substantial changes in this edition are (1) the use of immunofluorescent immunoglobulins in the elucidation of immunological mechanisms, and in the examination of renal biopsies; (2) the identification of increasing numbers of histological lesions in immunological diseases of the kidneys; (3) the increasing accumulation of knowledge about calcium, phosphorus and nitrogen metabolism in chronic renal failure: (4) the increase in knowledge about the control of sodium reabsorption, and the relation of sodium metabolism to hypertension in renal failure; (5) the results of maintenance dialysis and renal transplantation; (6) the ubiquity of phenacetin nephropathy; and (7) the usefulness of a suprapubic aspiration of urine and the localisation of the site of infection in urinary infections. I have therefore had to rewrite many chapters while trying to prevent the book from becoming longer. This has not been easy. For instance the description of glomerular nephritis from the clinical point of view is becoming increasingly difficult. It is now impossible to simplify the correlation between the various overlapping clinical syndromes and the now increasingly precise histological findings without a gross distortion of known accepted facts. The section on immunological disturbances of the kidney has therefore grown substantially. I am most grateful to Dr. Liliane Morel Maroger for her invaluable advice in rewriting this part of the book.

I am indebted to Miss Josephine Storey and Mrs. C. Hobbs for their help with the manuscript and to Mrs. A. Besterman for the 22 new figures which she drew.

London

H. E. de W.

1973

PREFACE TO THE FIRST EDITION

THE purpose of this book is to present an outline of renal structure and function of the normal and diseased kidney. It is intended for students, but I hope it may also be useful to others who wish to know more about the subject.

At the beginning there is a short description of normal structure and function; and the methods used to obtain information about each are discussed. There then follows a description of the four main syndromes which occur in renal disease, i.e. the nephrotic syndrome, acute renal failure, chronic renal failure, and the acute nephritic syndrome; there is also a section on the relationship between disturbances of renal function and electrolyte disorders. The second half of the book consists principally of an account of renal diseases, including the renal manifestations of some generalised diseases. These are discussed in terms of the patterns of functional disturbance which have been described in the previous sections. Unless, therefore, the reader is already familiar with the subject it is best that he should start at the beginning or at least read the sections on the four syndromes and electrolyte disturbances before those on specific renal disorders.

For the sake of clarity, I have to confess that I have over-simplified many controversial subjects and in some instances given only one explanation where several exist. I have not attempted a comprehensive classification of renal disease, for in the present state of knowledge I doubt whether it is possible to arrive at a classification whose subdivisions are at the same time mutually exclusive and collectively exhaustive. Renal tuberculosis, hydronephrosis, calculi, renal tumours and certain other predominantly surgical conditions have been excluded.

I am indebted to the many workers and writers who have preceded me and I should like particularly to mention the following sources of information: Homer Smith's textbooks of renal physiology; A. C. Allen's histological textbook, "The Kidney"; A. M. Fishberg's "Hypertension and Nephritis"; T. Addis' "Glomerular Nephritis"; R. W. Lippman's "Urine and the Urinary Sediment"; G. W. Pickering's "High Blood Pressure"; as a guide to more detailed reading there is a list of references at the end of each section.

I am grateful to Drs. B. E. Miles, R. R. McSwiney, D. M. Nutbourne, F. del Greco, R. D. Grainger, A. Herxheimer, Mr. K. E. D. Shuttleworth, Mr. R. D. de Vere, and Miss I. Maureen Young for their generous help with the manuscript and for giving me the benefit of their advice. I am also indebted to Drs. A. C. Dornhorst and M. S. R. Hutt, and Mr. M.Williams for their most helpful comments and for scrutinising the proofs. I wish to thank Miss J. Dewe and Miss P. Leicester for the patience and care with which they drew Figs. 1, 2, 4, 5, 6, 71 to 74, and Figs. 51, 53 to 60, and 68, respectively; and Mr. A. L. Wooding and Mr. B. Kentish for the photographs of the figures. I am also glad to acknowledge the help of Mr. F. A. Tubbs, Miss M. E. Warner, Miss M. Matthews and Miss M. Studart in checking the references, and that of Miss J. Buchanan for her investigations on may behalf.

I am indebted to Drs. W. J. Griffiths, R. R. McSwiney, J. R. Colley and W. W. Holland for Figs. 9 and 38.

H. E. de W.

London

CONTENTS

1

Structure of the Kidney

A KIDNEY contains about 1,000,000 nephrons. Each nephron is a thin tube approximately 20–50 μ wide and 50 mm long with one end closed and the other opening into a collecting duct. The total length of the tubules in the two kidneys is about 70 miles, or more than the distance between London and Brighton. The blind upper end of each nephron lies in the cortex, invaginated and expanded by a cluster of capillaries (the glomerulus); next to the glomerulus the tube is coiled into a compact mass (the proximal tubule); it then plunges straight towards the hilum of the kidney, sometimes reaching into the medulla

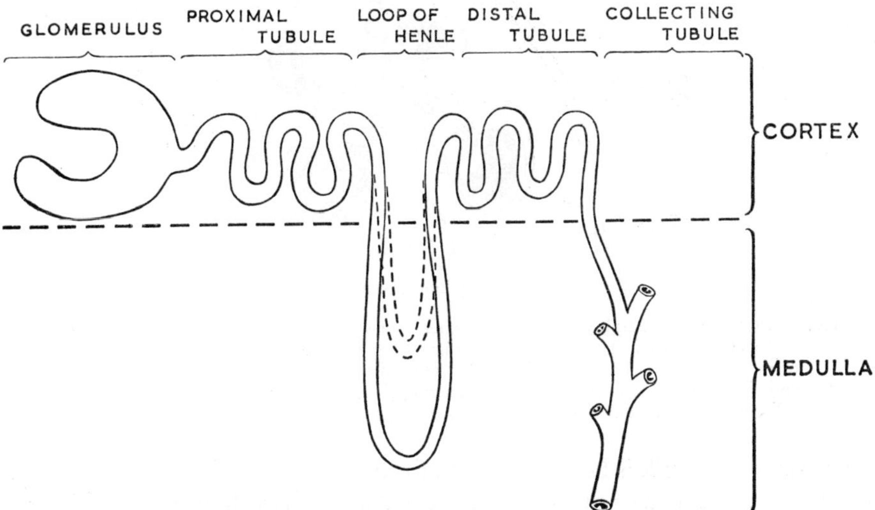

FIG. 1.1. Schema of the structure of a nephron and its distribution between the cortex and medulla.

for a variable distance; it turns back in a tight hairpin bend (the loop of Henle) and once again lies in a coil (the distal tubule) next to its own glomerulus. Finally, it straightens out and together with several other distal tubules joins a collecting duct, either in or near the medulla. Several collecting ducts join together and empty their contents into larger tubes called the papillary ducts which open directly on the surface of the papillae (Fig. 1.1). The proximal tubules of the nephrons which lie in the superficial parts of the cortex are half the length of the proximal tubules of the nephrons which lie more deeply. There are approximately four long nephrons to one short nephron.

Most of the proximal and distal tubules lie in the cortex, while the loops of Henle and the collecting ducts form the bulk of the medulla.

Glomerular Structure

The glomerulus is composed of 4–6 capillary loops which spring from the afferent arteriole and end in the efferent arteriole; they lie within a space whose peripheral wall is known as the glomerular capsule (or Bowman's capsule). This cluster of capillaries shares a central stalk of mesangial cells (Fig. 1.2). The

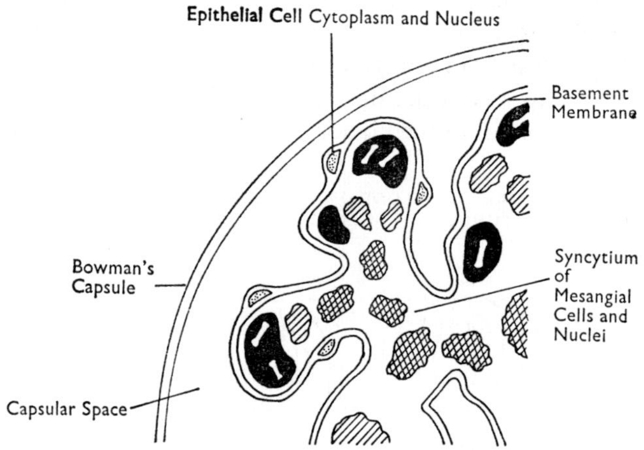

FIG. 1.2. Glomerulus. High magnification schema of a portion of the glomerulus to show that the lumens of the glomerular capillaries are situated at the periphery of a group of mesangial cells. The inner surface of the capillary is formed from a prolongation of endothelial cell cytoplasm while the peripheral outer surface is covered by epithelial cell cytoplasm; basement membrane lies between.

outer part of the stalk is hollowed out to form the lumens of the capillary loop. The total surface area of the glomerular capillaries of two human adult kidneys is about 1·5 square metres. The wall of each capillary loop consists of a sandwich of epithelial cell cytoplasm, basement membrane and endothelial cell cytoplasm. The endothelial cell nuclei can only be distinguished from the mesangial cell nuclei by electron microscopy. The mesangial cell is of mesenchymal origin. In normal circumstances it gives rise to the endothelial cells.

Electron microscopy reveals that the cytoplasm of the epithelial cells is divided into numerous thin extensions which lie in contact with the basement membrane covering the capillary loops (Fig. 1.3). The surface of the loops is therefore covered by a large number of interdigitating "foot" processes. Between these processes there is a thin (70 Å) membrane of epithelial cytoplasm. Similarly, the cytoplasm of the endothelial cells, where it forms the inner surface of the capillary loop has round punched out areas approximately 600 Å wide where the thickness of the cytoplasm is also about 70 Å. The basement membrane has a thickness of 800 Å. Glomerular filtrate has therefore to pass not only through the basement membrane but also through thin layers of both epithelial and endothelial cytoplasm. The basement membrane has a homogeneous marzipan–like structure. The mesangial cells have walls which can only be detected by electron microscopy. Between the mesangial cells there lies mesangial matrix which consists of a homogeneous ground substance in which is embedded fine fibres, similar to, but not identical to basement membrane. The matrix appears

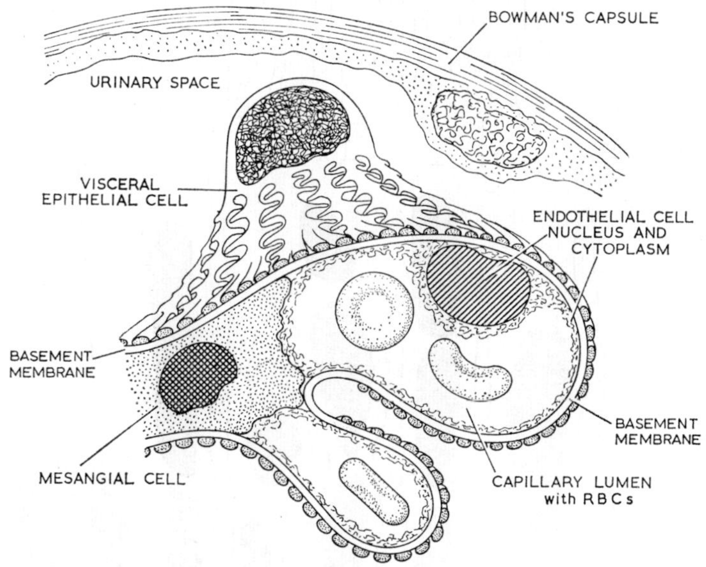

FIG.. 1.3 Glomerular capillary loop. Schema of the electron microscopy appearances.

to be manufactured by the mesangial cells. In normal kidneys there are only small quantities of matrix present.

It is also noticeable that there is no basement membrane between the perforated cytoplasm of the endothelium cell and the cytoplasm of the mesangial cell. The lumen of the capillary and the blood that it contains are therefore in contact with the cytoplasm of the mesangial cell. These dispositions are of some importance when considering the structural abnormalities that take place when the kidney is diseased. In some diseases the mesangial cells may multiply, large masses of mesangial cell cytoplasm may be formed and the mesangial cells may give rise to fibrocytic cells and collagen. It is possible that such mesangial changes are due to abnormal substances travelling directly from the lumen of the capillary into the mesangial cell cytoplasm.

Structure of the Tubule

The outer surface of the nephron is covered by a continuous layer of basement membrane. The proximal tubule is composed of irregularly cuboidal cells with coarse granular cytoplasm and ragged inner margins (the brush border). The cells of the descending thin limb of the loops of Henle are extremely thin and flat and have clear cytoplasm, whereas about two-thirds of the ascending

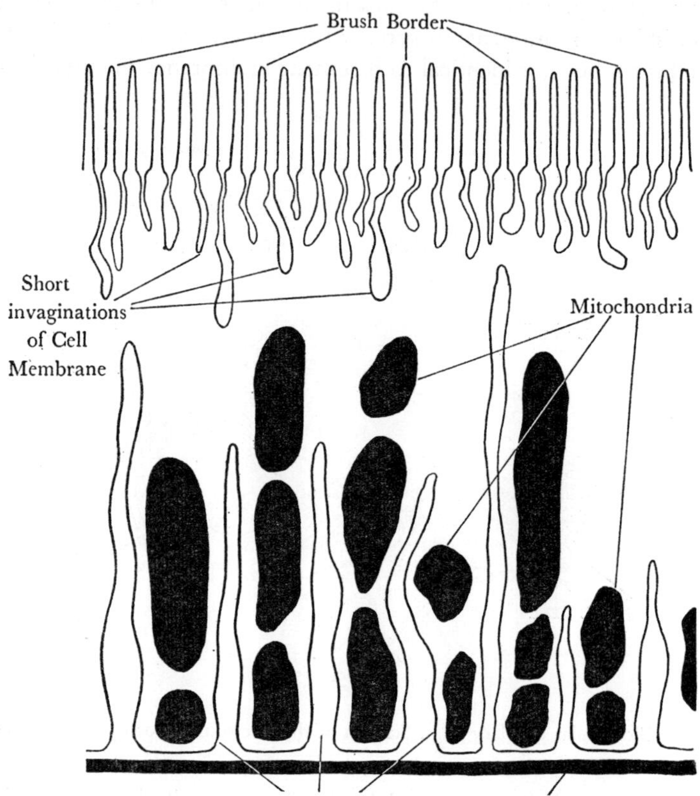

Fig. 1.4. Tubule. Schema of the electron microscopy appearances of a proximal tubule cell; the nucleus has been omitted.

limb is composed of cuboidal cells and is known as the thick part of the ascending limb. The length of the loops varies greatly; those that originate from glomeruli near the cortico-medullary junction are the longest and penetrate deeply into the medulla. The cells of the distal tubules are cuboidal but they are smaller than those in the proximal tubules; they have clear cytoplasm and sharp margins.

With the electron microscope the brush border of the proximal tubule cells is seen to consist of multiple projections of cell cytoplasm about $1\,\mu$ long covered by surface membrane. Between these projections invaginations of the surface membrane penetrate into the cell cytoplasm and extend towards the mitochondria. These projections and invaginations increase enormously the area of contact between the tubular fluid and the contents of the cells. The membrane of the surface which lies next to the peritubular venous capillaries is also invaginated into a number of pockets which lie between the basal mitochondria (Fig. 1.4). The cells of the distal tubules can readily be distinguished from those found in the proximal or collecting tubule, but it has been shown that cells with the appearances of those found in the distal tubule extend down into the collecting tubules. This is in keeping with the fact that some of the functions which are characteristic of the distal tubule also take place in the collecting tubule.

Lobules and Lobes

The nephrons are arranged in bundles called lobules. Each bundle is not unlike a mushroom. The renal cortex, consisting of glomeruli, proximal and distal tubules are the expanded overlapping head of the mushroom, while the medulla and papilla which contain the loops of Henle and collecting ducts are the stalk. The kidney consists therefore of a collection of mushroom like lobules closely apposed to each other. The "head" of each lobule lies just under the renal capsule, its sides dipping down away from the capsule. In other words the renal cortex lies not only on the surface of the kidney but at intervals, it also extends a short distance away from the capsule towards the renal pelvis. This is very obvious on a good intravenous pyelogram when the opacified cortex appears as an arcade. The lobules are themselves grouped into multiples called lobes.

Cortico-medullary Junction

At the junction of the cortex with the medulla there is a thick, wide-meshed fibrous net to which the renal pelvis is attached and through which the medulla and pyramids project. The vessels and lymphatic channels lie outside the lumen of the pelvis and have to travel up to the cortico-medullary junction before they can enter into the renal parenchyma.

Renal Vasculature

About 26 per cent of kidneys have multiple renal arteries, i.e. they have an artery arising from the aorta or the iliac artery in addition to the main renal artery. The renal artery divides into five segmental arteries (Fig. 1.5). It is important to note that, apart from the two poles, separate arteries supply the anterior and posterior surface of the kidney. In an ordinary antero-posterior view therefore angiography will reveal abnormalities of the arterial supply of the two poles, but isolated lesions of the arteries to the rest of the kidney may be obscured by overlying kidney substance to which the arterial supply is normal. The segmental arteries divide into interlobar arteries which, at the

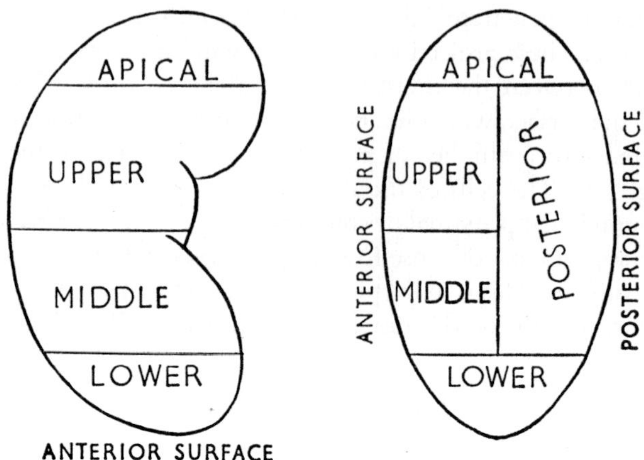

FIG. 1.5. Segmental distribution of renal arterial supply.

corticomedullary junction divide into the arcuate arteries. Contrary to original descriptions, these are only linked together by capillary connections (Fig. 1.6). The intralobular arteries branch off at right angles to the arcuate arteries, and penetrate straight into the cortex, where they give rise to short afferent glom-

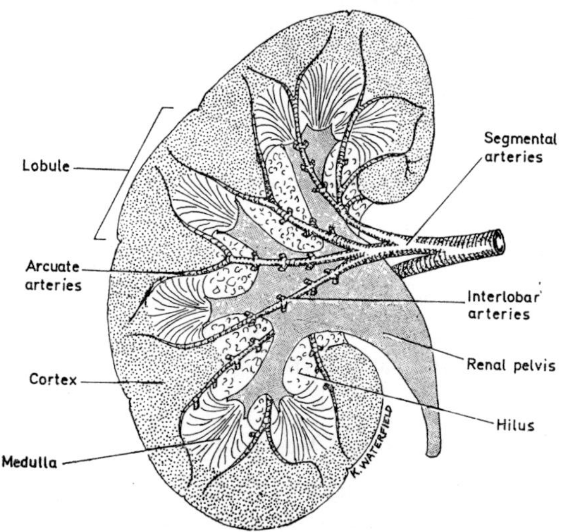

FIG. 1.6. Renal blood supply related to renal lobes.

erular arterioles, so that even the most distal glomerulus receives its afferent arteriole direct from a relatively large artery. The smooth muscle of the afferent arteriole ceases as the arteriole joins the area of the juxtaglomerular apparatus. Beyond the glomerulus the blood flows into the efferent arteriole and then into a capacious intercommunicating plexus of capillaries situated between the tubules (the peritubular venous capillaries) which empties into the intralobular veins (Fig. 1.7). The endothelial cytoplasm of the peritubular venous capillaries has the same electronmicroscopic appearance as that of the endothelial cells in the glomerular capillaries. It contains multiple round areas approximately 600 Å wide in which the thickness of the cytoplasm is reduced to 70 Å, an arrangement which must facilitate the transport of substances to and from the blood.

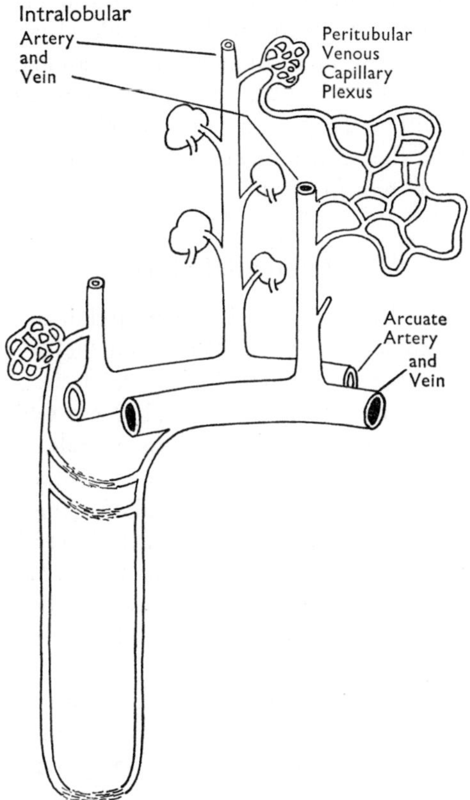

FIG. 1.7. Schema illustrating the renal circulation of the cortex and medulla.

The blood supply to the medulla passes through those glomeruli which are nearest to the medulla; these are sometimes known as juxtamedullary glomeruli. Their blood supply is quite different from other glomeruli. Instead of the blood flowing through an afferent arteriole which enters the glomerulus, breaks up into capillaries and then emerges as an efferent arteriole, the afferent and efferent arteriole form one large continuous vessel which contains smooth muscle throughout and in which there is little evidence of renin secretory activity. The lumen into the glomerular capillaries opens directly on one side of this arteriole in such a way that a proportion of the blood which flows to the medulla does not pass through glomeruli (Fig. 1.7).

The blood to the medulla courses through two distinct systems. One consists of compact bundles of long tubes of capillary thickness which carry the blood down to, and away from, the apex of the pyramids; these are the descending and ascending vasa recta. The other system consists of a thick network of fine capillaries, it is situated in the outer half of the medulla; the same area as that occupied by the thick parts of the ascending limbs of the loop of Henle. The venous blood from the medulla empties into the arcuate veins. The striking feature of the medullary circulation is that the blood in the long bundles of vasa recta is forced to flow in a counter-current fashion. It follows that the vasa recta with their capillary-like walls not only act as conduits for blood, but because the blood within them is in equilibrium with the interstitial fluid, there is imposed upon the environment of the medulla the physical properties of a counter-current system (p. 112).

Interstitial Space

The cortex is almost free of connective tissue and in an ordinary histological preparation the peritubular venous capillaries and the tubules are contiguous, which suggests that there is no interstitial space. It is by no means certain however that this is true in life. Sections from kidneys which have been frozen instantaneously, after being excised from living animals, show that there exists a clear area around each tubule, between the tubule and the peritubular capillary. It is also well established that the blood that drains from a kidney which has just been excised from a living animal has a much lower haematocrit than the haematocrit of that animal's arterial or venous blood. It is probable that the extra plasma lies in the clear areas around the tubules. Usually these spaces are not visible, for the plasma they contain escapes with the blood in the capillaries via the cut renal artery and vein.

The presence of an interstitial space in the medulla is certain, for the many parallel tubes that it contains are separated by a lagging of connective tissue which is particularly thick towards the apex of the pyramids.

The flow of lymph in the interstitial spaces of the cortex probably takes place in the capacious peri-arterial spaces. These must form relatively unyielding tunnels within which the pulsations of the arteries intermittently compress the adjoining lymphatics to ensure a flow of lymph.

Juxta-glomerular Apparatus

In each nephron the first part of the distal tubule rises from the medulla and comes to lie near the glomerulus of that nephron (Fig. 1.8). At this point the afferent and efferent arterioles to the glomerulus are in close contact with the distal tubule. The area where this contact takes place is called the juxta-glomerular apparatus. At this point the cells of the afferent arteriole contains cytoplasmic secretory granules of renin. The distal tubular cells next to the granular cells of the afferent arteriole are columnar with their nuclei placed near the lumen of the tubule. In the space between these specialised arteriolar and tubular cells there lies a third type of cells which form a lace-work pattern, known as lacis cells, they also extend into the intercapillary area of the glomerulus and resemble mesangial cells. Electron microscopy studies suggest that the granular cells of the arterioles, the lacis cells and the mesangial cells of the glomerulus are related to each other and to smooth muscle. This hypothesis

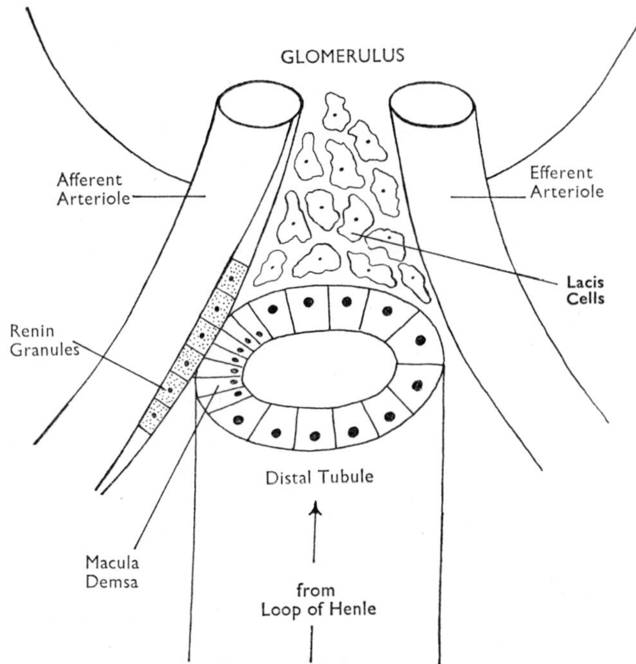

FIG. 1.8. Schema of juxta-glomerular apparatus.

strengthened by the finding that in cultures of human glomeruli the mesangial cells contract intermittently, and all do so synchronously. Smooth muscle cells in culture do the same. In addition immunofluorescent studies have shown that anti-muscle immunoglobulin adheres to mesangial cells.

Renal Nerves

The innervation of the kidneys comes from both the sympathetic and the vagus via the splanchnic nerves. The sympathetic supply is usually from T6 to T12. Within the renal parenchyma there is a widespread distribution of nerves and it is possible to trace nerve fibres until they reach and envelop the tubules as well as the capillaries. There are no ganglia in the kidney. Adenergic nerve fibres are present in relation to interlobar, intralobular, and arcuate arteries, and the afferent arteriole. They are never found in the glomerulus, efferent arteriole and the tubule.

BIBLIOGRAPHY

Boijsen, E. (1959). "Angiographic studies of the anatomy of single and multiple renal arteries." *Acta radiol. (Stockh.)*, suppl. 183.

Bowman, W. (1842). "On the structure and use of the Malpighian bodies of the kidney, with observations on the circulation through that gland." *Phil. Trans. Roy. Soc.*, **132** (1), 57.

Gruber, C. M. (1933). "The autonomic innervation of the genito-urinary system." *Physiol. Revs.*, **13**, 487.

Hall, B. V. (1954). "Further studies of the normal structure of the renal glomerulus." *Proc. VIth Ann. Conf. on the Nephrotic Syndrome*, Nov. 1956. National Nephrosis Foundation, New York.

Jacobsen, N. O., Jørgensen, J., and Thompsen, A. C. (1966). "An electron microscopic study of small arteries and arterioles in the normal human kidney." *Nephron*, **3**, 17.

Latta, H., Mannsbach, A. B., and Cook, M. L. (1962). "Relations of the centro-lobular region of the glomerulus of the juxta-glomerular apparatus." *J. Ultrastructure Res.*, **6**, 547 and 562.

Mayerson, H. S. (1963). "The lymphatic system with particular reference to the kidney." *Surgery*, **116**, 259.

Moffat, D. B., and Fourman, J. (1963). "The vascular pattern of the rat kidney." *J. Anat. (Lond.)*, **97**, 285.

Mueller, C. B., Mason, A. D., and Stout, D. G. (1955). "Anatomy of the glomerulus." *Amer. J. Med.*, **18**, 267.

de Muylder, C. G. (1952). "The 'Neurility' of the Kidney." Blackwell Scientific Pubs., Oxford.

Oliver, J. (1939). "Architecture of the Kidney in Chronic Bright's Disease." Paul B. Hoeber, Inc., New York and London.

Osathanoudh, V., and Potter, E. L. (1966). "Development of human kidney as shown by microdissection. *Arch. Path.*, **82**, 391 and 403.

Page, I. H., and McCubbin, J. W. (1968). Structure of the juxta-glomerular complex. "Renal Hypertension." Year Book Medical Publishers Inc., p. 40.

Peirce, C. E. (1944). "Renal lymphatics." *Anat. Rec.*, **90**, 315.

Rhodin, J. A. G. (1971). "Structure of the Kidney. Diseases of the Kidney." Ed. by Strauss, M. B., and Welt, L. G. J. & A. Churchill, London.

Suzuki, Y., Churg, J., Grishman, E., Manther, W., and Dachs, S. (1963). "The mesangium of the renal glomerulus." *Amer. J. Path.*, **43**, 555.

Swann, H. G., and Norman, R. G. (1970). "The periarterial spaces of the kidney." *Texas Rep. Biol. Med.*, **28**, 3, 317.

Swann, H. G., Valdivia, L., Ormsby, A. A., and Witt, W. T. (1956). "Nature of fluids which functionally distend the kidney." *J. exp. Med.*, **104**, 25.

Trump, B. F., Tisher, C. G., and Saladino, A. J. (1969). Nephron in health and disease. "The Biological Basis of Medicine." Academic Press, London and New York, p. 387.

2

Tests of Renal Structural Integrity

THE following methods are used to obtain information about the anatomical and histological structure of the kidney:

Clinical Examination of the Abdomen.
Straight X-ray of the Abdomen.
Intravenous Pyelography.
Renal Tomogram.
Renal Scintigram.
Retrograde Pyelography.
Renal Arteriogram.
Isotope Renogram.
Renal Biopsy.

Clinical Examination of the Abdomen

Obviously this is most helpful in thin patients and may give information about the presence of a tumour, hydronephrosis and polycystic kidneys; if the kidneys are readily palpable it is usually easy to decide whether or not they are much larger than normal. To obtain the best results from this examination it is essential that the patient move his diaphragm well down with each inspiration, while relaxing the anterior abdominal muscles. Some patients seem unable to do this, but may be taught to do so by being told to place their hands palm downwards on the surface of their abdomen while they practise. Tenderness in the renal angle or over the kidney anteriorly indicates that there is inflammation which may be due either to infection, infarction or an allergic reaction.

A distended bladder is often an invaluable clue to the presence and cause of renal failure.

Straight X-ray of the Abdomen

Such an X-ray is less revealing than an intravenous pyelogram, but it has certain advantages. It can be performed at short notice and it causes no discomfort. Often the outline of the kidneys may be distinguished so that their size, shape and position can be determined, and it may also be possible to decide whether there are any shadows consistent with the presence of calculi or renal calcification.

Intravenous Pyelography (I.V.P.)

This is achieved by the rapid intravenous administration of sodium diatrizoate (Hypaque), or a mixture of sodium and methylglucamine diatrizoate (Urografin) or a mixture of sodium and methylglucamine iothalamate (Conray), at a time when the rate of urine flow is minimal. These substances consist of dense molecules containing three radio-opaque iodine atoms which are filtered through the glomerulus, a very small amount is also secreted into the tubular fluid by the proximal tubules. When there is a considerable concentration of these substances in the tubular fluid the renal parenchyma becomes faintly visible, while their presence in the urine causes the calyces, pelves and ureters to be densely shadowed.

Intestinal gas and movements, faeces and fat may considerably obscure and confuse the results. An aperient should be taken the preceding evening and, if it has failed to act, a small enema should be given. It is best to allow the patient to be up and about for 24 hours before the examination, and a low-residue diet and no medicine containing bismuth or similar radio-opaque substances should be taken for at least two days previously. Intestinal gas can sometimes be dispelled by an injection of aqueous vasopressin or neostigmine methyl-sulphate.

The density of the pelvic shadow is dependent upon the following:

(1) The concentration of radio-opaque dye in the blood perfusing the glomeruli.
(2) The number of glomeruli and therefore the rate of glomerular filtration.
(3) The proportion of water which is removed from the glomerular filtrate as it travels down the tubule, thus concentrating the radio-opaque dye.
(4) The antero-posterior depth of urine through which the X-rays have to penetrate.

The optimum concentrations in the blood are obtained with 1 ml/kg body weight of 60 per cent sodium diatrizoate when the glomerular filtration rate is greater than 25 ml/min, and with 2 ml/kg body weight when the glomerular filtration rate is below 25 ml/min. Larger quantities increase the amount in the tubular fluid, but because of the accompanying osmotic diuresis their opaqueness to X-rays may be reduced. Nothing can be done to increase the number of nephrons, but it is probable that noxious stimuli (see below), including perhaps the radio-opaque substances themselves may decrease the function of the nephrons by renal vasoconstriction.

To increase the amount and depth of the urine in the pelves and ureters they are sometimes forcibly distended by partially obstructing the lower ureters by compression of the lower abdomen with an inflatable rubber balloon. This is best done about 5–10 min after the injection of the contrast solution, when its concentration in the pelves has reached a plateau. When renal function is normal the rate of urine flow is reduced as much as possible by fluid deprivation or the administration of vasopressin tannate in oil.

The main value of an I.V.P. is that it demonstrates the size and configuration of the pelves and calyces; it is helpful in determining the size, shape and position of the kidneys; it is particularly useful in first suggesting that there may be unilateral parenchymal disease. Occasionally distortion of a calyx is best seen on a lateral or oblique view. If the radio-opaque substance is given rapidly and films are taken at 15 sec, 1, 2 and 3 min intervals after the injection, additional information can be obtained which is useful in the detection of those occlusions of the renal arteries which are sufficient to cause hypertension; this manoeuvre must be performed without ureteric compression.

An intravenous pyelogram gives very misleading information about renal function. Small diseased kidneys with little renal function can sometimes give dense pyelograms, and absent or faint unilateral or bilateral shadows may be found when the kidneys are normal. Occasionally there may be no shadow during the first I.V.P., yet a normal shadow is seen a few days later during a second. The reason for these transient anomalies are not always clear. Occasionally they are due to a transient hypotension or ureteric obstruction. It is also possible that the apprehension and discomfort, which are an unavoidable part of intravenous pyelography, may sometimes be responsible. The patient has to remain in one position on a hard X-ray table for a considerable time and for some of this time he may endure a severe compression of the lower abdomen. Much less stress is known to cause a brisk rise in urine-flow from inhibition of anti-diuretic hormone secretion, or an osmotic salt diuresis (pp. 62, 126).

I.V.P. in patients with renal failure. Patients suffering from renal failure must not be dehydrated for this will make little difference to the concentration of the urine while it will often aggravate the renal failure. It is therefore imperative that all those concerned with the I.V.P. be specifically told not to deprive such patients of fluid. In addition to the usual technique it is most useful to include tomography (see below). Films are usually taken 20–30 min after the contrast medium has been administered, but it may be necessary to take films intermittently for up to 24 hours to obtain all the available information. The renal outline and the renal substance can nearly always be visualised so that obstruction of the urinary tract is almost invariably demonstrated or can be excluded, however severe the renal failure, even in patients who are oliguric or anuric. The ability to detect urinary tract obstruction is probably the most useful contribution an intravenous pyelogram can make in renal failure.

The dangers of giving large amounts of contrast media are minimal, if the patient is not deprived of fluid. Patients suffering from renal failure due to myelomatosis however may be an exception and great care should be taken with such patients.

Renal Tomograms

This technique is most useful when a patient presents with advanced renal failure of unknown cause. It is also useful in seeing whether calcification is within or simply overlying the kidneys. If an injection of contrast medium is given immediately before taking the tomogram, renal cyst can be diagnosed with a high degree of accuracy.

Renal Scintigram

After the administration of an Hg^{203} labelled diuretic, the mercurial salt and its label enter the cells of the proximal tubule where it remains for a certain time. It is then possible to delineate the outline of the kidneys by scanning the renal areas with a scintillation counter. The technique does not disturb the patient. Its main use is in finding out the position of the kidneys, detecting major differences in outline and size and in picking up local areas of renal disease when they are of sufficient size, such as tumours, cysts and areas of infarction. It is sometimes useful in detecting small amounts of viable kidney tissue which have not been revealed by any other tests.

Retrograde Pyelography

A radio-opaque solution is introduced directly into the pelvis of the kidney after cystoscopy and ureteric catheterisation. Sodium diatrizoate (25 per cent) or sodium acetrizoate (15 per cent) is injected under considerable pressure to distend the pelvis and ureter; this is done after the patient has recovered from the anaesthetic so as to avoid overdistension. It is a dangerous procedure when the urinary tract is obstructed for it may cause a severe urinary infection.

The information to be derived from a retrograde pyelogram is obviously confined within the borders of the pelvis, calyx and ureter. The need for retrograde pyelography has considerably diminished since the ureters, pelvis and calyces have been so well demonstrated with the large amounts of contrast media which are now given routinely for intravenous pyelography.

Renal Aortography and Arteriography

A radio-opaque substance is injected directly into the abdominal aorta at a point just above the origin of the renal arteries; 20–40 ml of 50 per cent sodium diatrizoate are administered via a catheter introduced through a femoral artery; the total volume is administered in 1 to 2 sec. The fluid travels into the renal arteries, capillaries and veins. Exposures are made at required intervals following the injection in order to demonstrate successively the filling of the arteries, veins and tubules (the nephrographic phase). It is a highly specialised technique which gives good pictures of the renal vascular tree. Its greatest use is to identify localised obstructions of the renal artery and its main branches. It can also reveal the presence of accessory arteries and is sometimes most useful in defining the existence of localised areas of disease in the renal parenchyma, and distinguishing between tumours and cysts. In principle the tumours being vascular become radio-opaque in contrast to cysts which do not cast a shadow, but there are anomalies. Aortography is also of help when the kidney has been injured. It is then used to assess the extent of vascular and parenchymal damage. To obtain good pictures of the vessels in the cortex it is necessary to introduce the dye through a catheter which has been threaded from the aorta directly into the renal artery. Serious complications after aortography or arteriography are rare, but include acute renal failure, and transient obstruction to the femoral artery.

Isotope Renogram

Para-amino-hippuric acid (PAH) is actively secreted by the proximal tubules into the tubular fluid, and it is then excreted in the urine (p. 32). If a single injection of I^{131} labelled PAH is given intravenously the concentration of PAH in the kidney rises within a minute to a peak and then falls gradually to control values in the next 10 to 20 min. If a detector is placed over the kidney and the intensity of radiation emitted from the I^{131} labelled PAH in that area is continuously monitored, it is possible to obtain a continuous graph of this process. The shape of the curve will clearly depend on (i) the rate at which the PAH reaches the kidney, i.e. the renal blood flow, (ii) the number and condition of proximal tubule cells which transport the PAH into the tubule fluid, and (iii) the rate at which the PAH is carried away from the kidney in the tubular fluid and urine. The technique is most useful in detecting and particularly in following the course of ureteric obstruction. There is a trap, however, in that the renogram appearances of obstruction are the same as those of acute renal failure. An isotope renogram is useful in following the progress of a transplanted kidney. At one time the isotope renogram was used extensively to try and detect localised abnormalities of the renal circulation such as renal artery stenosis. For this purpose, however, it should never be used as the only screening procedure; it should be one of a battery of tests, for it is liable to give false negative results in up to 25 per cent of patients with renal artery stenosis.

Renal Biopsy

A renal biopsy can be performed in two ways. Either the biopsy needle can be inserted through the intact skin when the biopsy sample is then obtained "blind". Or the biopsy needle is inserted into the kidney under direct vision through a deep formal surgical approach in the patient's flank. There is little doubt that in centres where renal biopsies are performed infrequently it is probably safer, and a satisfactory sample of renal tissue is more likely to be obtained more frequently, if the biopsy is performed under direct vision. This technique has the additional advantage that haemorrhage into the perirenal tissues can be prevented. On the other hand, in order to perform an open biopsy the patient has to be anaesthetised and he has to suffer the discomforts and possible complications of an abdominal operation.

In most centres, therefore, where renal biopsies are frequently needed it is customary to use the blind technique. The biopsy is usually performed with the patient in the prone position. Some experts prefer to have the patient in an operating theatre where it is certainly more convenient. A general anaesthetic is rarely given unless the patient is particularly nervous or very young. A sand-bag is placed under the abdomen, or if the patient is on an operating table, the bridge is raised. The kidney is usually found either by reference to a previously performed intravenous pyelogram, though sometimes a straight X-ray of the abdomen is sufficient, or by direct visualisation or television screen. A fine exploring needle is inserted through the renal angle and the structures down to the kidney infiltrated with local anaesthetic. When the needle is thought to be near the kidney the patient is asked to hold his breath, the syringe containing the local anaesthetic is disconnected from the needle and the patient is now asked to take one or two deep breaths. In the absence of a television screen the needle is probably in the kidney if that portion of the needle outside the skin swings through a wide arc with each respiration. This is sometimes misleading if the patient is fat or oedematous and it must be remembered that the needle will also swing if it is in the liver. Whether or not the needle swings, it sometimes rotates on its long axis on respiration. This is an almost certain indication that it is in the kidney. The fine needle is then withdrawn and the procedure repeated with the biopsy needle when an attempt is then made to bring a fragment of the kidney to the surface.

Experience greatly improves performance. Apart from the recurring difficulty of bringing the piece successfully to the surface, there are certain patients who present special difficulties. For instance, those with extensive spinal deformities such as spondylitis deformans or lumbar scoliosis, and those with ascites or pregnancy. There is general agreement that the contraindications to renal biopsy are (1) the presence of only one kidney, (2) a tendency to bleed, and (3) the presence of a hypernephroma, a large renal cyst, a perinephric abscess, or hydro- or pyonephrosis, and (4) an uncooperative patient. Some workers would also include a high blood urea (greater than 100 mg/100 ml), and malignant hypertension, unless the blood pressure is controlled during and for a few hours after the biopsy is performed. If the patient is being treated with an artificial kidney it is usual not to do a biopsy for two days before and one day after a dialysis because of the heparin which is used during the dialysis.

After the biopsy the patient is placed on his back and told to remain in that position uninterruptedly for at least 12–18 hours. This is more likely to produce haemostasis than reliance on a tight abdominal bandage. The patient is also given a large drink of water to induce a diuresis. This not only diminishes the possibility of clot formation if there is haematuria but more quickly demonstrates its presence and extent. The serious complications of biopsy are preponderantly those of haemorrhage either into the renal pelvis or into the retroperitoneal space. Microscopical haematuria always occurs, and direct observation of the retroperitoneal tissues during an open renal biopsy also shows that there is always a perirenal haematoma. It is generally considered, however, that a "complication" has occurred only when either the haematuria is macroscopic, particularly if there is clot formation, or if the retroperitoneal haemorrhage is sufficiently large to cause pain in the flank and a fall in haemoglobin. Gross haematuria occurs in about 5–10 per cent of cases, and perirenal haematoma in about 2 per cent. Occasionally macroscopical haematuria persists for several days, and there are a few instances of a delayed onset of haematuria. Blood transfusions have been used in about 2 per cent of cases. Other complications include pain during the biopsy which is usually in inverse relationship to the patient's nervousness. A sharp but unimportant pain is produced if the ileo-inguinal nerve is transfixed as it emerges from the border of the sacrospinalis, while a dull ache radiating into the iliac fossa indicates that a retroperitoneal haemorrhage is forming. A few patients complain of a transient pain in the back after the biopsy. Comparisons of renal functional capacity before and after the biopsy have demonstrated that unless there is ureteric obstruction from a clot there is no disturbance of function. Serial renal aortograms have been performed in a few patients after renal biopsy. They have revealed a disturbing number of transient intrarenal arterio-venous shunts which may take several months to resolve.

A renal biopsy is clearly the only method of making an exact histological diagnosis during life. The information which has been obtained in this way has been of the greatest value in throwing light upon the natural course of renal disease. And even in the present era of therapeutic helplessness in regard to many renal diseases there are an increasing number of occasions when an exact histological diagnosis is of importance in deciding the patient's future treatment.

BIBLIOGRAPHY

BRITTON, K. E., and BROWN, N. J. G. (1971). "Clinical Renography." Lloyd-Luke, London.

EMMETT, JOHN L. (1967). "Clinical Urography." Second Edition, Vols. I and II. W. B. Saunders Company, Philadelphia and London.

FOSTER, R. S., SHUFORD, W. H., and WEENS, H. S. (1965). "Selective renal arteriography in medical diseases of the kidney." *Amer. J. Roentgenol.*, **95**, 291.

FRY, K. I., and CATTELL, W. R. (1971). "Radiology in the diagnosis of renal failure." *Brit. med. Bull.*, **27**, No. 2, 148.

GARNETT, E. S. (1967). "A trial of the radio–isotope renogram." *Brit. J. Urol.*, **36**, 332.

GREEN, B., and SOWERBUTTS, I. G. (1956). "A comparative study of the value of sodium acetrizoate (Diaginol) 50 per cent, and sodium diatrizoate (Hypaque) 45 per cent, in intravenous urography." *Brit. J. Radiol.*, **29**, 161.

JOEKES, A. M., and RELLAN, D. R. (1965). "Radioactive renography in diagnosis and treatment of acute obstructive renal failure." *Lancet*, ii, 96.

KIRKLAND, J. A. (1959). "Massive albuminuria following aortography." *Lancet*, **2**, 1144.

MAXWELL, M. H., CONICK, H. C., WITTA, R., and KAUFMAN, J. J. (1964). "Use of rapid sequence pyelogram in the diagnosis of renovascular hypertension." *New Eng. J. Med.*, **270**, 213.

MAYO, M. E., HILTON, P. J., JONES, N. F., LLYOID-DAVIES, R. W., and CROFT, D. N. (1971). "^{131}I Hippuran renogram in acute renal failure." *Brit. med. J.*, **2**, 516.

MURRAY, R. S., and TRESSIDER, G. C. (1957). "Renal angiography." *Brit. med. Bull.*, **13**, 61.

RHYS, DAVIES, E. (1970). "Renal scintiscanning, a review." *Postgraduate Medical Journal*, **46**, 52.

SELDINGER, S. I. (1953). "Catheter replacement of the needle in percutaneous arteriography; a new technique." *Acta radiol. (Stockh.)*, **39**, 368.

SHERWOOD, T. (1971). The physiology of intravenous urography. "Scientific Basis of Medicine Annual Review," p. 336.

VAN WAES, P. F. G. M. (1972). "High dose urography in oliguric and anuric patients." Excerpta Medica, Amsterdam.

WESTPHAL, R. D., RISSER, J. R., MOTZIN, D., ERICKSON, E. E., and MORGAN, M. C. (1962). "Delineation of human kidneys by scintillation scanning." *Amer. J. Roentgenol.*, **87**, 1.

WHITE, R. H. R. (1963). "Observations on percutaneous renal biopsy in children." *Arch Dis. Child.*, **38**, 260.

3

Structural Changes (Histological) in Response to Disease

THE various ways the glomerulus, tubule or interstitial space may react to disease are limited. And many of the responses can occur in association with more than one renal disease. Structurally, therefore, individual diseases are recognised more often by a pattern of structural disturbance than by any specific change. This explains why to the beginner the histological appearances of most renal diseases all look so much the same. The similarity of the more obvious individual changes is more easily recognised than is the difference between their collective patterns. The analogy with function is relatively close. There are very few abnormalities of function which occur in only one form of renal disease, but patterns of abnormalities can be discerned in certain diseases more often than in others. In the present climate of knowledge it is accepted that functional changes can be studied and discussed separately from the diseases which cause them. The first part of this section attempts to do the same for the structural changes which result from disease. The second part discusses the use of immuno fluorescence, and the third the relation between the histological changes and renal function.

Glomerulus

Epithelial cells

These cells line the inside of Bowman's capsule and the outer surface of the glomerular capillaries. Those lining Bowman's capsule may proliferate and form "crescents" which are gradually replaced by basement membrane-like material. Crescents are seen most conspicuously but are by no means confined to patients suffering from rapidly progressive glomerular nephritis (p. 266).

The epithelial cells on the outer surface of the capillary loop may swell or lose their foot processes. The swellings are due to the ingestion of large macromolecules and occur with proteinuria. The loss of foot processes is only seen with the electron microscope, it may be focal or general and is also related to proteinuria. Both these changes are most evident but are not limited to patients who have a nephrotic syndrome. Sub-epithelial cell deposits are discussed later.

Endothelial cells and the capillary lumen

Endothelial cells may proliferate and/or swell. These changes may occlude the lumen of the capillary, a result which may also be produced by intraluminal

"

aggregation of platelets and leucocytes, or the insinuation of mesangial cytoplasm between the basement membrane and the endothelial cell (see below). The lumen may also be occluded by sub-endothelial deposits. Occlusion of the capillary by endothelial cell swelling and some proliferation occurs in toxaemia of pregnancy, while in acute glomerular nephritis it may be caused by several of the changes described above.

Mesangium

Mesangial cells are highly phagocytic and their function has been described as one of "garbage disposal". Nearly all conditions which affect the glomerulus are associated with some structural change of the mesangial cells. The most

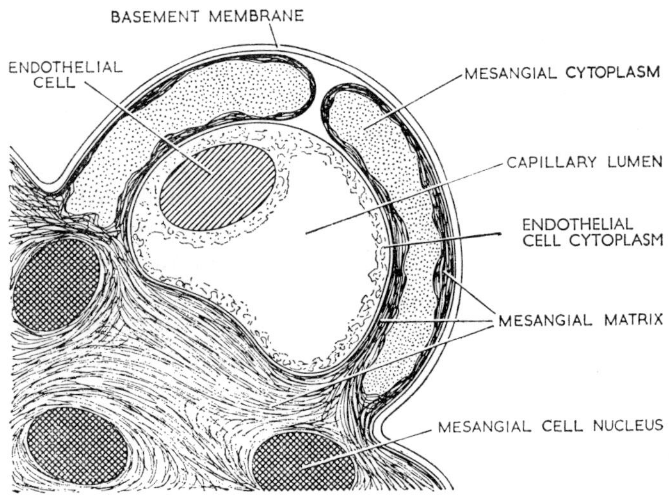

FIG. 3.1. Diagram of light microscopy appearances in membrano-proliferative glomerular nephritis. For the sake of simplicity the epithelial cell and its cytoplasm, on the outer surface of the basement membrane, have not been illustrated.

conspicuous is that of proliferation and particularly the formation of deposits of mesangial cell cytoplasm or matrix. Small changes cause what has been described as mesangial stalk "thickening", a change which is often seen after acute glomerular nephritis (p. 259). More pronounced changes include either focal nodules of mesangial matrix such as are seen in diabetes, or diffuse masses of matrix which occupy most of the glomerular tuft as in the "lobular" form of persistent glomerular nephritis. Later the mesangial proliferation disappears while the mass of matrix remains as large acellular areas. These changes can occur without, initially, any involvement of the capillary loop.

In other circumstances the mesangial cells may proliferate and send out cytoplasmic extensions between the endothelial cell and the basement membrane. These may extend peripherally so that the capillary loop is surrounded. The wall of the capillary is then considerably thickened and consists of four layers, the epithelial cell, the basement membrane, the mesangial cytoplasm and matrix and the endothelial cell (Fig. 3.1). Eosin stains the whole wall a diffuse pink including the mesangial cell cytoplasm and matrix, while P.A.S. and silver selectively stain only the fibrils of the matrix, and the basement membrane. As the mesangial cytoplasm infiltrates itself between the endothelial cells and the basement membrane the fibrils of matrix tend to condense on either side of the cytoplasm. With P.A.S. stain therefore, there is what looks like a split basement membrane surrounding a clear space. The space contains non-P.A.S. staining mesangial cell cytoplasm. This particular abnormality of the mesangium has been called a "membrano-proliferative" change, a term which does not immediately evoke the appearances which have just been described. It is seen in persistent glomerular nephritis (p. 266) and systematised lupus crythematosus (p. 285).

Basement membrane

Basement membrane surrounds the periphery of a capillary loop, but where the capillary faces the mesangium there is no basement membrane, the lumen of the capillary being in direct contact with the mesangial matrix through the perforations of the endothelial cell cytoplasm (Fig. 1.3). Nevertheless as both basement membrane, and the mesangial cytoplasm and matrix which lie next to the lumen react to disease in much the same way they can be considered together. The basement membrane appears to be altered in all diseases of the kidney, except for that form of glomerular nephritis which is associated with a nephrotic syndrome but in which no histological changes can be detected in the renal biopsy

The basement membrane and adjoining mesangial matrix may be uniformally thickened, or have focal excrescences, or erosions; they may also be the site of various deposits. Extensive relatively uniform thickening of the basement membrane may occur in diabetes and nephrosclerosis while focal erosions are found in acute glomerular nephritis. Focal excrescences of varying sizes, and various extravagant shapes are found in most prolonged immunological disturbances of the kidney such as chronic glomerular nephritis and lupus erythematosus. The commonest deposits to be found in relation to the basement membrane consist of focal and diffuse masses of material which contain various substances known to be involved in immunological reactions. They may be sub-epithelial or sub-endothelial. Focal sub-epithelial deposits are characteristic of acute glomerular nephritis and are known colloquially as "humps" (Fig. 3.2). Diffuse sub-epithelial deposits cause those changes which are described under the term extra-membranous glomerular nephritis. In this condition the basement membrane, at first, appears normal but silver stains demonstrate that it extends upwards at relatively regular intervals for a short distance between the deposits (Fig. 3.3). The appearance of the basement membrane is thus like that of a comb with short irregular teeth, the deposits lying between the teeth. Later the deposits increase in size until they become incorporated into a thickened

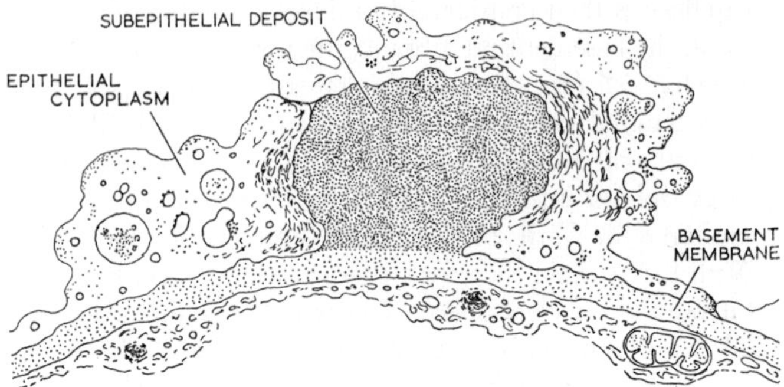

FIG. 3.2. Diagram of electron microscopy appearance of a hump-like extra-membranous deposit in acute glomerular nephritis.

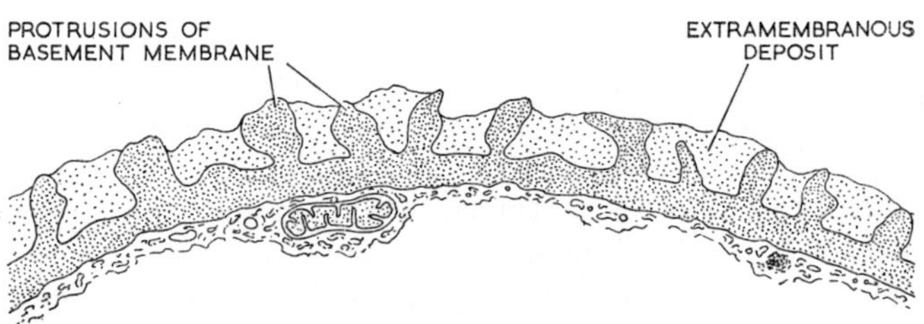

FIG. 3.3. Diagram of the electron microscopy appearances of the deposits and the basement membrane in extra-membranous glomerular nephritis

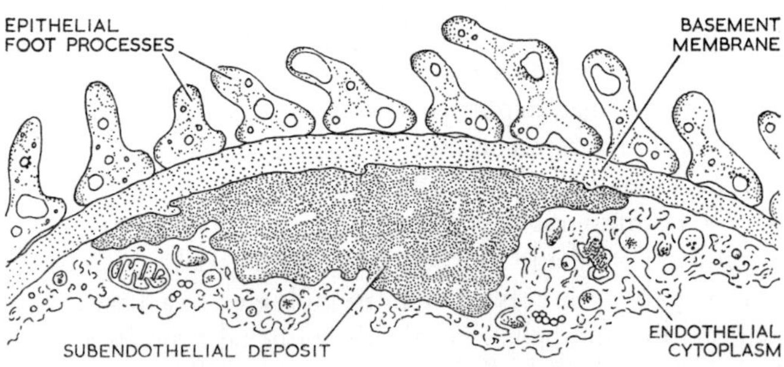

FIG. 3.4 Diagram of the electron microscopy appearances of a sub-endothelial deposit.

basement membrane which may then totally surround them. Deposits can sometimes be found within the basement membrane, this is particularly characteristic in systematised lupus erythematosus. Sub-endothelial deposits (Fig. 3.4) occur in a wide variety of conditions including lupus crythematosus (p. 285), diabetic nephropathy (p. 344) and pre-eclampsia (p. 355). Large focal accumulations may give rise to what have been called "wire loop" lesions which have only been described in lupus erythematosus. Sub-epithelial and sub-endothelial deposits of fibrin and amyloid may also be laid down. Fibrin deposits are found particularly in diseases in which there is intravascular coagulation.

Tubules

On light microscopy there are only a limited number of histological changes which can be discerned, and they are of relatively little help in identifying the disease process with which they are associated. Electron microscopy however has revealed that, at the level of the organelle, there are a large number of changes which can be detected.

The so-called hyaline droplet degeneration is seen in a wide variety of renal diseases. It consists of numerous eosinophilic droplets within the cytoplasm of the tubule cell. It is usually due to the tubule cell having absorbed a large

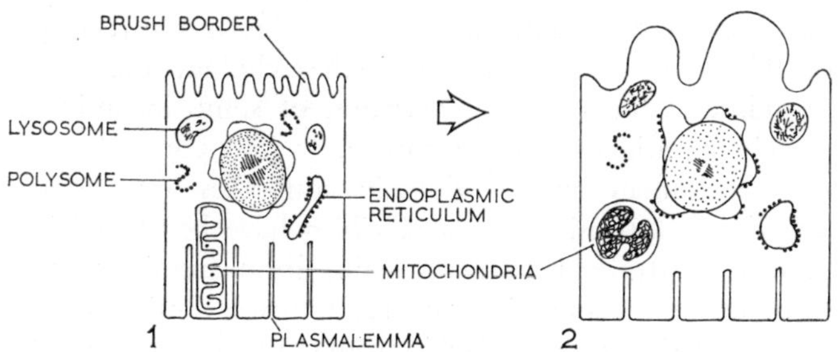

Fig. 3.5. Diagram of electron microscopy of tubular damage. (Trump, Tisher and Saladino, 1969. "The Biological Basis of Medicine".)

quantity of protein from the tubule fluid. The protein is ingested into lysosomes at a rate greater than the lysosomes can dispose of protein, so that the droplets consist of distended lysosomes filled with proteinaceous material. Pale unstainable vacuolations of the tubule cell are found after the administration of sucrose, manitol and glucose. Again these vacuoles are due to the rapid accumulation of these substances into the cells at a rate greater than the digestive powers of the lysosomes so that they become distended. Hypoxia, hypokalaemia, certain nephrotoxins, partial occlusion of the renal vein and hydronephrosis may cause a sub-lethal injury to the tubule cells leading to an increased number of pale vacuoles which are also due to distended lysosomes. Sometimes these contain fat or necrotic debris such as mitochondria. The vacuoles associated with hypokalaemia are particularly large, and in man are found within the proximal tubules. Tubule cells may also become calcified.

Many disease processes, and some nephrotoxins such as mercury or Amphotericin B may directly inhibit the sodium pump of the tubule cell. Sodium then accumulates within the cell, water is drawn into the cell and the cell swells. This change has been described as that of "cloudy swelling" or "hydro degeneration" (Fig. 3.5). Up to a point this change is compatible with prolonged survival. Prolonged injury may give rise to tubular atrophy, a feature which is seen in all forms of renal disease. The tubule may then appear as a shrivelled mass surrounded by a thick collar of P.A.S. positive basement membrane. Acute necrosis of the tubules may occur from acute ischaemia or nephrotoxic poisons. In those sites in which the necrosis does not involve the basement membrane the flat necrotic tubular epithelium regenerates rapidly.

The nucleus of the tubule cells may swell when the sodium pump is inhibited. Otherwise the nuclearplasm may show inclusion bodies such as virus particles in cytomegalic inclusion disease, or dense accumulations due to poisoning with heavy metals such as bismuth or lead.

Immunofluorescent Staining

The development of this technique has made it possible to detect the presence of certain substances such as antigens and antibodies in the renal parenchyma which are not there normally. The first step in the technique consists of repeatedly injecting an animal with a pure preparation of some intrinsic or extrinsic substance which is antigenic to the animal. In this connection it must be remembered that human immunoglobulin antibodies are antigenic to the experimental animal. Intrinsic substances which have been used include IgG, IgM, IgA, IgE, IgD, B_1C complement, renin, fibrin, insulin, some nucleoside fractions of DNA and neoplastic antigens. Extrinsic antigens include those obtained from malarial parasites, schistosoma, the leprosy bacillus and the Australia antigen. The animal develops circulating antibodies to the particular antigenic substance which has been injected. The antibodies are then extracted from the blood and labelled with a fluorescent stain. This preparation can now be used to detect the presence of that antigenic substance in a section of kidney from a patient. A renal biopsy is performed and a section is made when it is freshly frozen. A drop of the liquid preparation containing the fluorescent antibody which has been obtained from the experimental animal is then placed on the surface of the frozen section. If the antigen against which the animal formed the antibody is present in the renal biopsy the fluorescent antibody will bind onto it and will adhere to the section. After a suitable interval the section is repeatedly washed to remove any unbound fluorescent antibody. The section is then examined under ultra-violet illumination. The sites in the section which contain the antigenic substance will be fluorescent against a dark background.

In this way it has been possible to demonstrate that in various renal diseases one or more of the various substances listed above are present within the renal parenchyma. It has therefore made it possible to infer which renal diseases are probably associated with a humoral immunological disturbance. And, when

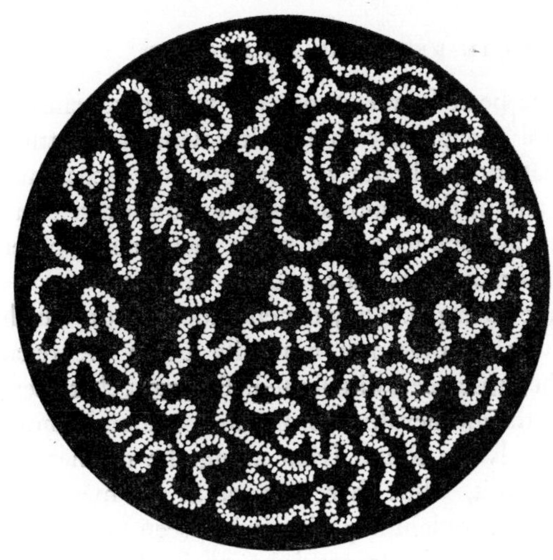

Fig. 3.6. Diagram of the appearances of immunofluorescent granular deposits along glomerular capillary walls.

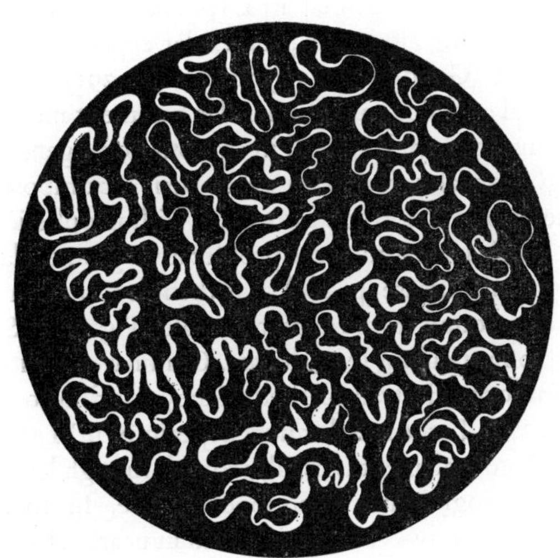

Fig. 3.7. Diagram of the appearances of immunofluorescent linear diffuse deposits along glomerular capillary walls.

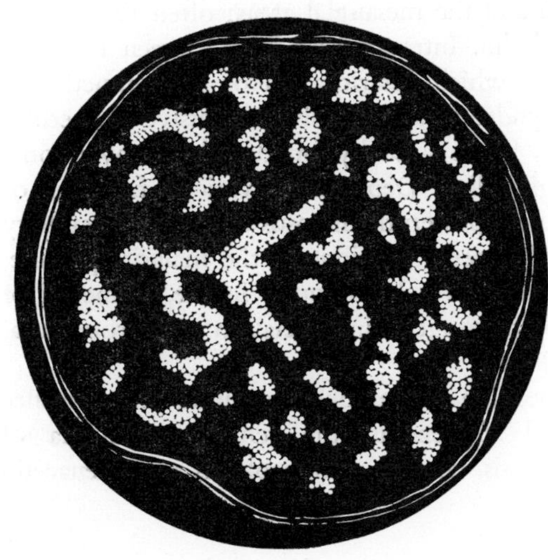

Fig. 3.8. Diagram of the appearances of immunofluorescent deposits in mesangial areas.

B

deposits of intravascular fibrin have been found, it has led to the conclusion that perhaps some of the structural changes are due to intravascular clotting which may itself cause inflammatory proliferative changes and ischaemia. Conversely the inability to detect any of these substances in various other renal diseases makes it possible that they are due to one or more mechanisms other than a humoral immunological disturbance, or intravascular clotting.

Some characteristic patterns have emerged. They depend not only on which particular substance is present, which should not normally be in the renal parenchyma, but also on the way the substance is distributed. The most characteristic patterns are almost all found in the glomerulus. For instance in membranous glomerular nephritis IgG is nearly always found lying along the glomerular capillary wall as a fine granular deposit, while there is none in the mesangial areas (Fig. 3.6). Whereas in Henoch–Schonlein nephritis IgA is seen predominantly in the mesangial areas (p. 290). In acute glomerular nephritis IgG is again found lying along the glomerular capillary wall but in a rather lumpy distribution. In Goodpasture's syndrome (p. 291), or in other syndromes in which the blood contains anti-glomerular basement membrane antibody, IgG is laid down along the capillary wall in smooth homogeneous lines (Fig. 3.7). Depositions of IgG are also found in renal vein thrombosis, embolic nephritis and in the nephrotic syndrome associated with neoplastic disease (p. 292).

IgA is seen in focal proliferative glomerular nephritis not associated with a systemic disease (p. 269), it is then deposited in the mesangial areas and is almost never found in the capillary walls (Fig. 3.8). Similar deposits of IgA are found in long standing liver disease. Granular deposits of IgM lying along the capillary wall occur in transplanted kidneys, and in focal sclerosing glomerular nephritis (p. 277). Large intraluminal deposits of IgM are also seen in macroglobulinaemia. B_1C complement is usually found, though less frequently, in association with the immunoglobulins mentioned above. In membrano-proliferative glomerular nephritis however B_1C is found in nearly all cases laid down in a coarse granular pattern both in the capillary wall and the mesangial areas; often there is no associated fixation of immunoglobulin. Intracapillary fibrin is seen in many conditions, particularly in those in which deterioration of renal function is most rapid such as Goodpasture's syndrome and rapidly progressive glomerular nephritis. In toxaemia of pregnancy fibrin is usually found without any accompanying deposition of immunoglobulins. Deposits of various fractions of DNA and IgG are present in diffuse lupus erythematosus both in the capillary wall and in the mesangial areas. Antigenic fractions of the malarial parasite, schistosomes, and the leprosy bacillus have been found in the glomeruli of patients suffering from infections by these agents in association with proteinuria, a nephrotic syndrome, or renal failure.

In contrast it has not been possible to demonstrate either the presence of immunoglobulin or abnormal antigens in the renal parenchyma of patients suffering from nephrosclerosis, chronic pyelonephritis and phenacetin nephropathy.

Relation Between the Structural Changes Found with Light Microscopy and Electron Microscopy, and the Findings Obtained with Immunofluorescence

Each one of these three techniques has something of individual importance to contribute. For instance in focal sclerosing glomerular nephritis electron microscopy can demonstrate intravascular deposits of fibrin which are too small to be detected with immunofluorescence. Alternatively immunofluorescent deposits have been detected in biopsies which appear normal on both light and electron microscopy. The routine use of a wide variety of immunofluorescent antibodies and the use of special preparations against certain unusual antigens such as those obtained from the malarial parasite and tumour cells has been of immense value in elucidating the probable aetiology of certain renal diseases. At the moment (1972), however, there are many confusing exceptions to the correlative patterns which are emerging. For example in a proportion of patients with mesangial proliferation no immunofluorescent staining can be detected, while others only show deposits of B_1C. Many patients with focal sclerosing glomerular nephritis have no immunofluorescent deposits. One thing is clear. It is that to examine renal biopsies with light microscopy only can be extremely misleading. On the other hand electron microscopy permits examination of only a small portion of the biopsy and is impractical for routine use. The technique of immunofluorescent staining is more practicable but the findings still demonstrate many unexplained inconsistencies.

Relation Between the Histological Changes Found with Light Microscopy and Renal Function

It is remarkable that glomerular filtration rate bears a much closer relation to the extent of tubular damage than to the extent of glomerular damage (Fig. 3.9). In other words it is not unusual to find patients with relatively unimpaired glomerular filtration rates in whom the renal biopsy demonstrates extensive glomerular damage with large eosinophilous deposits, but in whom the extent of tubular damage is minimal; the reverse is seen, in both acute and chronic renal failure. This phenomenon is difficult to explain. Perhaps the finding of a low glomerular filtration rate with damaged tubule and normal glomeruli is less paradoxical than it appears. Though it is clear that the substances used to measure glomerular filtration rate do so adequately when the tubule wall is normal it does not follow that they do so when the tubule wall is damaged. There is evidence which suggests that filtered substances which do not pass through a normal tubule wall may diffuse out of a damaged tubule. It is possible therefore that in some renal diseases the apparent glomerular filtration rate may be much lower than the true rate of filtration through the glomeruli, because the substance used to measure glomerular filtration rate (e.g. creatinine) has leaked from the lumen of the tubule into the interstitial spaces and back into the blood. The glomerular filtration rate of a nephron with

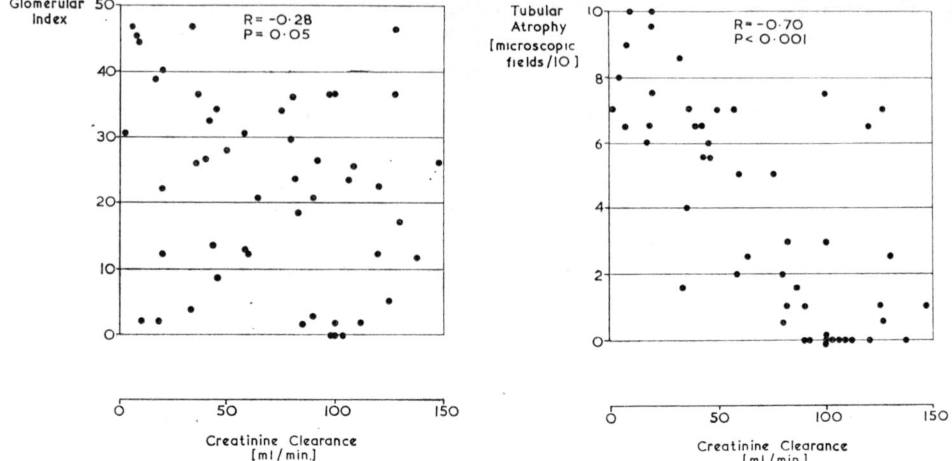

FIG. 3.9. (a) Correlation between creatinine clearance and glomerular damage and (b) between creatinine clearance and tubular atrophy. (Risdon, Sloper and de Wardener, 1968, *Lancet*.)

a relatively normal glomerulus could also be depressed by tubular damage if that damage led to obstruction of the tubular lumen.

BIBLIOGRAPHY

BERGER, J., YANEVA, H., and ANTOINE, B. (1969). "Applications de l'immunofluorescence à la pathologie rénal II) Étude immuno-histochimique des lésions glomerulaires." *J. Urol. Nephrol.*, **75**, 269.

BERGER, J., YANEVA, H., and HINGLAIS, N. (1971). Immunofluorescence des glomérulonéphrites. "Actualités Néphrologiques de l'Hôpital Necker." Ed. med. Flammarion, Paris, p. 17.

BURNS, J., and MacIVER, A. G. (1971). "Immuno-electron microscopy of the glomerular basement membrane in 'Goodpasture's Syndrome'." *Rev. Europ. Etuds. Clin. et Biol.* **16**, 48.

DUFFY, J. L., CLINQUE, T., GRISHMAN, E., and CHURG, J. (1970). "Intraglomerular fibrin, platelet aggregation and sub-endothelial deposits in lipoid nephrosis." *J. Clin. Invest.*, **49**, 251.

JENNINGS, R. B., and EARLE, D. P. (1968). In "Structural Basis of Renal Disease" (E. L. Becker, ed.). Harper and Row, New York, p. 271.

JØGENSEN, F. (1966). "The Ultrastructure of the Normal Human Glomerulus." Munksgaard, Copenhagen, p.15.

McCLUSKEY, R. T. (1970). "Evidence for immunologic mechanisms in several forms of human glomerular diseases." *Bull. N.Y. Acad. Med.*, **46**, 769.

McCLUSKEY, R. T., VASSALI, P., GALLO, G., and BALDWIN, D. S. (1966). "An immunofluorescent study of pathogenic mechanisms in glomerular diseases." *New Eng. J. Med.*, **274**, 695.

MOREL-MAROGER, L., LEATHEM, A., and RICHET, G. (1972). "Glomerular abnormalities in non-systemic diseases: Relation between light microscopy and immunofluorescence in 433 renal biopsies." *Amer. J. Med.*, **53**, 170.

RISDON, R. A., SLOPER, J. C., and DE WARDENER, H. E. (1968). "Relationship between renal function and histological changes found in renal-biopsy specimens from patients with persistent glomerular nephritis." *Lancet*, **2**, 363.

TRUMP, B. F., TISHER, C. C., and SALADINO, A. J. (1969). The nephron in health and disease. "The Biological Basis of Medicine." Edited E. E. Bittar and N. Bittar. Academic Press, London and New York, **6**, 387.

4

Introduction to Renal Function

and some Theoretical Considerations Concerned in Testing its Integrity

THE function of the kidney is to assist in keeping the volume and composition of the extracellular fluid within normal limits; it is also concerned with the maintenance of a normal blood pressure and erythropoiesis.

The composition and volume of the extracellular fluid is controlled by glomerular filtration, and tubular reabsorption or secretion. In a day approximately 180 litres of almost protein-free fluid is filtered through the glomerular capillaries into the glomerular space, from whence it passes into the tubule. As this filtrate travels down the tubule various substances are either subtracted or added to it, so that eventually only about 1 litre emerges as urine; this is the water and solutes which the body needs to discard. The renal mechanisms involved in regulating the blood pressure and erythropoiesis are obscure; they are discussed in Section 11 (p. 118) and Section 10 (p. 115).

In normal circumstances every glomerulus is continuously being perfused with blood; there is no evidence that the intermittency of glomerular circulation described in the frog is present in man. The rate of blood flow is adjusted by alterations in the afferent and efferent glomerular arterioles. Such changes must influence the glomerular capillary pressure and in turn the rate of glomerular filtration. Alterations in glomerular filtration rate are, within wide limits, affected by changing the rate of filtration in each glomerulus. There is no evidence that new nephrons are opened up when glomerular filtration rate increases, and complete closure of some glomeruli only occurs when glomerular filtration rate is suddenly reduced below 50 per cent.

Normally approximately 120 ml of filtrate are separated from the 600 ml of plasma that pass through the kidneys each minute. The ratio glomerular filtration rate : renal plasma flow is known as the filtration fraction. It can be seen that in health it is about 0·2. In disease it may vary from 0·1 to 0·3, but it is clear that, as might have been expected, the relationship between the rate of renal plasma flow and the glomerula filtration rate remains relatively close.

Glomerular filtrate contains all the diffusible ultrafiltrate substances present in plasma and, ignoring a slight difference caused by the plasma proteins, they are present in the same concentrations. There is also some indirect evidence that the filtrate contains small concentrations of protein, probably less than

30 mg/100 ml; though this is a relatively insignificant concentration, it nevertheless amounts to a filtration of about 50 g of protein in 24 hours.

Theoretical Considerations

The contents of the urine are selected from the plasma by a wide variety of mechanisms. It follows that the methods used to measure the efficiency of these mechanisms also vary. For instance, it will be shown in Section 5 that one of the best methods for testing the kidney's ability to control the sodium content of the extracellular fluid is to place the patient on a salt-free diet, and then to observe whether the kidney is able to diminish the excretion of sodium. Such a method is obviously unsuitable for measuring the kidney's ability to control the extracellular fluid concentration of substances which, regardless of intake, are continuously being manufactured by the body, e.g. urea and creatinine.

It has been found empirically that the most convenient gauge of the kidney's ability to control the extracellular fluid concentration of substances such as urea and creatinine is to calculate the quotient

$$\frac{\text{amount excreted in the urine per min (mg/min)}}{\text{concentration in the plasma (mg/ml)}} \quad \text{or} \quad \frac{UV}{P}$$

where U = the concentration in the urine (mg/100 ml), V = the urine volume per min (ml/min), and P = the plasma concentration (mg/100 ml). This quotient can of course be calculated for any substance which is present in the plasma and the urine, but it is of no value if the result is greatly influenced by factors unrelated to renal function (e.g. diet). It is useless, for example, to calculate the quotient for sodium for in a normal person it may vary by more than 100 per cent during a single day. The quotients for urea and creatinine, however, are relatively constant for their urinary excretion throughout the day is far more uniform.

The quotient UV/P is inevitably expressed as ml/min (i.e. (mg/min)/(mg/ml) = ml/min) and is conventionally referred to as a "clearance". This curious term derives from an extension of the fact that the result of dividing the amount excreted in the urine by the plasma concentration gives the least volume of plasma which could have contained the amount excreted. It follows that the quotient can therefore be considered as representing the volume of plasma which must be completely "cleared" to provide the amount appearing in the urine. The concept of a clearance is only a particular way of thinking about the quotient UV/P, it is obviously unrelated to what is actually happening in the kidney, for there is no evidence that some of the plasma is stripped of certain of its contents while the remainder emerges unchanged. The disadvantages of the word "clearance" are the tortuous explanations and frequent misconceptions to which it gives rise.

Measurement of Glomerular Filtration Rate

The most precise measurement of glomerular filtration rate is obtained with inulin, for after passing freely through the glomerulus it travels down the tubule without any being subtracted or added by the tubule cells. The quantity that is excreted in the urine in one minute is therefore the same as that which is filtered. But it is known from puncture of the glomerular capsule by micro-pipettes that the capsular fluid (i.e. the glomerular filtrate) is identical to plasma ultrafiltrate. Therefore the quantity of inulin present in the urine must, as it passes through the glomerulus, be accompanied by a quantity of water sufficient to keep the inulin concentration in the capsular space the same as in the plasma. This volume is clearly that of the glomerular filtrate; it is estimated by calculating the least volume of water (i.e. plasma) that can have contained the amount of inulin excreted in the urine, i.e. UV/P. The inulin clearance is thus a measure of glomerular filtration rate. For instance, if the plasma concentration of inulin is 10 mg/100 ml, and 10 mg of inulin is excreted in the urine in one minute, it is clear that if inulin is not reabsorbed or secreted by the tubule cells, 100 ml of water is passing through the glomerular filter in one minute.

For similar reasons the creatinine clearance is also used as a measure of glomerular filtration rate, but it is not so exact as inulin for a small quantity of creatinine is secreted into the tubular fluid by the tubules.

Measurement of Renal Plasma and Blood Flow

The renal plasma flow (R.P.F.) can theoretically be calculated by the Fick principle using any substance excreted in the urine, provided that the renal arterial (RA), and renal venous (RV) plasma concentrations, the urine flow (V), and the urine concentration (U) of that substance are known:

$$\text{R.P.F. (ml/min)} = \frac{\text{UV (excretion per minute)}}{\text{RA} - \text{RV (arterio-venous difference)}}$$

From this renal blood flow (R.B.F.) can be calculated from the arterial haematocrit (Hct):

$$\text{R.B.F.} = \frac{\text{R.P.F.}}{1 - (\text{Hct}/100)}$$

It will be seen below that this laborious procedure is seldom necessary, but it can be performed by obtaining samples of arterial blood from the femoral artery, while renal venous blood is obtained via a catheter introduced through an antecubital or femoral vein.

Clearly a substance that is almost completely excreted by the kidney and therefore has a large RA − RV difference will give more accurate results than one like sodium which has an insignificant RA − RV difference. An almost ideal substance is para-amino-hippuric acid (PAH) which is infused intravenously until a steady plasma concentration is achieved.

If the plasma PAH level is less than 5 mg/100 ml about 90 per cent of the PAH reaching the kidney is promptly excreted in the urine (except in cases of advanced renal failure). In general, therefore, it is not necessary to catheterise the renal vein to sample the renal venous blood, for it can be assumed that RV is negligible (i.e. RV=0) or:

$$R.P.F.=\frac{UV}{RA}$$

In other words the clearance of PAH is a measure of renal plasma flow.

Furthermore, since the *peripheral* venous plasma concentration of PAH is almost identical to that in the arterial blood, it is also unnecessary to sample arterial blood, and the whole technique is greatly simplified.

In clinical work PAH clearances are hardly ever estimated. There is a relatively rigid relationship between the renal blood flow and the glomerular filtration rate, and it is easier to estimate filtration rate than renal blood flow. The simplest way to perform a PAH clearance is to inject 12 ml 20 per cent PAH mixed with 6 ml 2 per cent xylocaine into the loose subcutaneous tissues of the axilla. The urine collection periods are begun 30–45 min later. Alternatively the use of small quantities of ^{125}I-Hippuran greatly simplifies the technique.

BIBLIOGRAPHY

GOLDRING, W., and CHASIS, H. (1944). "Hypertension and hypertensive disease." Commonwealth Fund, New York. (For inulin and para-amino-hippuric acid clearance techniques.)

GUTMAN, Y., GOTTSCHALK, C. W., and LASSITER, W. E. (1965). "Micropuncture study of inulin absorption in the rat kidney." *Science*, **147**, 753.

PITTS, R. F. (1963). "Physiology of the Kidney and Body Fluids." Year Book Medical Publishers Inc., Chicago.

RAM, M. D., EVANS, K., and CHISHOLM, G. D. (1967). "Measurement of effective renal plasma flow by the clearance of ^{125}I-Hippuran." *Lancet*, ii, 645.

SMITH, H. W. (1956). "Principles of Renal Physiology." Oxford University Press, New York.

5

Tests of Glomerular Functional Integrity

THE mean hydrostatic pressure in the glomerular capillary in the rat, in which it has been measured directly, is considerable. It is approximately 60 cm H_2O. The effective filtration pressure, which is the hydrostatic pressure less the plasma protein osmotic pressure is therefore about 14 cm H_2O. The permeability of the glomerular capillary wall is also higher than capillaries elsewhere. This combination of a relatively high capillary hydrostatic pressure and permeability accounts for the high rate of filtration which occurs across the glomerular capillary wall. It has been mentioned earlier that in man approximately 600 ml of plasma pass through the glomeruli per minute from which are filtered about 120 ml of fluid that is almost free of protein and blood cells. Glomerular integrity can thus be studied by measuring glomerular filtration rate and by examining the urine for the presence of protein, cells and casts.

Glomerular Filtration Rate

The four methods most widely used to obtain an indication of the glomerular filtration rate are, in descending order of accuracy:

1. Inulin clearance.
2. ^{51}Cr EDTA clearance.
3. Creatinine clearance.
4. Urea clearance.
5. Plasma concentrations of creatinine and urea.

Inulin Clearance

An inulin clearance is a protracted procedure, many blood samples are needed and, as urine is collected at short intervals, relatively large errors due to incomplete bladder emptying may occur which can only be avoided with certainty by catheterisation. For these reasons glomerular filtration rate, except for research purposes, is hardly ever determined by inulin clearance. For clinical purposes an inulin clearance can most easily be performed after an intravenous injection of 90 ml of 10 per cent inulin. The urine collections are begun 30 min later.

^{51}Cr EDTA Clearance

Ethylenediaminetetracetate (EDTA) is handled by the kidney in almost the same way as inulin. The clearance of EDTA can therefore be used to measure glomerular filtration rate. It has an enormous advantage over inulin, however, for it can be labelled with ^{51}Cr which is a gamma emitter. ^{15}Cr EDTA is a stable substance while ^{51}Cr has a usefully long half life, is relatively innocuous and is rapidly eliminated in the urine. All the advantages of using a gamma emitting isotope can therefore be used to measure glomerular filtration rate. ^{15}Cr EDTA clearance can either be determined in the usual way from the quotient UV/P during the administration of ^{51}Cr EDTA by a continuous intravenous infusion, or it can be calculated from the fall in plasma concentration of ^{51}Cr EDTA 2 hours after a single intravenous injection. The latter, though indirect, avoids the hazards inherent in trying to collect a timed sample of urine.

Creatinine Clearance

This remains by far the most convenient method of obtaining a fairly accurate estimate of glomerular filtration rate. The clearance of pure creatinine however is slightly greater than that of inulin, indicating that some creatinine is actively secreted by the tubules. The amount of creatinine that is actively secreted is related to the level of plasma creatinine. With advancing renal failure therefore the discrepancies between the clearance of creatinine and inulin increases. When the plasma creatinine is about 4 mg/100 ml the creatinine to inulin clearance ratio is 1·4. At higher levels this effect diminishes so that at plasma creatinine concentrations around 10 mg/100 ml the ratio has fallen to 1·2. Nevertheless at these plasma levels of creatinine the glomerular filtration rate is so small that such discrepancies are of no moment.

The clearance of creatinine is a much more convenient determination to make than that of inulin, for creatinine is already present in body fluids; its plasma concentration being remarkably steady throughout the 24 hours. Creatinine clearance tests can therefore be performed over long periods without the necessity of continuous intravenous administration; and because the plasma concentration is so constant only one sample of blood need be taken for a 24-hour collection of urine. Such long periods minimise inaccuracies caused by incomplete bladder emptying or slipshod timing of the duration of urine collection; they also diminish the effect of transient emotional reactions on renal function.

Procedure for a 24-hour creatinine clearance

The basic requirements are a 24-hour collection of urine and one sample of blood taken at any time during this period. But because an accurately timed collection of urine is so incredibly difficult to obtain, it is perhaps worth while describing some of the difficulties which are encountered. A 24-hour collection of urine can start at any convenient hour, e.g. 9 a.m.; at this time the patient is asked to empty his bladder and this urine is discarded; for the next 24 hours all the urine that is passed is collected into one container and the collection ended when the patient is asked to empty his bladder for the last time 24 hours after the collection period began, e.g. at 9 a.m., this urine being included in the 24-hour collection. It is clearly of no importance if the actual duration of the collection period is a few hours more or less than 24, so long as it is accurately timed. The volume of the urine is then measured and the rate of urine flow per minute is calculated by dividing this volume by the number of minutes which the collection period has lasted. A convenient slogan is that the urine collection should be "timed to the nearest minute and measured to the nearest ml". A small screw-topped bottle full of this urine, and another containing the blood sample, are then sent together to the laboratory for creatinine estimation and calculation of the clearance.

This simple manoeuvre may be vitiated by the following accidents. (1) Unless the patient has been warned, urine may be passed during defaecation and thrown away; (2) unless urine is placed immediately into a large container it may be lost and not included in the 24-hour collection; (3) occasionally the urine passed at the beginning of the collection period is included in the total collection; though the patient may have four or five hours urine in his bladder; (4) it is not unknown for a 24-hour collection to cease when the container into which it is being collected is full, regardless of the time the collection began; beware, therefore, of a 24-hour collection bottle filled to the brim. Many of these troubles can be avoided by making the patient responsible for his own urine collection.

Urea Clearance

The clearance of urea used to be the most widely used test of renal function. Its value depends on the fact that urea clearance is directly related to the glomerular filtration rate. As a guide to the rate of glomerular filtration, however, it is inferior to the creatinine clearance. Its main disadvantages are: (1) The clearance of urea is considerably less than the rate of glomerular filtration; (2) this discrepancy varies with the rate of urine flow; and (3) the ward procedure involved in a urea clearance makes it very vulnerable to technical inaccuracies.

In normal subjects, when the urine flow is greater than 2 ml/min urea clearance is about three-fifths of the glomerular filtration rate; at lower urine flows it is less. This relationship is illustrated in Fig. 5.1. It suggests that though there is every reason to believe that urea is filtered through the glomerulus at the same rate as inulin and creatinine, for urea is a small highly diffusible molecule, a great deal must be reabsorbed as it passes down the tubule. At urine flows above 2 ml/min the amount reabsorbed is constant and is about two-fifths of the quantity which has been filtered, and as the urine flow becomes less so gradually more urea is reabsorbed. In an average man, therefore, the urea clearance at urine flows above 2 ml/min is $3/5 \times 120 = 72$ ml/min; such a clearance (obtained at urine flows greater than 2 ml/min) is sometimes called the maximum urea clearance. For traditional reasons this absolute figure is sometimes converted into a percentage, i.e. a urea clearance of 37 ml/min is reported as being $37/72 \times 100 = 50$ per cent of normal. The merit of this system is that one does not have to remember the normal urea clearance, but why this dispensation to feeble memories should be extended to urea clearance is not certain. It probably dates from the time when clinicians were considered to be unable to grasp absolute figures.

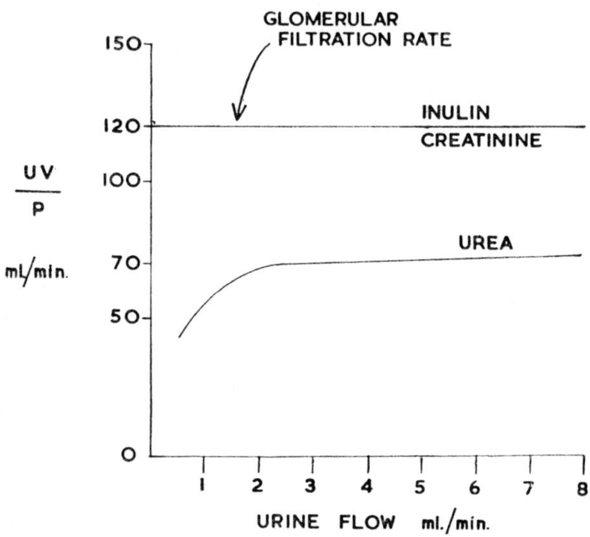

FIG. 5.1. Schema showing the relationship between the clearances of inulin, creatinine and urea to the urine flow and to each other.

When the urine flow is less than 2 ml/min urea clearance varies with the rate of urine flow, but in normal subjects if the clearance is then multiplied by the square root of the rate of urine flow, a figure is obtained which approximates to an average of 54 ml/min, regardless of the rate of urine flow. This mathematical jugglery is called a "standard urea clearance"; it is a manoeuvre which adjusts all the true clearances measured at rates of urine flow below 2 ml/min as if they had been estimated at a standard urine flow of 1 ml/min. The results are again expressed as a percentage. This rigmarole has probably caused more confusion about the nature of renal function in those not familiar with the subject than any other of the many mathematical obscurities which so often enshroud the kidney. It is obvious that a "standard urea clearance" is *not* a clearance and that the use of the word "standard" in this context is misleading. For clinical purposes these complications are best avoided by doing urea clearances at rates of urine flow above 2 ml/min.

Procedure for a urea clearance

Plasma levels of urea may fluctuate, and urea clearances vary with the urine flow, so that clearances have to be performed over short periods. It is customary to perform them in the morning when the patient is in a fasting state. In order to raise the urine flow above 2 ml/min two glasses of water are given about half an hour before the beginning of the first period when the bladder is emptied and the urine discarded. An hour later the bladder is emptied again, the urine is saved and a sample of venous blood is taken. Finally the urine is collected once more after a further hour. The volume of the two urine collections is measured and a sample of each collection is then sent, together with blood, to the laboratory for urea estimation and calculation of the clearance. The point of having two collection periods is to enable a comparison to be made between these two clearances so that the accuracy of the urine collection may be gauged.

Serious errors will occur if the bladder cannot be emptied properly or if those concerned with noting the duration of the urine collection period are horologically amoral. Occasionally the test may be influenced by the emotional reactions of the patient to having to empty his bladder at predetermined intervals, or to having to submit to venepuncture.

There is a point in the laboratory technique which sometimes causes confusion. The urea clearance is usually expressed as a "blood" clearance, i.e. UV/B (as opposed to UV/P). This is possible because urea is freely diffusible into red cells, and the concentration of urea in whole blood is almost identical to its concentration in plasma. Blood urea estimations can therefore be performed on spun red cells, leaving the supernatant plasma available for other estimations.

Plasma Concentrations of Urea and Creatinine as a Guide to the Rate of Glomerular Filtration

Normal plasma urea concentrations vary between 15–35 mg per 100 ml, the lower values tending to be found principally in children, and during pregnancy: normal plasma creatinine concentrations vary between 0·15–1·4 mg per 100 ml. If the clearance of these substances parallels the rate of glomerular filtration it is clear that when the filtration rate falls their plasma concentrations will rise. It would seem simpler therefore, when trying to gauge the state of the glomerular filtration rate, to be guided by an estimation of these plasma concentrations instead of having to perform clearances. Unfortunately the relation between glomerular filtration and plasma concentration is such that these concentrations are only of limited usefulness in this respect. The reasons for this are given below.

The plasma concentrations of urea and creatinine depend on their rate of production and elimination. If their route of elimination is via the glomerular filtrate and their daily production is relatively constant, then a fall in glomerular filtration rate will cause their plasma concentrations to rise until a new equilibrium is reached. Conversely, if glomerular filtration rate remains constant and the rate of urea or creatinine production increases, their plasma concentrations will also increase. The connection between glomerular filtration, the production of urea and creatinine, and their plasma concentrations are analogous to the situation that obtains when fluid is being poured into a funnel. The height of the level of the fluid in the funnel depends on the diameter of the funnel's outlet and the rate at which the fluid is being delivered into the funnel. The level rises until it has become sufficiently high above the outlet to force the fluid out as fast as it is being poured in at the top. If the outlet is then partially

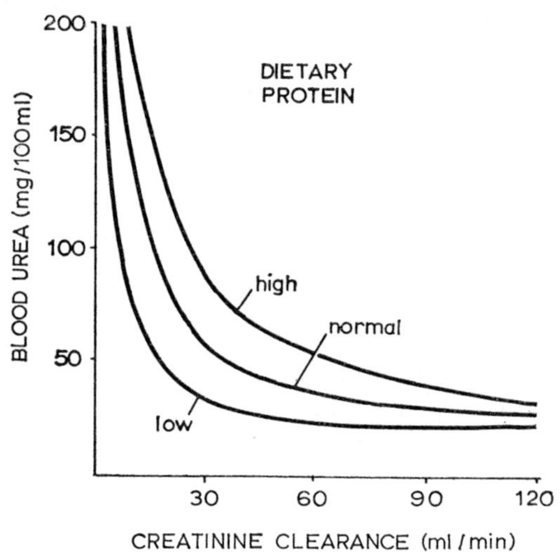

FIG. 5.2. Schema of the relationship between glomerular filtration rate (creatinine clearance) and the blood urea at varying levels of protein intake.

occluded or the rate of delivery into the funnel is increased the level of fluid in the funnel rises higher until a new equilibrium is reached. The supply of liquid into the funnel represents the production of urea and creatinine; the height of liquid in the funnel their plasma concentrations; and the diameter of the outlet the rate of glomerular filtration. When each new equilibrium is reached the rate of elimination equals the rate of production.

The relationship between the blood concentration of urea and the glomerular filtration rate is illustrated in Fig. 5.2. It can be seen that as the glomerular filtration rate diminishes there is at first only a small absolute rise in blood urea so that when the filtration rate is down to half its normal value the blood urea is still only 35–50 mg per 100 ml. Further reductions in filtration rate, however, produce large absolute changes.

The implications behind this relationship are: (1) Plasma concentrations of urea and creatinine show little absolute change until, functionally, the patient has lost one kidney; (2) when the glomerular filtration rate is low a small additional reduction in filtration rate will produce large changes in plasma concentrations. The latter is particularly striking in a patient with a moderate degree of renal failure and a blood urea of 50–60 mg per 100 ml who develops cardiac failure, or who has a haemorrhage; the blood urea may then rise to 150–200 mg per 100 ml due to a superimposed decrease in glomerular filtration rate of only 10–20 ml/min.

It is clear that if the blood urea concentration is greater than 60 mg per 100 ml, or the plasma creatinine above 2 mg per 100 ml, there is probably severe depression of glomerular filtration rate; but values below these are

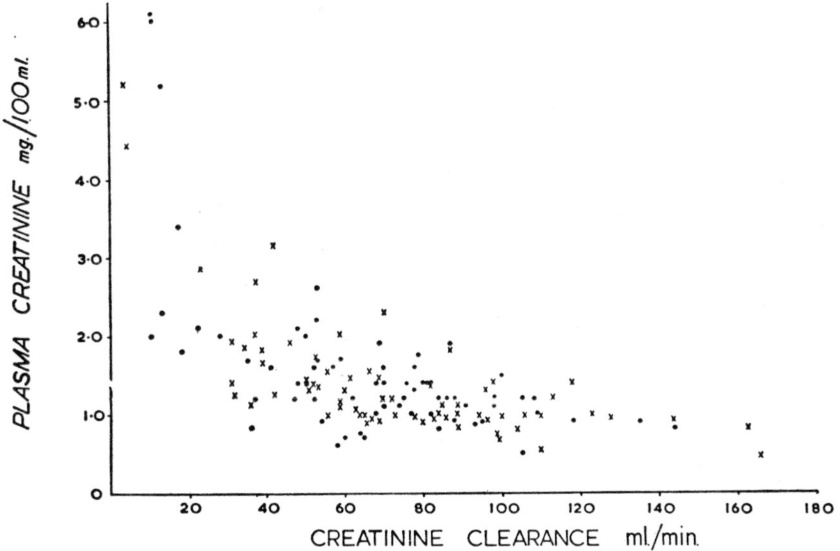

FIG. 5.3. The relationship between plasma creatinine concentration and the creatinine clearance in 140 patients. It can be seen that at any one clearance the plasma creatinine concentrations are widely scattered. For instance, there are several clearances below 50 ml/min with normal creatinine concentrations (i.e. below 1·4 mg/100 ml).

indifferent indications of glomerular function (Fig. 5.3). This is not only because at these lower concentrations large disturbances of glomerular filtration cause small absolute changes in plasma concentrations, but also because such small changes may be due to other factors than alterations in filtration rate. This is particularly applicable to urea, for (1) its rate of elimination in the urine is not only related to the glomerular filtration rate but also to the urine flow, and (2) its rate of production is profoundly affected by dietary protein content and endogenous protein catabolism. Fig. 5.2 illustrates the effect of high and low protein diets on the relation between blood urea and glomerular filtration rate in normal subjects. It shows that with low protein intakes the level of blood urea may remain within the normal range though there is a substantial

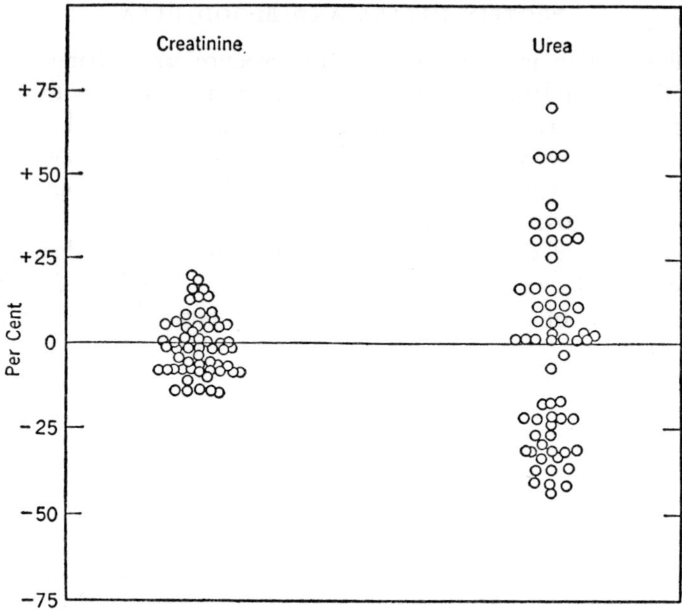

FIG. 5.4. Serum concentration of creatinine and urea. The percentage variation from the average serum concentrations of creatinine and urea in normal men on diets containing 0·5 to 2·5 g of protein per kg body weight. It is apparent that the creatinine concentrations vary less than those of urea. (Addis, 1949, "Glomerular Nephritis", Macmillan, New York.) See also Fig. 5.5.

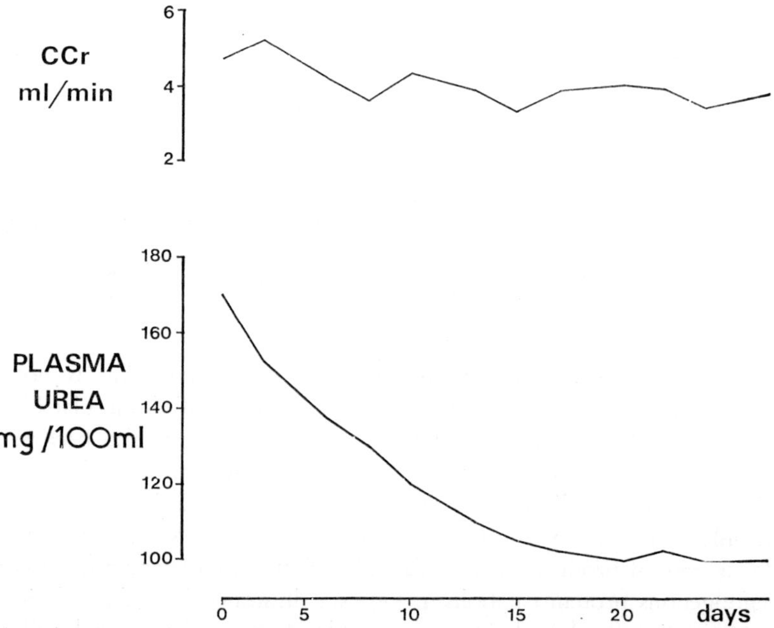

FIG. 5.5. The effect of a 20 g protein diet on the blood urea and creatinine clearance in a patient suffering from advanced renal failure. There is a profound fall in blood urea though there has been a fall in creatinine clearance.

fall in glomerular filtration rate (the impaired production of urea in liver disease may also cause a similar effect) Fig. 5.5 illustrates this point in a patient with advanced renal failure (creatinine clearance of 5 ml/min). Conversely, a high protein diet (Fig. 5.4), will raise the blood urea to pathological levels though the glomerular filtration rate is normal or unchanged. These factors also influence the plasma concentrations of creatinine but to a much smaller extent (Fig. 5.4) for the rate of creatinine production is mainly a function of the size of the muscle mass and is little influenced by protein intake. On the other hand when patients with small muscle masses develop renal failure they have plasma creatinines which are misleadingly low, e.g. plasma creatinine of 2·0 mg/100 ml with a glomerular filtration rate of 12 ml/min.

Finally, plasma concentrations of both urea and creatinine are often misleading because they lag behind changes in glomerular filtration rate. This is most obvious during the first few days of acute renal failure when there may be a gross reduction in glomerular filtration rate with initially a relatively small rise in blood urea or creatinine.

Conclusion

In a patient in whom renal disease is suspected the finding of a substantial rise in blood urea or creatinine is nearly always good evidence of a severe reduction in glomerular filtration rate. If the patient has been on a low protein diet however, an estimation of the plasma concentration of urea may be grossly misleading (e.g. blood urea of 70 mg per 100 ml with a glomerular filtration rate of 10 ml/min); in these circumstances the creatinine concentration permits a much more accurate assessment of the filtration rate. With plasma concentrations in or near the normal range it is necessary to estimate a 24-hour creatinine clearance or preferably a ^{51}Cr EDTA clearance before it can be decided whether there is any impairment of filtration rate.

The only advantage of a urea clearance is that when the glomerular filtration rate is below approximately 10 ml/min, then an accurate urea clearance estimated over a short collection period is close to the inulin clearance regardless of the rate of urine flow. In addition, an abnormally low urea/^{51}Cr EDTA clearance ratio indicates an increased back diffusion of urea through damaged tubules.

Once it has been established that the patient is suffering from renal failure further progress is followed by repeated measurements of plasma urea and creatinine. Plasma urea gives information about protein metabolism and glomerular filtration rate, while plasma creatinine mainly gives information about glomerular filtration rate. If both are measured it is therefore possible to follow what is happening to protein metabolism and renal function separately. This is particularly important when eventually the patient is placed on a low protein diet. The blood urea may then stay around 150 mg/100 ml obscuring the fact that renal function continues to deteriorate.

Proteinuria

It is probable that glomerular filtrate contains 10–20 mg per 100 ml of protein, and that the relative lack of protein in the urine is due to its being reabsorbed by the tubules. The normal 24-hour protein excretion is 0–90 mg. In theory, therefore, the presence of protein in the urine means either that an increased amount has escaped from the glomeruli or that less has been reabsorbed by the tubules. But though diminished tubular reabsorption may occur, proteinuria is usually due to changes in the glomeruli.

It is best to test for proteinuria by precipitation either by boiling or by the addition of salicyl sulphonic acid. "Stick" tests such as Albustix do not detect Bence Jones protein (p. 384) and should therefore not be used in a ward. The normal low protein concentration of the urine is not apparent with these tests; otherwise they are relatively delicate and with 25 per cent salicyl sulphonic acid a protein concentration of 0·2 g/l is evident as a "trace", and 5·0 g/l will give a heavy flocculent precipitate. For clinical purposes it is traditional to comment on the proteinuria in a semiquantitative manner, a barely perceptible precipitate being called a "trace" and a heavy precipitate $+ + + +$, with $+$ to $+ + +$ in between. This is more useful if the concentration (i.e. specific gravity) of the urine is measured at the same time, for the rate of protein excretion is relatively constant throughout the 24 hours and is related to the glomerular filtration rate, whereas the concentration of protein fluctuates with urine flow. In other words, the finding of $+$ of protein in a dilute urine indicates a much greater rate of protein loss than a similar finding in a concentrated urine. The only accurate way to measure the extent of proteinuria is to measure the amount of protein excreted in 24 hours.

In general one may say that persistent proteinuria does not occur with disease of the lower urinary tract; neoplasms of the urinary tract, however, will sometimes give rise to intermittent or persistent proteinuria; and with severe exudative or haemorrhagic lesions there may be protein $+$, but this will only occur when the pus and blood are visible macroscopically. It is essential to realise that it is the presence of protein in the urine which is the important abnormality; and that the rate of protein excretion is of secondary importance. Advanced renal failure may be associated with only a trace of protein in the urine. Proteinuria is almost always present when there is disease of the renal parenchyma, and though there are many transient and unimportant causes of proteinuria, it should not be dismissed, particularly if it is persistent. In women a trace of protein may be caused by contamination with vaginal discharge.

Starch electrophoretic separation of urinary proteins distinguishes some of the proteins being excreted. They are the same as those present in the plasma, although their relative concentrations are different, for their rate of urinary excretion seems to be related to molecular size. The loss, therefore, of albumin and α_1 globulin is usually much greater than that of α_2 globulin, a distribution which is characteristic in the nephrotic syndrome. Occasionally the pattern may be different; in acute nephritis the urinary proteins are in the same proportions as those in the plasma, while in myelomatosis a small globulin may appear without albuminuria. The pattern of protein excretion is best measured quantitatively by distinguishing the proteins either by specific immunochemical techniques or by their molecular weights on a Sephadex G.200 column.

Urinary Deposit

Red and white cells and hyaline casts are found in normal urine. In order to determine accurately the extent of white and red cell excretion it is necessary to measure their rate of excretion per unit time.

The subject empties his bladder as completely as possible, the time is carefully noted, and the urine discarded. Three to four hours later, the bladder is emptied once more, the time again noted and the urine kept. In women it is necessary to avoid including cells from the urethra and introitus. The urine is therefore collected in two containers. The concentration of cells is measured only in the urine that is excreted into the second container; the rate of excretion is then calculated by multiplying this concentration by the total volume, i.e. the volume of urine in both containers. In men it is only necessary to avoid preputial contamination. Within two hours the specimen is thoroughly shaken, precipitated phosphates dissolved by adding a few drops of glacial acetic acid, and 10 ml is measured into a graduated centrifuge tube. After spinning at 2,000 r.p.m. for 5 min, 9 ml of the supernatant is discarded and the remaining 1 ml thoroughly mixed with a Pasteur pipette. The cells in a drop of this fluid are then counted in 2 mm^3 of the ruled area of a Fuchs–Rosenthal counting chamber under 1/6 objective. Only unequivocal polymorphs in which the lobes of the nuclei can be distinguished are counted, disrupted and degenerated cells are not included. The results are calculated as follows, and expressed either as the number of red cells or the number of leucocytes cells excreted per hour.

$$N = \frac{500 \times C \times V}{10\ T} = \frac{50\ CV}{T},$$

where C = actual number of cells counted, V = volume of specimen in millilitres, T = time in hours over which the specimen was formed, and 500 = the factor to convert 2 mm^3 to 1 ml. The cells are more easily recognised if the urine is not too concentrated; it is useful therefore, to see that the patient passes about 200–400 ml of urine in the three to four hours of the collection period.

With this technique an excretion of white cells greater than 200,000 per hour is abnormal; the average normal excretion is about 50,000 per hour with a range of 0 to 200,000/hr though occasionally normal subjects have rates between 200,000 and 400,000/hr. The rate of excretion of red cells is approximately the same. This is a relatively laborious technique which again suffers from those recurrent difficulties which are associated with trying to obtain a timed sample of urine. It has been found, however, that a close approximation to the red or white cell excretion rate can be obtained by simply measuring the *concentration* of red or white cells in a drop of uncentrifuged urine (Fig. 5.6). Again a counting chamber is used but it is not necessary to time the urine collection or to spin the urine. When there are more than 10 white or red cells per mm³ the white or red cell excretion rate is abnormally high, whereas if

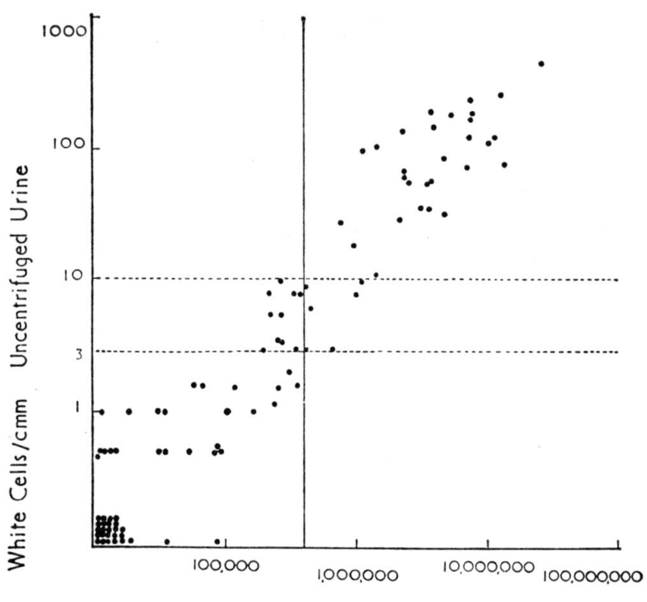

Fig. 5.6. Comparison of the white cell concentration measured in uncentrifuged urine (white cells per mm³) with the white cell excretion rate calculated from counts made on centrifuged urine (white cells per hour). The vertical line is at 400,000 cells per hour. The horizontal lines at 3 and 10 cells per mm³. (Little, 1964, *Brit. J. Urol.*)

there are less than three per mm³ it is normal; when the result lies between 3 and 10 per mm³ it is best to repeat the test. These criteria apply to children and adults; in infants less than 10 white cells per mm³ is considered to be normal.

There are two other ways in which the white cell content of the urine has been gauged in the past. One consisted of anecdotal remarks such as "scanty white cells", "a moderate number of white cells" and the now famous "white cells seen". This technique is only of use when the white cells are very numerous. In the other method a sample of urine is spun for 10 min, a drop of the deposit is then placed on a plain glass slide and covered by a cover slip. The numbers of cells seen per high power field (usually with a 1/6 objective) is then reported. Fig. 5.7 compares the number of white cells seen per high power field in each of 155 urines against the white cell excretion rate. It is clear that this technique is only useful when there are more than five cells seen per high power field when it can be safely assumed that there is a high urinary excretion of white cells. When there are less than five cells per high power field the excretion rate may be normal or raised. As this technique is more complicated and less reliable than the one in which a drop of unspun urine is examined in a counting chamber there is no good reason why it should linger.

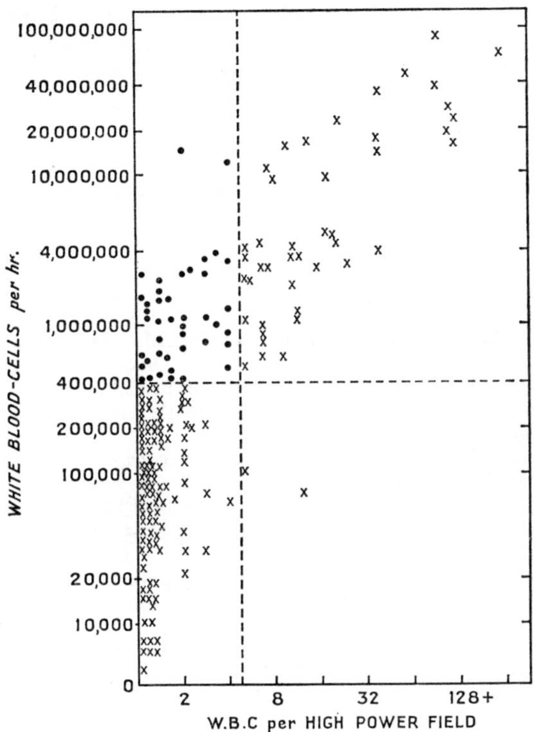

FIG. 5.7. Urinary white cell excretion rate compared with the number of cells seen per "high power field" examination of the same urines. The horizontal line is at 400,000 cells per hour; the vertical line is at five cells per "high power field". O = urine with high w.b.c. excretion but with less than five cells seen per "high power field". (Little, 1962, *Lancet*.)

It is important to note that there is a misleading relationship between the colour of the urine and the concentration of red cells it contains. For instance, frank haematuria, i.e. the macroscopic appearance of red cells in the urine sufficient to cause an acid urine to be brown or an alkaline urine to be red is, produced by only 0·2 ml of blood in 500 ml of urine.

Many different types of casts may be seen—blood, granular, hyaline waxy, and broad—the most important diagnostically being granular and blood casts. All are basically formed by the precipitation of a mucoprotein secreted by the tubule into which are imbedded either the red cells that are leaking through the diseased glomeruli, or the degenerated tubule cells that are flaking off the walls of the nephron. Hyaline casts are transparent, without any cells attached to their surfaces; they are of no importance clinically. Blood casts are characterised by a diffuse orange-yellow colour which is the haemoglobin from haemolysed red cells; these casts tend to break into short stumpy rectangular masses which are easily overlooked. Granular casts contain either relatively intact red cells or desquamated tubular cells. The highly significant fact about blood and red cell granular casts is their indication, beyond any shadow of doubt, that the haemoglobin and red cells they contain must have originated from the renal parenchyma and not from the lower urinary tract.

BIBLIOGRAPHY

BLANEY, J. D. (1965). "Estimation of the glomerular filtration rate." *J. clin. Path.*, **18**, 511.

BRAUDE, H., FORFAR, J. O., GOULD, J. O., and MCLEOD, J. W. (1967). "Cell and bacterial counts in the urine of normal infants and children." *Brit. Med. J.*, **4**, 687.

CHANTLER, C., GARNETT, E. S., PARSONS, V., and VEALL, N. (1969). "Glomerular filtration rate measurement in man by single injection method using ^{51}Cr-EDTA." *Clin. Sci.*, **37**, 169.

DICKER, S. E. (1956). "Standard renal clearances in mammals. Modern views on the secretion of urine—Cushny Memorial Lectures." J. & A. Churchill, London.

DONATH, A. (1971). "The simultaneous determination in children of glomerular filtration rate and effective renal plasma flow by the single injection clearance technique." *Acta Paediat. Scand.*, **60**, 512.

FRANCOIS, B., POZET, N., RATTANACHANE, B., and TRAEGER, J. (1971). "L'estimation de la filtration glomerulaire par l'EDTA ^{51}Cr." *Nephron.*, **8**, 147.

GOLDRING, W., and CHASIS, H. (1944). "Hypertension and Hypertensive Disease." Commonwealth Fund, New York. (For inulin and para-amino-hippuric acid clearance techniques.)

HEATH, D., KNAPP, M. S., and WALKER, W. H. C. (1968). "Comparison between inulin and ^{51}Cr labelled EDTA for the measurement of glomerular filtration rate." *Lancet*, ii, 1110.

HILTON, P. J., ROTH, Z., LAVENDER, S., and JONES, N. F. (1969). "Creatinine clearance in patients with proteinuria." *Lancet*, **2**, 1215.

LAVENDER, S., HILTON, P. J., and JONES, N. F. (1969). "The measurement of glomerular filtration rate in renal disease." *Lancet*, **2**, 1216.

LITTLE, P. J. (1964). "A comparison of the urinary white cell concentration with the white cell excretion rate." *Brit. J. Urol.*, **36**, 360.

LITTLE, P. J. (1965). "Diagnostic criteria of pyelonephritis." *J. clin. Path.*, **18**, 556.

MCQUEEN, E. G. (1966). "Composition of urinary casts." *Lancet*, **1**, 396.

ROWE, D. S., and SOOTHILL, J. F. (1961). "Serum proteins in normal urine." *Clin. Sci.*, **21**, 75.

SHANNON, J. A. (1935). "The renal excretion of creatinine in man." *J. clin. Invest.*, **14**, 403.

SHANNON, J. A., and SMITH, H. W. (1935). "The excretion of inulin, xylose and urea by normal and phlorizinised man." *J. clin. Invest.*, **14**, 393.

SMITH, H. W. (1956). "Principles of Renal Physiology." Oxford Univ. Press, New York.

TOBIAS, G. J., MCLAUGHLIN, R. F., and HOPPER, J. (1962). "Endogenous creatinine clearance." *New Eng. J. Med.*, **266**, 317.

WINDBERG, J. (1959). "Determination of renal concentration capacity in infants and children without renal disease." *Acta paediat. Upsala*, **48**, 318.

WINDBERG, J. (1959). "The 24-hour true endogenous creatinine clearance in infants and children without renal disease." *Acta paediat. Upsala*, **48**, 443.

6

Tubular Function and
Tests of Tubular Functional Integrity

THE functions of the tubule are to reabsorb, or prevent the reabsorption of the contents of the tubular fluid, and to secrete into the tubular lumen substances which are either circulating in the peritubular venous capillaries or which are formed by the tubule cell. These processes are under the control of many hormones, some plasma and intracellular electrolyte concentrations, and the hydrostatic, plasma protein, and gas pressures in the peritubular capillaries.

The principal function of the proximal tubule is to reabsorb about 80 per cent of the total solids and water from the glomerular filtrate. The solids are reabsorbed in unequal proportions so that while proteins and glucose, for instance, appear to be almost completely reabsorbed (Fig. 6.1), sodium chloride and urea are only partly reabsorbed, and there is no reabsorption of creatinine. Reabsorption from the proximal tubule takes place in such a way that the fluid in the proximal tubule always remains isomotic to arterial blood. The pH of

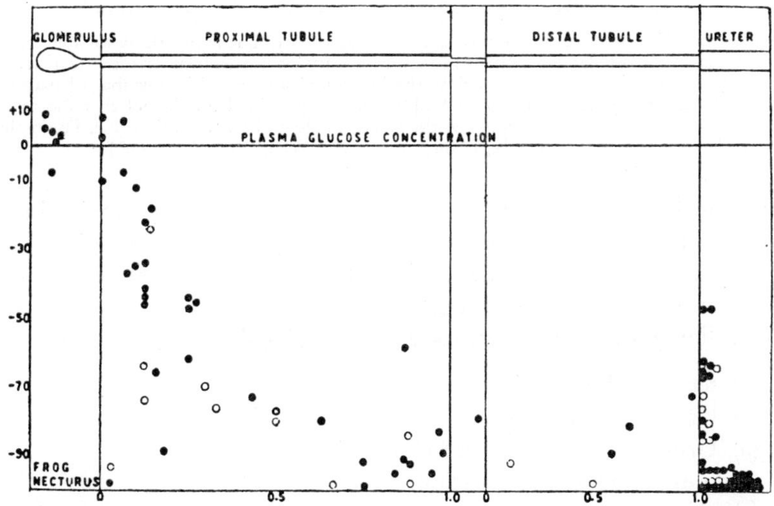

FIG. 6.1. Site of glucose reabsorption. Difference in glucose concentration between plasma and fluid collected with a micropipette from various levels of the renal tubules of normal Necturi and frogs. Zero on the ordinate represents plasma, figures above and below zero represent percentage differences from plasma. (Walker and Hudson, 1937, *Amer. J. Physiol.*)

the fluid, however, may change, and when the urine is acid the process of acidification begins in the proximal tubule (Fig. 6.2). The main function of the loop of Henle is to make the interstitial fluid in the medulla *hypertonic* and the tubular fluid that emerges from it, into the distal tubule, *hypotonic*; these changes permit the concentration of the final urine to be modified over a wide range (see below). The hypotonic tubular fluid which flows into the distal tubule contains considerable quantities of sodium chloride and waste products and has a pH

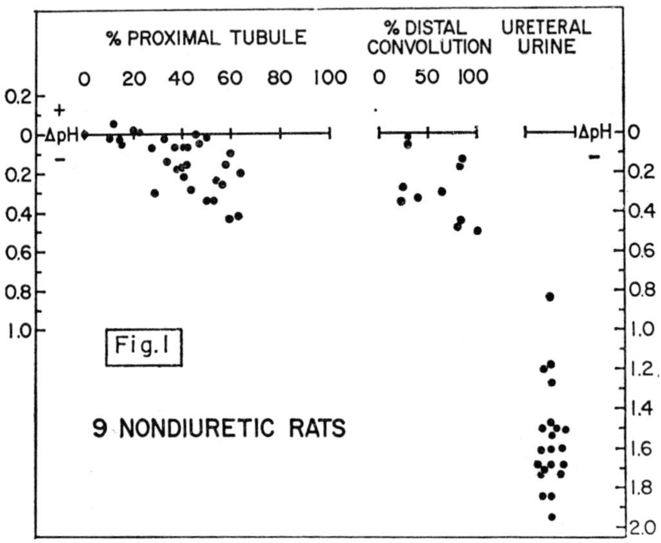

FIG. 6.2. Localisation of urine acidification in the rat kidney. The points show the difference in pH of the tubular fluid obtained in various parts of the nephron or the ureter, from that of arterial blood. Points below the horizontal line = pH below that of plasma. Note that the fluid begins to be acidified in the proximal tubule but that the main increase in acidity occurs between the distal tubule and the ureteric urine, i.e. in the collecting tubule. (Gottschalk, Lassiter and Mylle, 1960, *Amer. J. Physiol.*)

which is much the same as that in the fluid emerging from the proximal tubule. The principal functions of the distal and collecting tubules are to adjust the pH, osmolality and electrolyte content of this fluid and to prevent or impede the reabsorption of the waste products.

The following tubular functions will be discussed:

1. Water excretion.
    (*a*) Urine concentration.
    (*b*) Urine dilution and water elimination.
2. Sodium and chloride excretion.
    (*a*) Tubular reabsorption.
    (*b*) Relation to volume control.
3. Hydrogen ion excretion.
    (*a*) Bicarbonate excretion.

    (*b*) Titratable acid and ammonia excretion.
    (*c*) Urine pH.
  4. Potassium excretion.
  5. Calcium excretion.
  6. Magnesium excretion.
  7. Phosphate excretion.
  8. Amino-acid excretion.
  9. Uric acid excretion.
10. Maximal tubular capacity to reabsorb glucose and secrete PAH.

WATER EXCRETION

The kidney's ability to modify the rate of urine flow is largely responsible for the constancy of the volume and osmolality of body fluids; and the rate of urine flow is mainly determined by the tubule's ability to control the concentration of the urine. In the following account the terms *hypertonic, isotonic* and *hypotonic* refer respectively to osmolalities which are greater than, equal to, and less than those of plasma. Osmolality can be defined as the concentration of particles in a solution. The highest urine concentration attainable is about 1,300 m.osmole/kg H_2O (S.G. 1·040) which is about four times greater than the concentration of plasma, approximately 300 m.osmole/kg H_2O (S.G. 1·008), while the lowest concentration is about 50 m.osmole/kg H_2O (S.G. 1·001).

The osmolality of the urine is mainly dependent on two interlocking factors, (i) the functional integrity of the loop of Henle, and (ii) the concentration of circulating antidiuretic hormone (ADH). The loop of Henle produces a *hypotonic* tubular fluid (Fig. 6.3) and a hypertonic interstitial fluid. Fig. 6.4 illustrates how this takes place. The ascending thin and thick limb of the loop of Henle which is persistently impermeable to water transfers sodium chloride (and perhaps urea) actively from its lumen into the interstitial fluid. The tubular fluid within the lumen thus becomes hypotonic and the interstitial fluid hypertonic. In addition the descending streams of fluid within the thin descending loop of Henle, and the capillary-like vasa recta, both of which are in osmotic equilibrium with the interstitial fluid, greatly increase this hypertonicity so that it becomes maximal towards the tip of the papillae. This effect is most easily understood if it is considered as a series of successive steps which tend to trap the sodium chloride in the interstititial fluid of the medulla. As the descending isotonic fluid (300 m.osmole/kg H_2O) first enters the area into which the ascending thick limb is pumping out sodium it becomes slightly hypertonic (e.g. 350 m.osmole/kg H_2O). The next step repeats the first. The now slightly hypertonic fluid continues downwards, and again more sodium and chloride is added to it by the ascending thick limb of the loop of Henle. There is therefore another rise in the osmolality of the fluid, but this time from slightly hypertonic (350 m.osmole/kg H_2O) to slightly more hypertonic (e.g. 400 m.osmole/kg H_2O). By a succession of such steps the osmolality at the tip of the papillae may

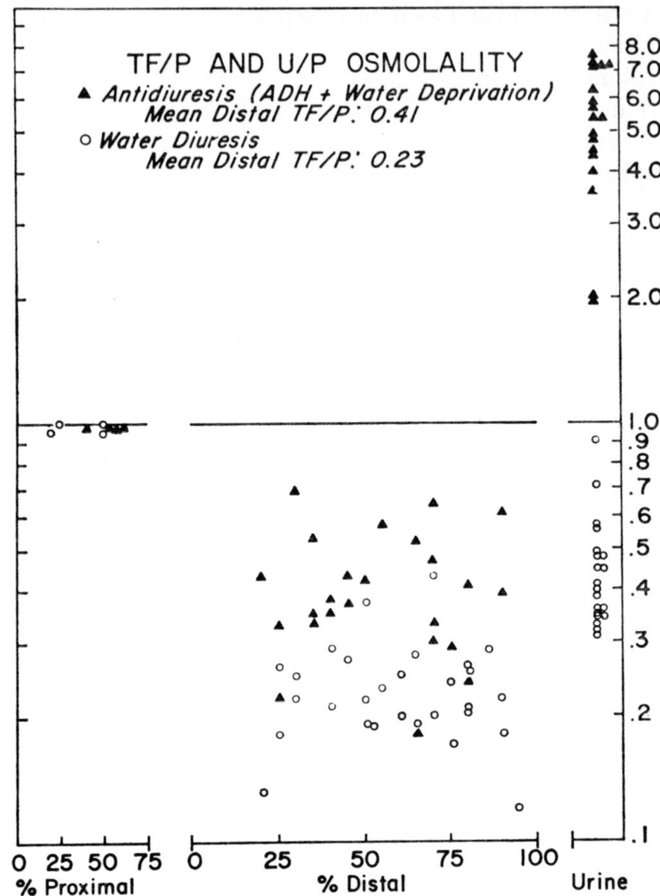

Fig. 6.3. Site of dilution and concentration of the urine in the dog. Each triangle or circle represents the results obtained in a sample of tubular fluid removed by micropuncture. The site of each micropuncture is represented along the horizontal axis as a percentage of the length of the proximal or distal tubule. The tubular fluid or urine/plasma osmolal ratio is indicated along the vertical axis. At the horizontal line 1·0 the tubule fluid is isosmotic with the plasma; above this line the urine is hypertonic, and below the line the fluid or urine is hypotonic. ▲ = results in dehydrated dogs; ○ = results in dogs having a water diuresis. It can be seen that the tubular fluid in the proximal tubule is always isosmotic whereas in the distal tubule it is always hypotonic whether the urine is hyper- or hypotonic. In the dehydrated animal the osmolality of the distal fluid is about 150 m.osmole/kg (plasma = 300 m.osmole/kg/H_2O), whereas in the dogs having a water diuresis it is approx. 75 m.osmole/kg/H_2O). (Clapp and Robinson, 1966, *J. clin. Invest.*) The results are similar in the primate.

rise to 1,300 m.osmole/kg H_2O. This phenomenon is known as a counter current multiplier. The osmolality of the medullary fluid is always hypertonic but the extent of this hypertonicity varies with the osmolality of the urine. When the urine is hypotonic it falls to approximately 400 m.osmole/kg and when the urine is hypertonic it rises to the same level as that of the urine, i.e. to a maximum of around 1,300 m.osmole/kg.

When the plasma ADH concentration is low, following a drink of water or disease of the neurohypophysis, the urine is hypotonic and is excreted in large volumes, and when the ADH concentration is raised following dehydration the urine is hypertonic and only small amounts are excreted. ADH alters the concentration of the urine by changing the permeability of the distal and collect-

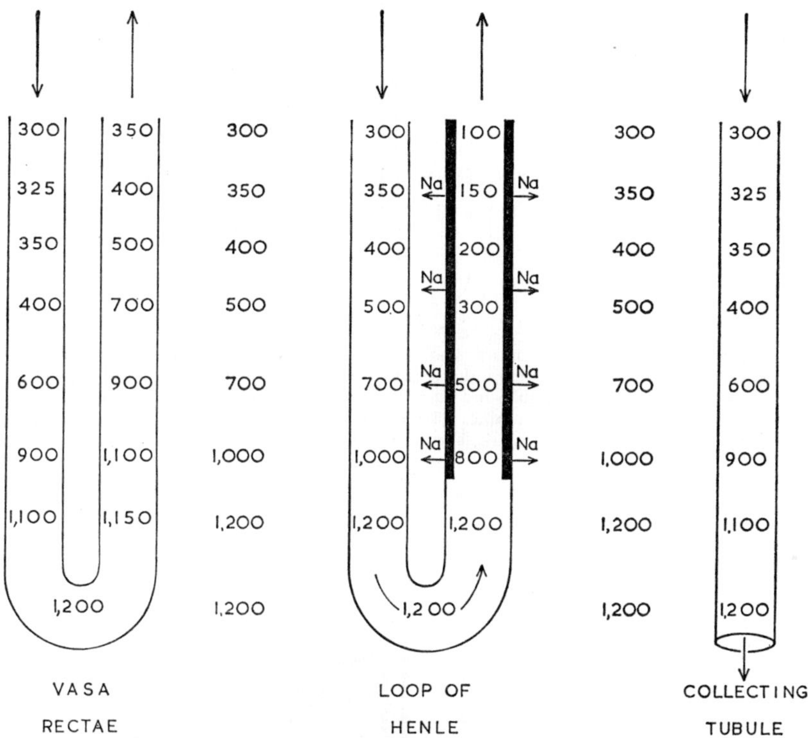

FIG. 6.4. Mechanism of urine concentration. The diagram illustrates the counter–current multiplier of the loop of Henle (p. 50) and the counter–current exchanger of the vasa rectae (p. 53). The first is responsible for the rise in medullary interstitial fluid osmolality, and the second ensures that this hyperosmolality is not dissipated by vascular irrigation.

ing tubule; the presence of ADH causing the permeability to increase. In this way when ADH is absent the impermeability of the distal and collecting tubules is intact, the hypotonic fluid which continuously emerges from the loop of Henle then remains hypotonic as it travels down, and hypotonic urine is excreted. This phenomenon is aided by the simultaneous fall in the osmolality of the interstitial fluid, in the medulla, which occurs when the concentration of circulating ADH is low.

When ADH is present and the "permeability" of the distal and collecting tubule is increased, the hypotonic fluid which emerges from the loop of Henle tends to come into osmotic equilibrium with the interstitial fluid on the other

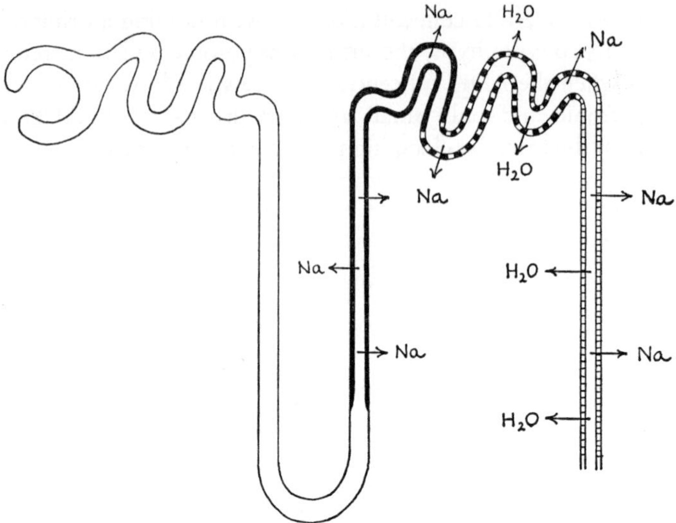

FIG. 6.5. Mechanism of urine concentration. Diagram of a nephron during the excretion of a hypertonic urine. Thick lines indicate sites where it is probable that the tubule wall is always relatively impermeable, and the lattice lines where, in the presence of antidiuretic hormone, it becomes permeable. The effect of the antidiuretic hormones on the permeability of the distal tubule is less marked than on the collecting duct.

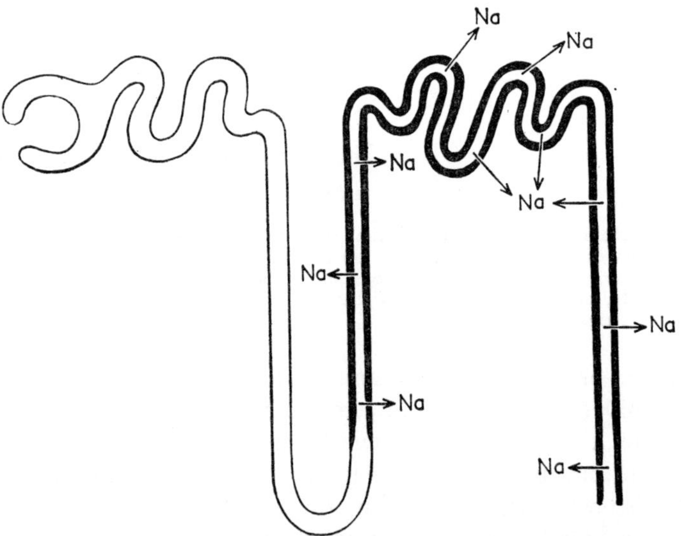

FIG. 6.6. Mechanism of urine dilution. Diagram of a nephron during the excretion of hyptonic urine. Thick lines indicate relative impermeability of the tubule wall. It is probable that most of the ascending limb of Henle and the first part of the distal tubule are always relatively impermeable whereas the wall of the second part of the distal and the whole of the collecting tubule only become permeable in the presence of antidiuretic hormone. (de Wardener, 1960, *J. Chron. Dis.*)

side of the tubule wall. As the fluid passes along the distal tubule therefore, where it is surrounded by the isotonic interstitial fluid of the cortex, it becomes less hypotonic and its volume is much reduced, but when it leaves the distal tubule, it is still hypotonic (150–200 m.osmole/kg) (Fig. 6.5). In the collecting duct where the interstitial fluid of the medulla is hypertonic this reduced volume of moderately hypotonic fluid from the distal tubule becomes hypertonic, so that hypertonic urine is excreted (Fig. 6.6).

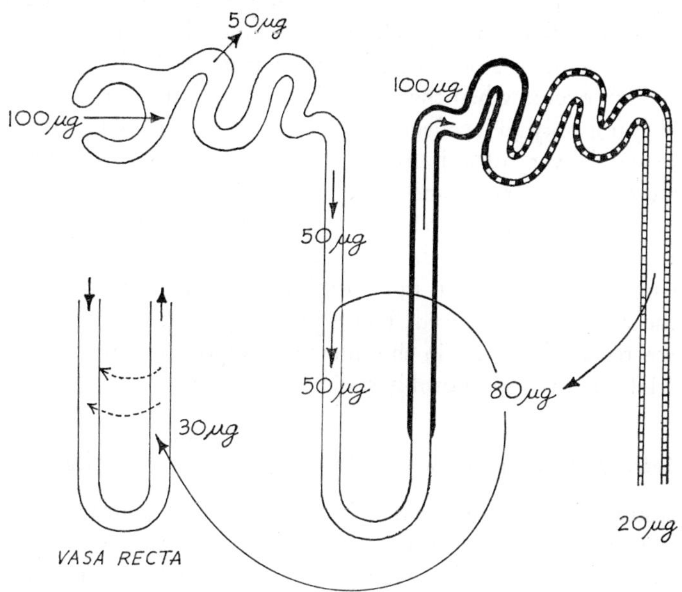

FIG. 6.7. Schema of the trapping of urea in the medulla during hydropenia. Of each 100 μg of urea that is filtered at the glomerulus 50 μg is reabsorbed in the proximal tubule. The remaining 50 μg passes down into the loop of Henle where it is joined by 50 μg which has come from the collecting ducts. 100 μg therefore goes into the distal tubule and collecting duct. 80 μg diffuses out of the collecting duct into the interstitial space and 20 μg is excreted in the urine. 30 μg of the 80 μg which diffuses out of the collecting duct is removed from the kidney by the vasa recta. (Diagram based on findings of Ullrich *et al.*, 1963, *Amer. J. Physiol.*)

All the evidence suggests that the permeability of the distal and collecting tubule also controls the passive reabsorption of urea from the tubular fluid and that this in turn influences the concentration of the urine. In the absence of ADH, when the urine is hypotonic, the reabsorption of urea is at its lowest and the excretion of urea is at its highest; whereas in the presence of ADH, when the urine is hypertonic, the movement of urea out of the tubular fluid into the hypertonic medullary interstitial fluid is at its highest, and the excretion of urea is at its lowest. The counter-current of fluids within the vasa recta and loop of Henle tends to trap the urea within the medulla (in the same way that it traps the sodium chloride) so that the concentration of urea rises towards the tip of the papillae, a mechanism known as a counter-current exchanger (Fig. 6.7).

This increases the osmolality of the medullary interstitial fluid and more water is then reabsorbed from the fluid in the collecting ducts. The osmolality of the urine then rises by an amount equal to the urea concentration in the medullary interstitial space. It follows that one of the factors responsible for the kidney's increased capacity to concentrate the urine on a high protein diet is the increased excretion of urea that then occurs.

In addition to its effect on the tubule's permeability to water and urea ADH has also been shown to increase the rate of active sodium transport in isolated membranes such as frog skin. If ADH has the same effect on the ascending limb of the loop of Henle it is possible that the increase in the hypertonicity of the medulla, which occurs when there is a rise in the concentration of circulating ADH, is due not only to its effect on the tubule's permeability to urea but also to an increased delivery of sodium into the medullary interstitial fluid.

It is intuitively understandable that the counter-current exchanger phenomenon of the vasa recta is likely to be more efficient at relatively low rates of blood flow. It is interesting therefore that when ADH is present and there is a need for as high a medullary interstitial fluid osmolality as possible, the flow of blood through the vasa recta is reduced. This is probably due to the constricting effect on the vasa recta of the rise in the interstitial fluid osmolality, caused by the effect of ADH on urea and possibly sodium transport.

Methods Used to Measure the Concentration of the Urine

It is customary to measure the concentration of the urine by its specific gravity, which is an indication of the weight of the solutes in solution. The kidney's capacity to concentrate however, is related to the concentration of particles in solution (i.e. the osmolality*) and not to their weight. This fact is most easily demonstrated by measuring the specific gravity of urine following an intravenous pyelogram when values of S.G. 1·060 may be found. Such values are much greater than any obtained following dehydration and are due to the excretion of large heavy molecules of radio-opaque substance; the particle concentration of such urine is within normal limits.

The concentration of particles, i.e. the osmolality of a solution, may be calculated from a determination of its freezing point or vapour pressure. These techniques are laboratory procedures, and it is fortunate that when urine contains only normal constituents, the correlation between specific gravity and osmolality is sufficiently close for specific gravity to be used as a clinical guide to the osmolality of the urine. This relationship is illustrated in Fig. 6.8, which

---

* The osmolality of a solution is an index of the number of particles it contains in 1 kg of water, whereas the osmolarity of a solution is an index of the number of particles contained in 1 litre of the solution. In biological fluids the two are very similar. Determinations of freezing point and vapour pressure measure osmolality, i.e. m.osmole/kg H_2O. Some years ago some of us failed to appreciate these facts and the term osmolarity was used when osmolality was measured. This explains why some of the diagrams in these pages, which have been taken from earlier papers mention osmolarity and m.osmole/l instead of osmolality and m.osmole/kg H_2O. It should be noted that in this context the symbol H_2O is often omitted, and osmolality described as m.osmole/kg.

also shows that if urine contains much glucose the specific gravity will be greater at a fixed osmolality, than in normal urine; and, conversely, if the urine contains much urea (a less dense molecule) the specific gravity will be lower.

Clinical hydrometers are convenient but relatively coarse instruments with which to measure specific gravity; it is important therefore that they should be

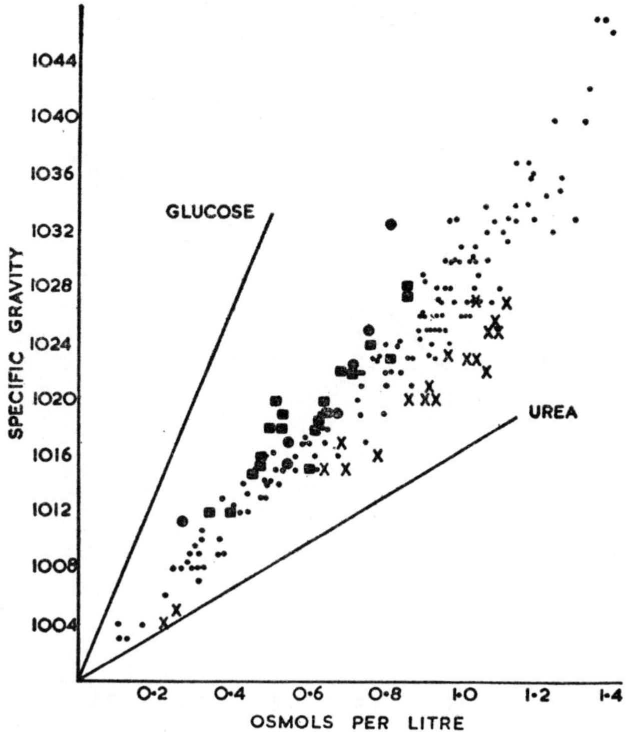

FIG. 6.8. Relationship between specific gravity and osmolality of urine. Different urines are shown as follows: with no sugar or protein (○), with +++ sugar (●), with +++ protein (■), after 25 g urea by mouth (×). Lines are also given showing the relationship between specific gravity and osmolality of glucose and urea solutions. (Miles and de Wardener, 1954, *Brit, med. J.*)

used with care. In order to check incorrect graduations clinical hydrometers should always be tested in water each time they are used; and, to avoid surface tension errors on the stem, the hydrometer should be spun and plunged well into the urine. Detergents should not be used for cleaning urine bottles or specimen glasses, for these lower surface tension and increase the measured specific gravity. And the specific gravity should never be measured in freshly passed warm urine, for hydrometers are standardised at a temperture of 16° C; for every 3°C above this temperature the specific gravity will appear to be 0·001 less than its true value, i.e. if a hydrometer is placed in urine at 37° C and shows a reading of 1·013 the true specific gravity is 1·020. An adjustment is also necessary when there is gross proteinuria; 0·001 is subtracted for every 5 g/l of protein.

Procedure Used to Test the Tubule's Ability to Concentrate Urine

This test can be performed by depriving the patient of fluid or by giving an injection of vasopressin tannate in oil. Before doing either, the specific gravity

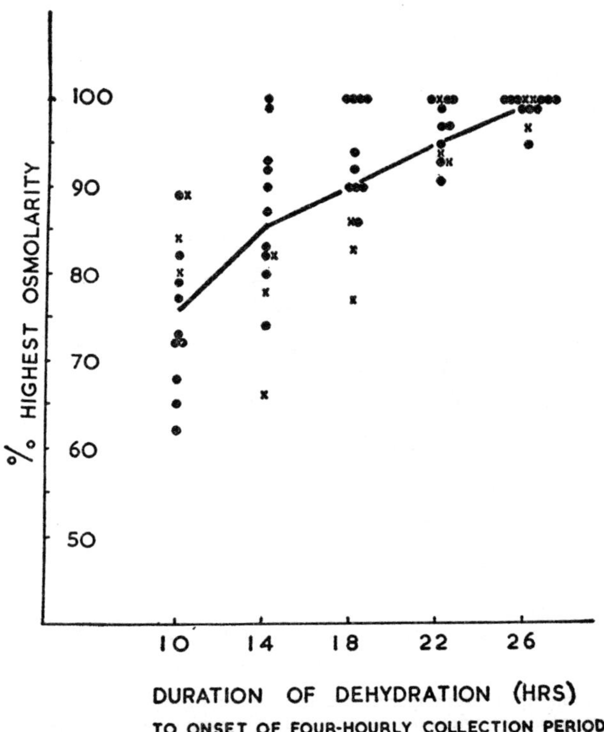

FIG. 6.9. The effect of progressive water deprivation on the urine osmolarity in 13 subjects. The osmolarity is expressed as a percentage of the highest osmolarity reached in each subject during 30 hours fluid deprivation. Urines were collected between 8 a.m. and 4 a.m. in cases marked with a dot, and between 8 p.m. and 4 p.m. in those marked with a cross. (Miles and de Wardener, 1954, *Brit. med. J.*)

of a sample of urine passed on waking should be measured, for if such a random sample is greater than 1·018 it is most unlikely that the maximum concentration achieved by fluid deprivation or vasopressin administration will be below normal.

FLUID DEPRIVATION. Fluid deprivation results in a rise of plasma osmolality and a shrinkage of the extracellular volume, both changes which are known to increase antidiuretic hormone production. The urine becomes concentrated but often does not approach its maximal value for 24–36 hours (Fig. 6.9). This is rather a long time to dehydrate patients and a convenient clinical compromise is to do the test over a period of 24 hours as follows. The period starts at 8 a.m. when the intake of all fluid, including ice creams, soups and fruit, ceases until 8 a.m. of the following day. The concentration of all urine samples passed during the last 12 hours of this period is estimated, and one of these should equal or be greater than S.G. 1·022. The normal range of urine concentration obtained

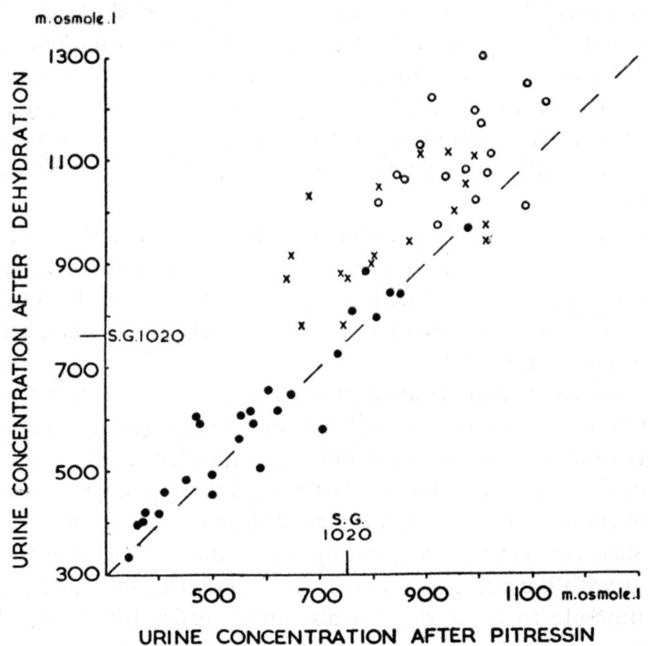

FIG. 6.10. Osmolarity of urine after 36–48 hours deprivation of fluid compared with that following an injection of vasopressin tannate in oil in 62 persons: (○) healthy persons, (×) patients convalescent from non-renal disease, (●) patients with renal disease. The diagonal line shows where the points would lie if deprivation of fluid and vasopressin tannate concentrated the urine equally. (After de Wardener, 1956, *Lancet*.)

with this procedure varies from S.G. 1·022 to S.G. 1·040. The highest figures are rarely seen in persons over the age of 20. Occasionally an apparent inability to concentrate is due to the test being performed during a diuresis caused by the spontaneous (and sometimes induced) excretion of oedema fluid.

Fluid deprivation is nearly always unpleasant for the patient, and occasionally, if a severe negative fluid balance develops because of an inability to concentrate, the test may even be dangerous. The test should always be terminated if the loss of body weight exceeds 4 per cent. For these reasons the test is hardly ever repeated, which greatly lowers its value. The test may also be vitiated by the patient's emotional reactions to having his kidneys "tested" and it may induce him to have an emotional diuresis.

C

VASOPRESSIN* TANNATE IN OIL. Fluid deprivation and its discomforts and disadvantages can be avoided by giving instead an injection of vasopressin tannate in oil. Theoretically one might expect the concentration of the urine to be the same whichever method were used. In practice the concentration following vasopressin is slightly less than after fluid deprivation; but for clinical purposes this is not important, as the discrepancy between the two techniques becomes smaller as the ability to concentrate diminishes (Fig. 6.10).

The test is best performed by combining a short period of fluid deprivation and an injection of vasopressin. Fluid deprivation begins at 6 p.m., at 8 p.m. an injection of 5 units of vasopressin tannate in oil is given subcutaneously and at 10 p.m. the bladder is emptied. Fluid deprivation ceases at 10 a.m., or sooner if the patient is distressed by thirst. In infants vasopressin should be used with care, for the large quantities of milk they normally imbibe can easily cause water intoxication.

With this method the highest specific gravity obtained should be 1·020 or above. The effect of vasopressin tannate in oil only lasts about 24–48 hours so that the test can be repeated at fairly frequent intervals, both to confirm earlier results and to follow the course of a disease. Intervals of one week between tests have been found satisfactory.

The use of vasopressin tannate in oil has one serious disadvantage. The vasopressin tannate is mixed with oil and after prolonged standing it settles at the bottom of the ampoule where it looks like an insignificant brown discoloration and is easily overlooked. To avoid its being left behind, those actually giving the injection should be aware of this fact, and that it is thus often necessary to warm and shake the ampoule vigorously before use, and occasionally to scrape the sediment with the point of a needle. The transfer of the oil and vasopressin from the ampoule to the syringe is also made easier by using a large-bore needle.

Interpretation of the Urine Concentration Test

In order to understand the result of a concentration test it is necessary to keep in mind the three factors which are directly concerned in concentrating the urine; they are:

1. The concentration of circulating antidiuretic hormone (ADH).
2. The ability of the tubules to respond to the antidiuretic hormone.
3. The rate of solute output.

The concentration of circulating ADH is regulated by both the amount of ADH produced by the neurohypophysis and the rate at which it is being destroyed at the periphery, particularly in the liver and kidney. As yet there is no

* Vasopressin is the name given to the antidiuretic substance obtained from the neurohypophysis of animals after death; there is no evidence that it differs from antidiuretic hormone (ADH), the substance secreted by the neurohypophysis during life. Pitressin is the name given by Parke Davis Ltd to the vasopressin preparations which they manufacture, e.g. Pitressin Tannate in oil.

evidence of any pathological condition in which there is an abnormal rate of ADH destruction; changes in the circulating level of ADH are therefore due to alterations in its production by the neurohypophysis. A wide variety of factors influences neurohypophyseal function including the osmolality of the extra-cellular fluid, the blood volume and certain disease processes involving the hypothalamus or the posterior pituitary.

The ability of the tubules to respond to ADH depends on the integrity of the

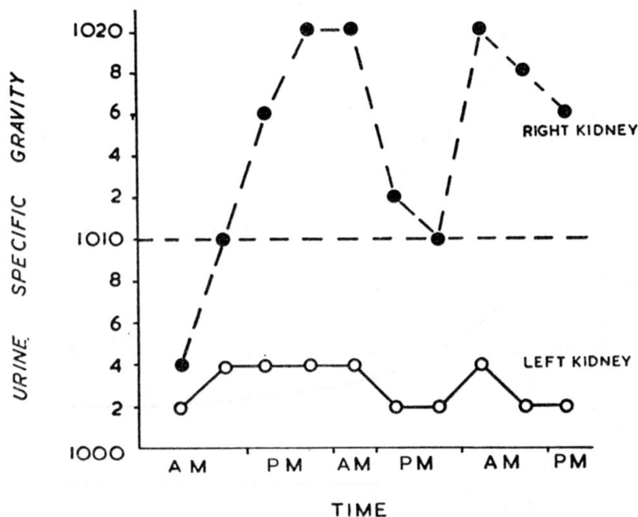

FIG. 6.11. The effect of a raised intrapelvic pressure on the ability to concentrate. The observations were made on a patient with a left-sided hydronephrosis due to a recent obstruction of the left ureter. The urine from the left kidney was obtained through a nephrostomy tube, and from the right kidney in the usual way. The hydronephrotic kidney continually excreted a strongly hypotonic urine, though the high concentrations of the urine from the right kidney indicated that there were adequate concentrations of antidiuretic substances in the circulating blood.

loop of Henle, the collecting tubule and the flow of blood through the vasa recta. The response may be impaired because of a congenital defect or an acquired disturbance; the latter may be reversible. The acquired disturbances which may be reversible initially include fever, urinary tract obstruction (Fig. 6.11), potassium deficiency, hypercalcuria, water intoxication, hypo-adrenalism, and occasionally certain acute phases of some generalised allergic diseases. In many of these conditions the urine may be persistently hypotonic even during dehydration or the intravenous administration of vasopressin; this is particularly characteristic of hypercalcaemia and potassium deficiency. Chronic pyelonephritis is also occasionally responsible for a state of fixed hypotonicity.

The rate of solute output. If a person is dehydrated for a considerable time so that the level of circulating ADH, and the concentration of the urine are high, and if at this time some substance is then administered which is promptly excreted by the kidney, there is not only a prompt increase in solute output, but also a rise in urine flow and *a decrease in urine concentration*. This phenomenon is called an osmotic diuresis and is illustrated by the curve A in Fig. 6.12. It can be seen that in these conditions of maximal ADH activity an osmotic diuresis is associated with a fall in urine concentration towards that of plasma, but that the urine concentration remains greater than plasma.

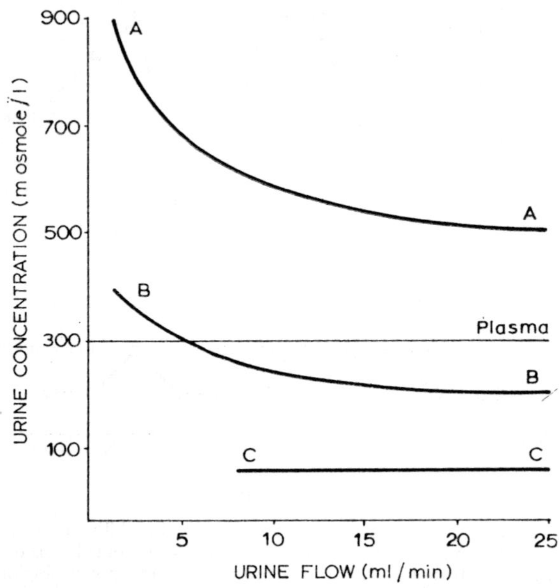

FIG. 6.12. Osmotic diuresis in the normal kidney; A was obtained in a normal subject during severe dehydration; B in a patient with diabetes insipidus during the infusion of minimal quantities of vasopressin and C in the same patient when no vasopressin was being given.

If on another occasion an osmotic diuresis is induced when the level of circulating ADH is less than during the experiment just described, similar changes in urine flow and concentration will take place, but the curve will be at a lower level; i.e. line B in Fig. 6.12. The lower the concentration of circulating ADH therefore, the lower the curve until, when there is no ADH in the circulation, an osmotic diuresis increases the urine flow but there is little or no associated change in the urine concentration, for it is already at its lowest (line C).

The increased rate of urine flow and fall in urine concentration during maximal ADH activity (line A) are mainly due to a fall in the osmolality of the interstitial fluid in the medulla. This is probably due to (i) an increased rate of flow through the loop of Henle which disturbs the counter-current system (p. 50), and (ii) the increased delivery of fluid to the collecting tubule which causes large quantities of water to be transferred into the medullary interstitial space. Lines B and C, however, are principally due to the increased delivery of hypotonic fluid from the loops of Henle into distal and collecting ducts the permeability of which is only partly altered, or unaltered by ADH. It is evident that a high solute excretion rate is not compatible with a high urine concentration however great the level of circulating ADH. The most important clinical example of an osmotic diuresis is that associated with the glycosuria of diabetes.

If the total solute output remains unchanged but the number of nephrons is reduced, the solute excretion rate for the remaining nephrons is increased and an osmotic diuresis occurs in each nephron. This is the situation that can be produced experimentally in animals by excising one kidney completely and about 50 per cent of the other. Though the remaining piece of kidney contains presumably normal nephrons such an animal is unable to produce concentrated urine. It is likely that similar conditions exist in many forms of renal disease associated with much parenchymatous destruction. If the patient is eating normally the total solute excretion rate must remain relatively unchanged, yet these solutes are being excreted through a considerably reduced number of nephrons. In such circumstances a diminished capacity to concentrate is probably due in part to the osmotic diuresis *per nephron* which must be taking place, rather than any particular inability of the tubules to respond to circulating ADH.

Procedure to Test the Tubule's Ability to Produce a Dilute Urine and Eliminate a Water Load

The test is started early in the morning and is performed in the fasting state. After emptying the bladder the patient is asked to drink water (20 ml per kg body weight) in about 10–20 min. It is inadvisable to ask the patient to drink this amount more rapidly, for in some cases this will induce nausea and vomiting with the release of large quantities of ADH; it is also advisable to sweeten the water with fruit juice. Urine is collected at hourly intervals for four hours and the concentration of each specimen and the cumulative total are measured. During these four hours a normal person should excrete 75 per cent or more of the amount ingested, and the concentration of at least one specimen should be below S.G. 1·004.

Apart from the risks of nausea and vomiting, this test is subject to other causes of inaccuracy. For instance, smoking may inhibit a water diuresis; or emotional reactions may cause either (i) an exuberantly high rate of urine flow unrelated to the patient's normal response to a water load; or (ii) an almost complete inhibition of the expected diuresis; an example of both of these is illustrated in Fig. 6.13.

In addition to renal disease a persistent impairment in the ability to excrete a water load can be caused by many other disturbances including hypoadrenalism, or an inverted diurnal rhythm.

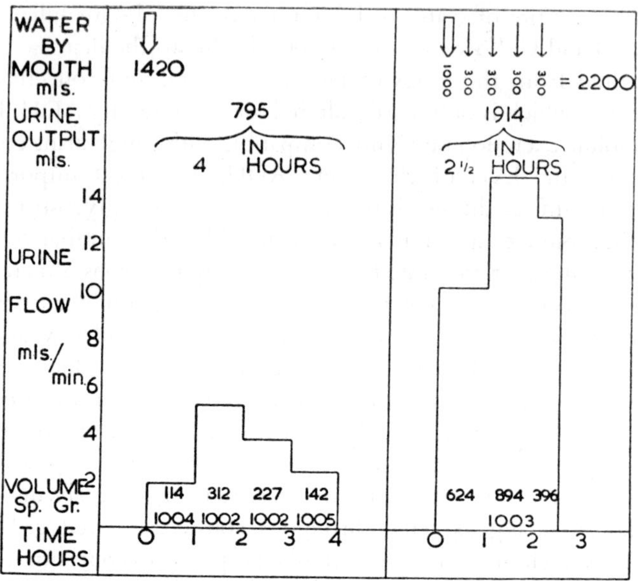

FIG. 6.13. The effect of a water load in an emotional subject. On the first occasion only 50 per cent of the amount ingested was excreted in the subsequent four hours, but the next time nearly 100 per cent was passed in only two and a half hours.

SODIUM EXCRETION

Sodium is the principal solid constituent of the extracellular fluid, the volume and osmolality of which are closely related to the amount of sodium it contains. In one hour a pair of normal adult kidneys filter and reabsorb rather more than 1,000 mEq of sodium. Or in other words 6 litres of physiological saline. Whereas less than 1 per cent of this amount, about 6 to 8 mEq, is excreted in the urine. The quantity of sodium which appears in the urine is almost entirely controlled by small adjustments in the amount of sodium reabsorbed by the tubule. Urinary sodium excretion appears to be little influenced by changes in glomerular filtration rate. Clinically this is very obvious, for patients with chronic renal failure do not develop oedema in spite of very low filtration rates.

Mechanisms of Sodium and Water Reabsorption

The first stage of sodium and water reabsorption, and by far the most important, occurs in the proximal tubule, where about two-thirds of the filtered sodium and water are reabsorbed. In the proximal tubule the tubular fluid remains isosmotic to plasma, and normally no gradient for sodium is established across the proximal tubular epithelium. Nevertheless, in certain experimental conditions it can be shown that sodium reabsorption can occur against a steep electrochemical gradient, which provides direct proof that sodium is actively pumped out of the proximal tubule. Additional evidence that sodium transport is an active process comes from the finding of a linear relationship between renal oxygen consumption and sodium reabsorption, so that about 20 to 30 mEq of sodium are reabsorbed per mole of oxygen.

In normal circumstances, therefore, the osmolality of the fluid in the proximal tubule is the same as that of the plasma. Thus it is not immediately obvious what makes water follow the sodium and move from the lumen of the

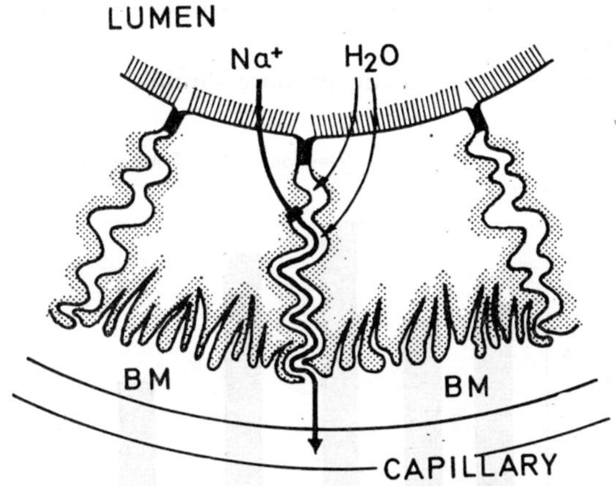

Fig. 6.14. Schema of sodium and water reabsorption through the intracellular channel in the proximal tubule. On the luminal side are the brush border, and the tight junction of the intracellular channels. The basal infoldings on the capillary side of the cell are shown opening into the basement membrane (BM). (de Wardener, 1969, *Brit. Med. J.*)

proximal tubule to the peritubular capillary; and, of course, if it is prevented from doing so sodium reabsorption eventually ceases. The following hypothesis to explain the movement of water has been put foward. It is based on the ultrastructural finding that the tubule cells are associated with two groups of long narrow channels (Fig. 6.14). One group consists of channels between the cells (the intercellular channels). These are partially blocked at their luminal end while the other end opens directly into the interstitial space on the basal and capillary side of the cell. The other groups of channels consist of deep unfoldings at the base of the cell (Fig. 1.4). Lining the intercellular channels and the basal infoldings there is a layer of adenosine triphosphatase, an enzyme which is closely connected with sodium transport. It has been proposed that sodium is actively transported from the inside of the cell into the intercellular channels and basal infoldings. This makes the fluid within them hypertonic. Water consequently flows across the walls of the channels down the osmotic gradient and into their lumen so that the sodium and the water in the channels are then swept towards their open end at the base of the cell towards the capillary. In this way there is a continuous movement of sodium and water, from the tubule lumen to the interstitial space in contact with the peritubular venous capillaries, through the intercellular channels and basal infoldings. Or, in other words, an isotonic solution passes from one isotonic solution in the tubule lumen to another isotonic solution in the interstitial space via a standing osmotic gradient built-up deep in the intercellular channels and basal infoldings.

Factors which Influence Sodium Reabsorption

The rate of reabsorption of sodium from the tubules is under the control of the hydrostatic and plasma protein osmotic pressures in the peritubular capillaries and by certain hormones.

A rise in peritubular hydrostatic pressure diminishes sodium reabsorption

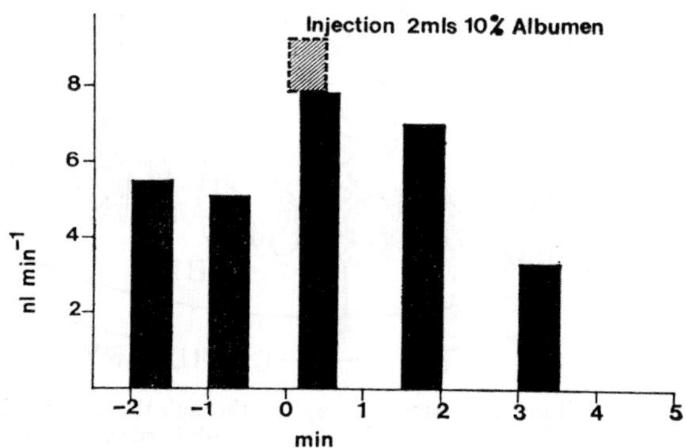

Fig. 6.15. The effect on sodium and water reabsorption of injecting 2 ml of 10 per cent albumin into the rat renal artery. The ordinate (nl min^{-1}) indicates water reabsorbed from a segment of nephron perfused constantly at 20 nl min^{-1}. There is a brisk increase in reabsorption. (T. Morgan, 1970, Supp. II to *Circulation Research*.)

whereas a rise in plasma protein osmotic pressure increases sodium reabsorption. The direction in which these factors influence the rate of reabsorption are those to be expected intuitively. Changes in hydrostatic pressure will occur with changes in the calibre of the afferent and efferent glomerular arterioles, and in the renal arterial or venous pressure. Changes in plasma protein osmotic pressure are directly related to changes in filtration fraction, for the filtration fraction is that proportion of water which is filtered at the glomerulus from the total plasma perfusing the kidney. It is evident therefore that the higher the filtration fraction the greater the concentration of plasma protein in the plasma leaving the glomerulus to perfuse the peritubular capillaries. These mechanisms have been distinguished by experiments such as those illustrated in Figs. 6.15, 6.16, 6.17.

Many hormones are known to effect tubular reabsorption of sodium including steroids (particularly aldosterone), adrenaline and nor-adrenaline, and angiotensin. Most if not all of these increase sodium reabsorption in the distal

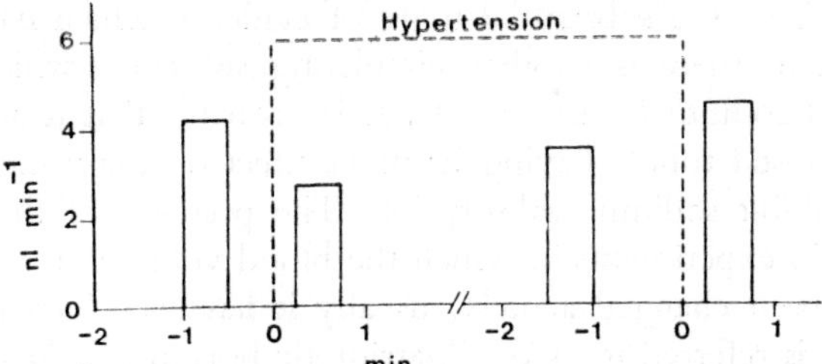

FIG. 6.16. The effect of hypertension on sodium and water reabsorption in a segment of nephron perfused at 20 nl min^{-1}. The rate of water reabsorption (nl min^{-1}) was measured immediately before and after producing acute hypertension by carotid and femoral artery ligatures. In the second part of the figure the rate of water reabsorption in a second nephron was measured before and after the release of the ligatures. (T. Morgan, 1970), Supp. II to *Circulation Research*.)

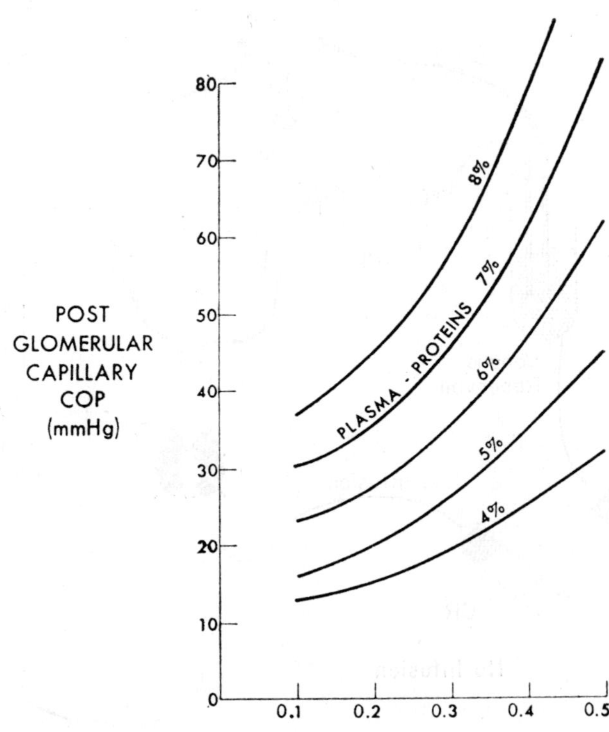

FIG. 6.17. Calculation of the effect of filtration fraction on post glomerular colloid osmotic pressure (COP) at various initial plasma protein concentrations. There is a greater rise in COP with increasing filtration fraction the higher the plasma protein concentration. (Brenner and Julia Troy, 1971, *Journal of Clinical Investigation*.)

C§

tubule. There is now a substantial body of evidence which has demonstrated that, in addition, there is another circulating substance which controls the reabsorption of sodium by the tubule. It is probable that it acts on both the proximal and distal tubule having its main effect on the proximal tubule. Its action is to inhibit sodium reabsorption. The presence of this substance has been revealed in experiments in which the blood volume or extracellular fluid volume have been changed acutely, usually it has been increased (Fig. 6.18). This substance is referred to as the "natriuretic hormone". At one time it was known as the "third factor". The nature and site of production of this hormone are not known. There are fragmentary pieces of evidence that it comes from the brain. It has been proposed, on the basis of experimental evidence, that the natriuretic hormone may be responsible for the adjustment in tubular sodium

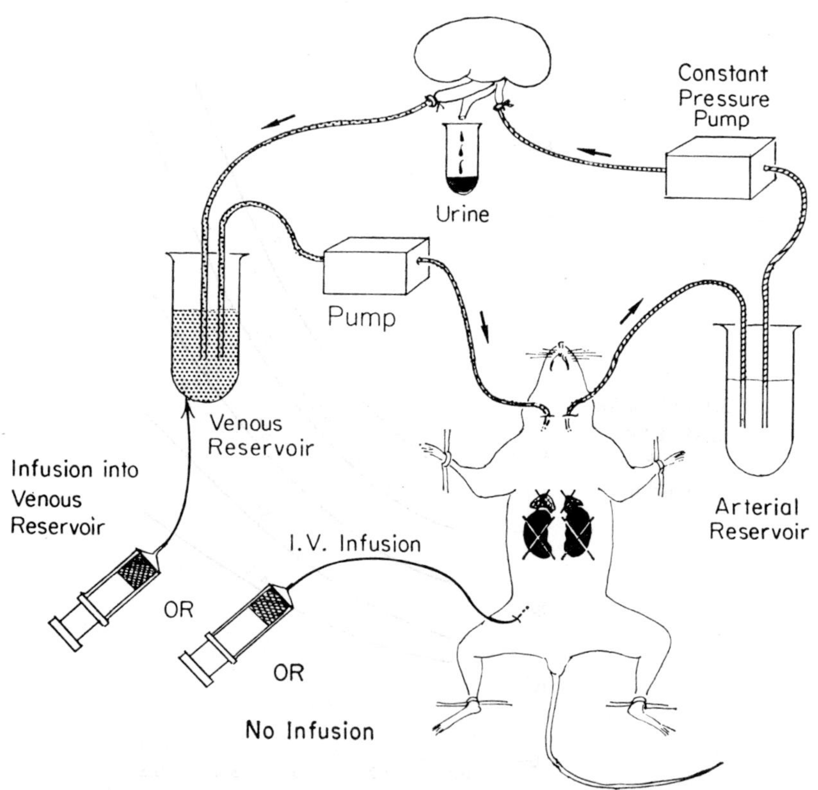

FIG. 6.18. Technique to distinguish the effect on urinary sodium excretion of an isolated rat kidney of either diluting the blood or expanding the blood volume of a rat. Infusion into the venous reservoir without changing the blood volume of the rat caused no change in sodium excretion of the isolated kidney. Intravenous infusion of the same solution into the animal caused an increase in sodium excretion of the isolated kidney. (Tobian, Coffee and McCrea, 1967, *Trans. Assoc. Amer. Phys.*)

reabsorption which takes place in chronic renal failure. In this condition the intake of sodium is usually normal, and yet the patient is not oedematous. Therefore as the number of nephrons diminishes the reabsorption of sodium by the surviving nephrons must decrease. And this often occurs in spite of a rise in the circulating concentration of aldosterone.

Among the many other factors which are known to influence the tubular reabsorption of sodium, there are, an osmotic diuresis, the renal nerves and possibly a redistribution of regional perfusion within the kidney. An osmotic diuresis always causes an increase in sodium excretion. This can sometimes be of great clinical importance, e.g. in diabetes mellitus. The renal nerves have been shown, in acute experiments, to alter tubular sodium reabsorption. Nevertheless patients who rely on a transplanted kidney for survival are in sodium balance. The hypothesis that urinary sodium excretion is controlled in part by changes in regional perfusion derives from the observation that when sodium excretion is low the blood flow to the nephrons with glomeruli near the medulla is also low, and vice versa. It is not at all certain whether this phenomenon is one of cause or effect. The original suggestions which were put forward to support the proposition that there was a causal connection have been difficult to support experimentally.

The Relationship Between Sodium Reabsorption and the Tubular Handling of Potassium, Hydrogen and Calcium Ions

Sodium reabsorption is related to the movement of potassium, hydrogen and calcium ions into and from the tubular fluid. Sodium reabsorption in the distal and collecting ducts is closely related to the tubular secretion of hydrogen ions and potassium ions. For instance, under conditions of intense sodium reabsorption (e.g. during sodium deprivation) the administration of sodium sulphate causes a precipitate fall in urine pH and a rise in tritatable acid excretion, together with a rise in potassium excretion. This is due to the positively charged sodium ions being actively reabsorbed from the tubule lumen while the negatively charged sulphate ions remain behind owing to their poor penetrative qualities. The electrical gradient which results is then responsible for a passive movement of hydrogen and potassium ions from the tubule cells into the tubule lumen. Such an intravenous infusion of sodium sulphate during sodium deprivation is a highly abnormal situation, but the urinary changes which it induces probably reflects the normal pattern of events, i.e. active sodium reabsorption from the tubule lumen into the tubule cells sets up a potential gradient along which chloride ions travel into the cell while hydrogen and potassium ions move in the opposite direction from the cell into the tubule fluid.

A close and parallel relationship between the urinary excretion of sodium and calcium ions can be demonstrated in acute experiments when the urinary excretion of one of them is acutely changed. It seems therefore that the mechanism of reabsorption for these two ions are related. Nevertheless in chronic situations the urinary excretion of the two ions is not related. For instance a person on a low calcium diet who is excreting small amounts of calcium does not become oedematous.

Procedure Used to Test the Tubules' Ability to Control Sodium Excretion

The efficiency of the tubules' ability to control sodium excretion can be tested either by increasing or decreasing the intake of sodium. An excess of sodium, however, is rarely given, for an inability to excrete a sodium load is more frequently due to extrarenal influences stimulating the tubules to retain sodium (i.e. cardiac failure, liver failure, etc.) than to renal disease itself. The dangers which follow an inability to excrete a sodium load may also be more sudden in onset, dangerous, and difficult to treat than those which may accompany sodium deficiency.

Reducing the intake of sodium is a more specific test of intrinsic tubular abnormality. The patient is placed on a normal ward diet containing about 100 mEq of sodium per day, and the daily urinary sodium excretion is estimated for a control period during which it should (in the absence of diarrhoea or much sweating) be approximately 15 mEq/day less than the intake (to allow for loss in sweat and faeces). The dietary intake of salt is then reduced to about 10 mEq/day, which is the content of the average hospital "salt-free" diet. Within 7–10 days urinary sodium excretion should also be down to 10 mEq per day.

The kidney's response to a low salt diet depends not only on tubular function but also on the many mechanisms which influence the tubule to retain salt. A more direct test of tubular ability to control salt excretion is obtained by keeping the patient on a normal diet and giving 2 mg of 9-α-fluorohydrocortisone twice a day for two or three days when the urinary excretion of sodium should fall below 10 mEq/day.

Apart from Addison's disease and severe glycosuria, an inability to conserve sodium is seen occasionally in many forms of chronic renal failure, e.g. polycystic kidneys; it also occurs sometimes during the diuretic phase of acute renal failure, and very rarely as a result of a primary disturbance of tubular function (Renal Tubular Acidosis, p. 237). In contrast, in chronic renal failure there may sometimes be an impaired ability to excrete a high intake of sodium.

CONTROL OF ACID-BASE BALANCE AND URINE ACIDITY

Plasma hydrogen-ion concentration is maintained close to pH 7·4 by a variety of mechanisms. The most important are the buffering capacity of the cells and the skeleton, and the control of the $B.HCO_3/H.HCO_3$ buffer system in the plasma (where B = metallic cations, i.e. sodium, potassium and calcium). In this system the level of carbonic acid is regulated by the excretion of CO_2 by the lungs, and the concentration of bicarbonate (mainly in the form of sodium bicarbonate) by the kidney's ability to excrete an acid or alkaline urine and to generate bicarbonate.

On a normal diet and with a normal ventilation the pH of the blood can only remain constant if about 40–60 mEq of hydrogen ions are excreted in the urine each day. This represents the net load which remains to be disposed of, when metabolism is normal. The kidney's ability to excrete hydrogen ions depends on the tubule's capacity to secrete both hydrogen and ammonia ions into the tubular fluid. In the urine the hydrogen ions are either (i) free, or potentially free in association with a buffer, or (ii) combined with ammonia in the form of ammonium.

The amount of alkali that must be added to acid urine to return the pH to that of plasma is a measure of the net quantity of free and potentially free hydrogen ions in the urine and is known as the titratable acid. The sum of the urinary titratable acidity and ammonium is a measure of the kidney's excretion of hydrogen ions, i.e. its contribution towards preventing the internal environment from becoming acid.

Tubular Control of Hydrogen Ion Secretion and Bicarbonate Reabsorption

Tubular fluid pH is consistently acid along the length of the tubule indicating that bicarbonate is reabsorbed by a process which involves hydrogen ion secretion. Direct reabsorption of bicarbonate would not be associated with these low pH values. The secretion of hydrogen ions into the tubular fluid that permits the excretion of free hydrogen ions is necessary for the reabsorption of sodium bicarbonate, and is responsible for generating fresh bicarbonate.

Hydrogen ion secretion from the tubule cell and bicarbonate reabsorption from the tubule lumen occur in both the proximal and distal tubule and are dependent on the intracellular production of free hydrogen ions. Throughout the nephron this is probably due primarily to the formation of carbonic acid from the hydration of carbon dioxide. Some of the carbonic acid then dissociates into hydrogen and bicarbonate ions, i.e.

$$CO_2 + H_2O \underset{\text{Carbonic anhydrase}}{\rightleftharpoons} H_2CO_3 \rightleftharpoons H^+ HCO_3^-$$

These additional hydrogen ions are available for transfer into the tubular fluid in exchange for the sodium ions which are being actively and independently transported from the tubule lumen into the cell. The positively charged hydrogen ions diffuse into the tubule lumen not only because of their higher intracellular concentration (consequent upon their continuous intracellular production) but also because of the electrical gradient caused by the simultaneous active transport of the positively charged sodium ions from the tubule lumen.

Most of the hydrogen ions which enter the tubular fluid combine with bicarbonate to form carbonic acid which then either diffuses back into the cell

(Fig. 6.19) or is dehydrated in the tubule lumen to carbon dioxide and water when the carbon dioxide then diffuses back into the cell. Once in the cell the carbonic acid or carbon dioxide are then reutilised or diffuse into the blood. The hydrogen ions which remain in the tubule fluid are finally excreted in the urine, either as free ions or in association with a buffer, particularly phosphate (Fig. 6.20), or they are combined with ammonia. The transfer of hydrogen ions from the tubule cell into the tubule fluid in the distal tubule can continue in the face of a steep rise in the concentration of hydrogen ions in the tubular fluid;

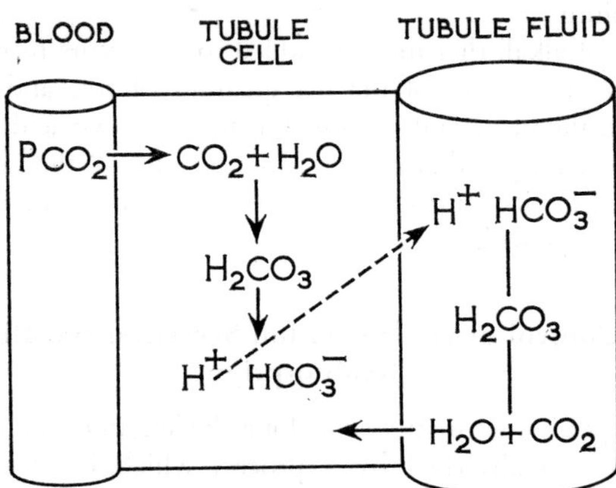

FIG. 6.19. Reabsorption of bicarbonate in tubule; control by PCO_2 in both proximal and distal tubule.

the highest concentration which can be sustained is about pH 4·3. At this point the further transfer of hydrogen ions depends on the supply of buffer or ammonia.

The intracellular formation and concentration of hydrogen ions in the tubule cells and their secretion into the tubule lumen is dependent on a variety of factors. In the proximal tubule it appears to be dependent on the ambient carbon dioxide tension (Fig. 6.19), whereas in the distal tubule it is also dependent on the carbon dioxide tension but it is also related to the intracellular content of carbonic anhydrase which accelerates the hydration of carbon dioxide. In addition, in the distal tubule, sodium reabsorption from the lumen of the tubule into the cell can cause potassium ions to flow from the cell into the tubule lumen as well as, or instead of, hydrogen ions. The relative intracellular concentration of these two ions probably determines in what proportions they are excreted in the urine. For instance, the increase in intracellular potassium concentration which is produced by the administration of potassium chloride diminishes distal tubular secretion of hydrogen ions and increases the urinary excretion of potassium. As a result less bicarbonate is reabsorbed, therefore more is excreted and there is a fall in plasma bicarbonate. Alternatively, if the cellular production of hydrogen ions in the distal tubule is inhibited by the administration of a carbonic anhydrase inhibitor such as acetazoleamide (Diamox) the reabsorption of sodium in the distal tubule will again be associated with a rise in potassium excretion and a diminution of hydrogen ion excretion. On this occasion, however, the increased potassium excretion is due to a decrease of intracellular hydrogen ion concentration and not to an increase in potassium concentration.

Bicarbonate reabsorption, like that of phosphate and sodium reabsorption, is closely related to glomerular filtration rate. In other words, changes in

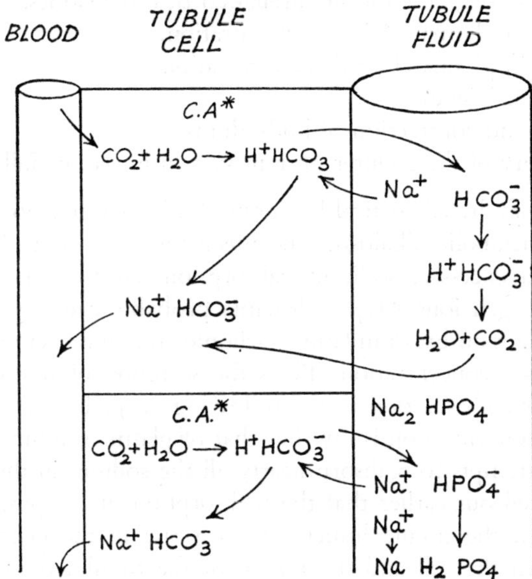

FIG. 6.20. Secretion of hydrogen ions in the distal tubule, and bicarbonate reabsorption and generation. Note that the excretion of titratable acid is chiefly in the form of acid phosphate, and that the formation of this salt is accompanied by the generation of fresh bicarbonate ions.

glomerular filtration of bicarbonate are accompanied by almost equal change in tubular reabsorption of bicarbonate with the result that the change in filtration produces little if any change in bicarbonate excretion. It is important that this phenomenon be remembered when studying the effect of various stimuli on tubular reabsorption, if such stimuli also produce changes in glomerular filtration rate. It is for this reason that in such studies changes in bicarbonate (and phosphate) reabsorption are related to a constant glomerular filtration.

Other Mechanisms Involved in the Control of Bicarbonate Excretion

It is clear from the above that one of the main factors which influences bicarbonate excretion is the secretion of hydrogen ions into the tubule lumen.

When a sufficient quantity is secreted into the tubule lumen all the filtered bicarbonate can be reabsorbed—if less hydrogen ions are secreted some of the filtered bicarbonate will not be reabsorbed and will therefore be excreted. It has also been pointed out that two of the factors which influence this tubular secretion of hydrogen ions are variations in Pco_2 and body stores of potassium. The secretion of hydrogen ions and therefore the reabsorption and excretion of bicarbonate are also influenced by:

1. Variations in the secretion of adrenal cortical hormones.
2. Variations in plasma calcium concentration.
3. Variations in plasma chloride concentration.
4. Potassium deficiency.
5. Expansion and contraction of body fluids.
6. The integrity of the counter-current system in the medulla.

Insufficiency of adrenal cortical hormones leads to a metabolic acidosis, and an excess to a metabolic alkalosis. The mechanisms are not clear. Perhaps a diminution or an excessive sodium reabsorption has a parallel effect on the secretion of hydrogen ions. Hypercalcaemia probably causes a rise in urinary hydrogen ion excretion by stimulating carbonic anhydrase activity.

Plasma chloride concentration affects the secretion of hydrogen ions and therefore bicarbonate excretion in the following way: let us assume that the plasma chloride concentration is low but that of plasma sodium is normal, and that the tubule attempts to reabsorb nearly all the sodium in the normal way. It has been pointed out earlier that the reabsorption of the positively charged sodium ions from the tubule lumen causes a rise in the electrical potential difference between the cell and the lumen of the tubule; the cell tending to become increasingly positive and the lumen increasingly negative. This potential gradient causes the negatively charged chloride ions to diffuse from the tubule lumen into the cell and the positively charged hydrogen ions to diffuse from the cell into the lumen. If the supply of chloride ions to the tubule lumen falls because of a fall in plasma chloride and if at the same time sodium reabsorption remains normal, it is clear that even if all the chloride ions diffuse back into tubule cell, the steepness of the potential gradient will remain higher than when the supply of chloride is normal. It is then inevitable that the passive flux of hydrogen ions from the tubule cell into the tubule lumen will increase and thus enhance bicarbonate reabsorption.

Expansion of body fluids profoundly inhibits sodium and therefore bicarbonate reabsorption. At one time it was considered that the tubule had a limited capacity to reabsorb bicarbonate, i.e. a Tm HCO_3 (page 73). This conclusion was based on experiments which were performed by raising the plasma bicarbonate progressively by the intravenous infusion of large volumes of sodium bicarbonate solutions. It has now been demonstrated that this apparent limitation of bicarbonate reabsorbed is an artefact produced by expanding the extracellular fluid volume with the bicarbonate solution. If the experiment is repeated in such a way that the rise in plasma bicarbonate is produced with a minimal expansion of body fluid there is no discernible limit to the tubule's capacity to reabsorb bicarbonate (Fig. 6.21). Conversely contraction of body fluid which causes excessive reabsorption of sodium is associated with excessive reabsorption of bicarbonate. In some instances this can give rise to a metabolic alkalosis with a raised plasma bicarbonate. This may occur with diarrhoea and vomiting, and with diuretics (except Spironolactone, Amiloride and Triamterene) when the alkalotic effect of sodium depletion is often reinforced by a simultaneous increase in potassium secretion leading to potassium deficiency, In potassium

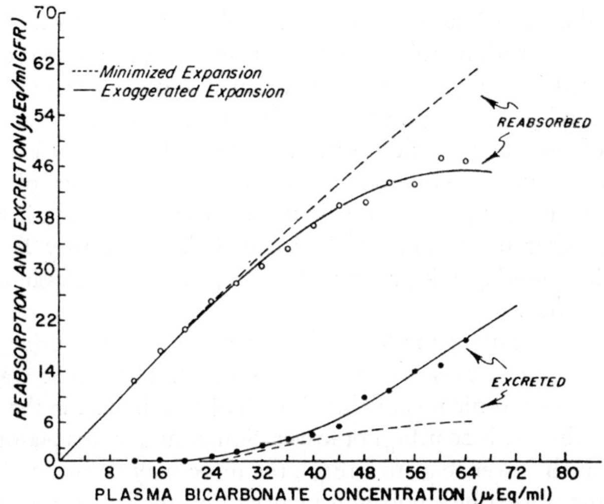

Fig. 6.21. The effect of extracellular fluid volume expansion on bicarbonate reabsorption in the rat. Bicarbonate reabsorption is depressed by extracellular fluid volume expansion. (Pukerson, Lubowitz, White and Bricker, 1969, *Journal of Clinical Investigation*.)

deficiency the diminution in the intracellular potassium of the tubular cells causes a diminution in tubular potassium secretion and a rise in hydrogen ion secretion.

The Pco_2 of an alkaline urine excreted by a normal person may be around 100 mmHg. The kidney's ability to excrete a urine with such a high Pco_2 is due to counter-current systems in the medulla which traps the carbon dioxide (p. 112). This phenomenon permits the presence in the urine of very high concentrations of bicarbonate and thus increases the kidney's capacity to excrete large amounts of bicarbonate.

Procedures Used to Detect the Presence of an Abnormal Handling of Bicarbonate by the Kidneys

One method is to estimate the tubules "maximal" capacity to reabsorb bicarbonate (Tm HCO_3, see p. 75). Though this is a spurious Tm, and is only apparent because of the way in which the plasma bicarbonate is increased during the test it is sufficiently reproducible to be used as a test of bicarbonate handling by the kidney. A low Tm HCO_3 is evidence of bicarbonate wastage due to diminished bicarbonate reabsorption in the proximal tubule. The patient should not be taking diuretics and should be emotionally at rest to avoid hyperventilation. A large intravenous infusion of sodium bicarbonate is given so as to raise the plasma bicarbonate to approximately 28–30 mEq/l. As bicarbonate reabsorption is related to glomerular filtration the maximal rate of bicarbonate reabsorption is then adjusted to a standard quantity of glomerular filtrate; it is usual to adjust to one litre of filtrate.

The normal maximal rate of bicarbonate reabsorption under these conditions is 26 to 29 mEq/l of glomerular filtrate. It is lowered in chronic renal failure. It is also reduced in many diseases, in particular those associated with hyperglobulinaemia when it is almost invariably associated with many selective disturbances of proximal tubule function (p. 241). Tm HCO_3 is low in some patients with essential hypertension without overt evidence of other renal functional abnormalities, it is also lowered when hyperventilation lowers Pco_2; on the other hand, Tm HCO_3 is raised in respiratory failure with a raised Pco_2, in vomiting with hydrochloric acid loss, in potassium deficiency and hyperadrenalism.

In chronic renal failure the leak of bicarbonate into the urine may be an important contributory cause of metabolic acidosis. The easiest way to spot a bicarbonate leak in chronic renal failure is to find bicarbonate in the urine when the plasma bicarbonate is 20 mEq/l or lower. Sometimes with a plasma bicarbonate which is much lower, e.g. 10 mEq/l, the urine may be free of bicarbonate. If, however, the plasma bicarbonate is increased by the intravenous administration of bicarbonate, bicarbonate is then observed to appear in the urine at plasma bicarbonate of between 15 and 20 mEq/l. This leak of bicarbonate in chronic renal failure is partly due to an insufficient secretion of hydrogen ions by the reduced number of nephrons (see below), and to the raised concentration of plasma parathyroid hormone which inhibits bicarbonate reabsorption.

The plasma bicarbonate tends to be low when the ability to reabsorb bicarbonate is reduced and raised when the ability to reabsorb bicarbonate is raised.

Acidosis

In chronic respiratory acidosis (e.g. emphysema) the rise in Pco_2 causes an increase in the concentration of hydrogen ions both in the plasma and the cells, including the tubule cells. This in turn increases the tubular secretion of hydrogen ions from the cells into the tubule lumen and thus causes a rise in both the urinary excretion of hydrogen ions and an increased intracellular generation of bicarbonate. The increased secretion of hydrogen ions into the tubule lumen ensures that all the filtered bicarbonate is reabsorbed, in addition, however some of the extra bicarbonate generated in the tubule cell also diffuses into the blood. The combination of total bicarbonate reabsorption, intracellular bicarbonate generation with diffusion into the plasma, and increased urinary hydrogen ion excretion causes a rise in plasma bicarbonate. The ability to reabsorb all the filtered bicarbonate increases in parallel with the rise in P_{CO_2} and remains complete with P_{CO_2} tensions of 80 mmHg and above

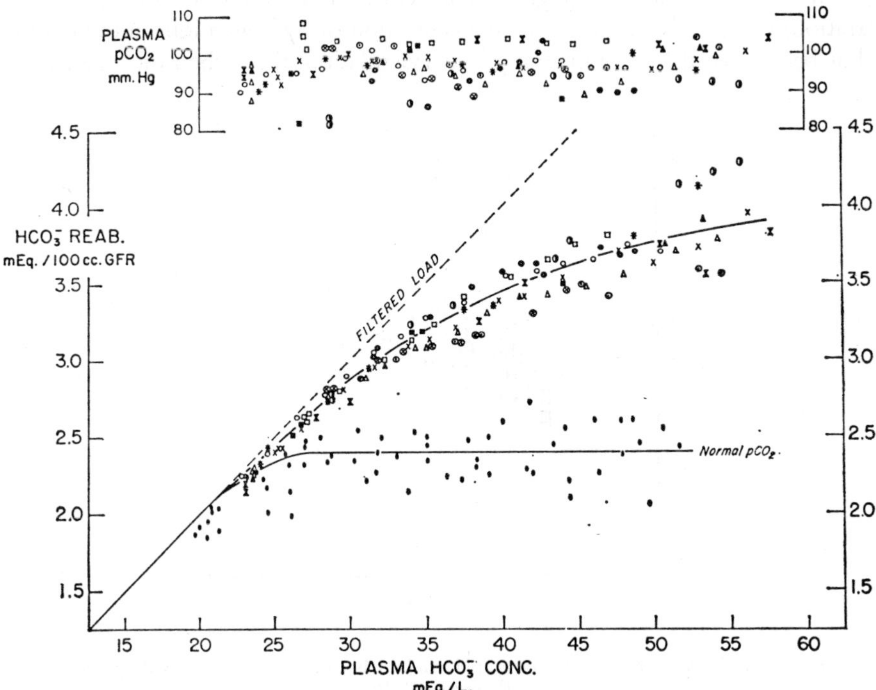

FIG. 6.22. Bicarbonate reabsorption in the dog. The effect of acute increases in P_{CO_2} during the progressive elevation of plasma bicarbonate by the intravenous infusion of $NaHCO_3$ in large volumes of water. The lower line = values obtained at normal P_{CO_2} between 35 and 45 mmHg. The upper curved line = values obtained when the P_{CO_2} was between 80 and 110 mmHg. It can be seen that the bicarbonate reabsorption is greater when the P_{CO_2} is raised. It is clear that at both concentrations of P_{CO_2} the capacity to reabsorb bicarbonate flattens out, but at different values. This flattening is due to the effect of the large expansion in body fluids caused by the sodium bicarbonate infusion which inhibits bicarbonate reabsorption (see page 73). (Schwartz, Falbriard and Lemieux, 1959, *J. clin. Invest.*)

(Fig. 6.22). The generation of extra bicarbonate and urinary excretion of hydrogen ions, however, are only sufficient to compensate for a rise of P_{CO_2} up to 60 mmHg. This can be seen in Fig. 6.24 where up to a rise in P_{CO_2} of 60 mmHg the accompanying rise in bicarbonate is sufficient to prevent a major change in plasma pH. Above a P_{CO_2} of 60 mmHg the urine remains free of bicarbonate but the rise in plasma bicarbonate is minimal and there is a sharp fall in plasma pH. The inadequacy of the urinary hydrogen ion excretion is particularly striking and is due to an impaired production of ammonia. It is probable that this impairment is due directly to the poisonous effect of the rise in Pco_2 on the tubule cell's capacity to form ammonia. In metabolic acidosis the ammonia production is much higher. The sustained rise in bicarbonate reabsorption is necessarily associated with a sustained diminution in chloride reabsorption. It results in a severe chloride loss and a low plasma chloride.

In a metabolic acidosis (e.g. diabetic ketosis or ammonium chloride administration) there is also an increased concentration of hydrogen ions in the plasma, but because of the accompanying hyperventilation, the carbon dioxide tension

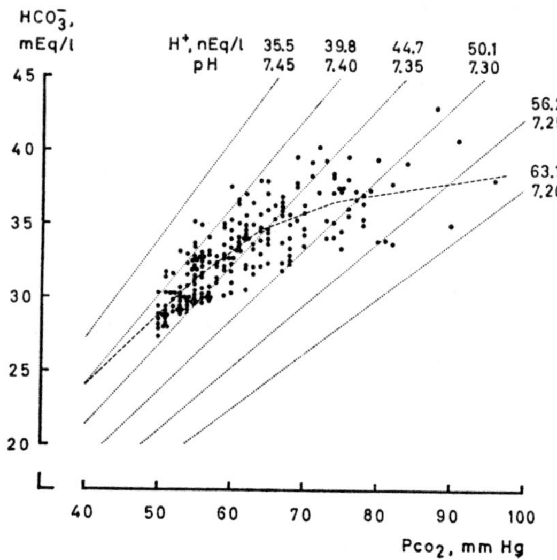

FIG. 6.23. The relation of arterial Pco_2, pH and bicarbonate in 210 patients with pulmonary insufficiency breathing air. (Refsum, 1964, *Clin. Sci.*)

is *reduced*. Nevertheless the tubules again increase the secretion of hydrogen ions and the reabsorption of bicarbonate. It appears therefore that in a metabolic acidosis the inhibitory effect of the reduced carbon dioxide tension on the intracellular production of hydrogen ions is swamped by the persistent rise in extracellular fluid hydrogen ion concentration which presumably causes a rise in intracellular hydrogen ion concentration. In normal man when the plasma bicarbonate concentration falls below 25 mEq/l the urinary excretion of bicarbonate rapidly diminishes. In the metabolic acidosis associated with renal disease, however, this compensatory mechanism may break down and in some patients bicarbonate excretion may continue down to plasma bicarbonate levels of about 20 mEq/l (see above). The maximum acidity which the tubule can sustain is approximately pH 4·6, which limits the kidney's ability to excrete large quantities of free hydrogen ions unless the urinary content of phosphate buffer is raised or there are large volumes of urine, as in diabetic ketosis.

Alkalosis

When there is a respiratory alkalosis (e.g. voluntary hyperventilation, left heart failure, or excessive artificial ventilation as in severe poliomyelitis) there is a fall both in the plasma hydrogen ion concentration and the carbon dioxide tension. Both these factors will decrease the availability of the hydrogen ions in the tubule cell so that less hydrogen ions are excreted and bicarbonate reabsorption is decreased; both of which will tend to reduce the alkalinity of the plasma. In *acute* respiratory alkalosis there is a simultaneous increase in the excretion of sodium and potassium. The rise in sodium excretion is due to a cardiovascular reflex which is not completely understood. The afferent limb of this reflex is a change in venous pressure in the left side of the heart. The rise in potassium excretion is due to a sudden rise in intracellular potassium concentration consequent upon the alkalosis.

In a metabolic alkalosis (e.g. sodium bicarbonate administration) there is also a fall in hydrogen ion concentration but, because of the accompanying hypoventilation, there is a *rise* in the carbon dioxide tension. The rise in carbon dioxide tension does cause a slight increase in bicarbonate reabsorption but, when the plasma bicarbonate concentration rises above 27 mEq/l bicarbonate reabsorption does not increase further and urinary excretion of bicarbonate then equals the increasing quantities which are filtered; if the glomerular filtration rate is normal this spill over prevents the concentration of plasma bicarbonate from rising steeply. In contrast to metabolic acidosis therefore, which is controlled entirely by tubular mechanisms, the ability of the kidneys to control a metabolic alkalosis is mainly related to the glomerular filtration rate. But tubular function is also involved for very large quantities of bicarbonate can only be excreted if the counter-current system in the medulla is sufficiently intact to matintain a high Pco_2 (p. 112).

Ammonia Excretion

Ammonia (NH_3) is formed in the tubule cells throughout the whole length of the nephron, with the exception of the thin part of the loop of Henle (Fig. 6.24). Ammonia is a base with no electrical charge which is highly soluble in lipids, for this reason it diffuses easily across cell membranes. When ammonia combines with a hydrogen ion, however, and becomes ammonium (NH_4^+) it is charged, has a low lipid solubility and only diffuses across cell membranes with some difficulty. The ammonia formed within the tubule cells diffuses passively from the cells into the tubular lumen on one side of the cell and the peritubular venous capillaries on the other. When the ammonia in the tubule fluid combines with a hydrogen ion and forms an ammonium ion it is trapped within the lumen and most of it remains there to be excreted in the urine. The formation of ammonium in the tubule lumen diminishes the intraluminal concentration of ammonia so that the diffusion of ammonia from the cell to the tubule lumen down a concentration gradient continues. On the other hand, if the secretion of hydrogen ions from the cell into the tubule lumen is diminished the formation of ammonium will be less and the intraluminal concentration of ammonia will rise; this in turn will reduce the rate of diffusion of ammonia from the cell to the lumen.

Ammonia is formed within tubule cells mainly from the action of glutaminase on glutamine, though other amino acids are also involved. This process is depressed by accumulation of intracellular ammonia and accelerated when the

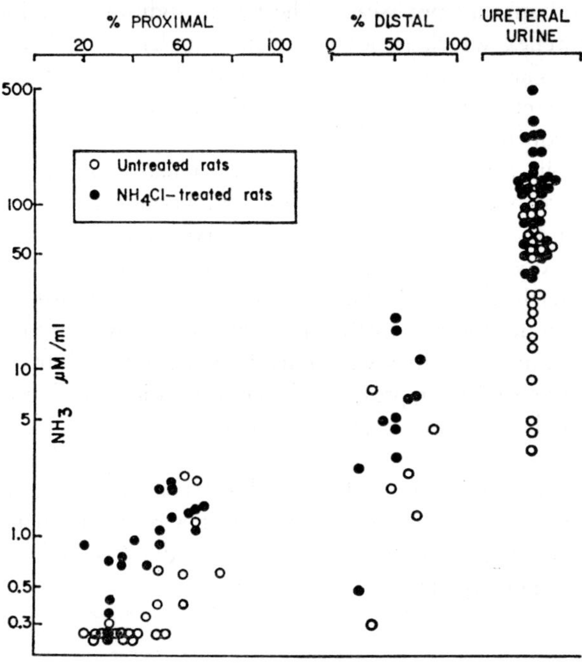

FIG. 6.24. Site of ammonia production in the rat nephron. (Glabman, Klose and Giebisch, 1963, *Amer. J. Physiol.*)

concentration falls; conversely, it is accelerated in potassium deficiency, perhaps because of the intracellular acidosis that then occurs which probably reduces the concentration of free ammonia. It is important to remember that free ammonia diffuses both into the tubule lumen and into the peritubular venous capillaries and that the amount that diffuses into the blood is therefore inversely proportional to that which is secreted into the urine. Clinically this is particularly relevant in patients with liver failure who develop oliguria or anuria.

Urinary ammonium excreted is inversely related to the pH of the urine and almost ceases when the urine becomes alkaline (Fig. 6.26). The increase in ammonium excretion, which occurs as the urine pH falls, is due in part to the increased formation of ammonia in the tubule cell mentioned above and due to the depletion of intracellular ammonia. But if the urine continues to be acid the

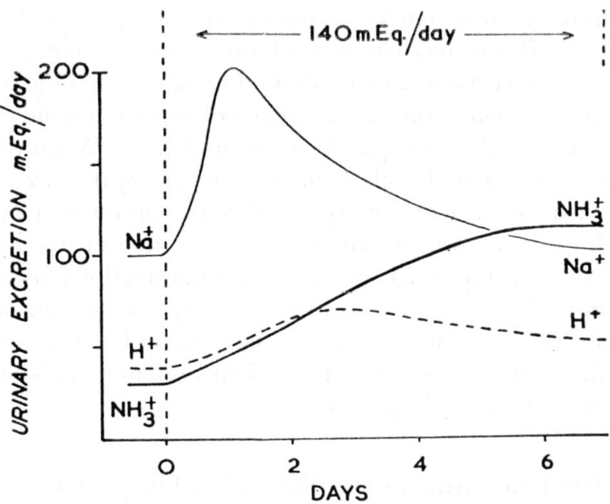

FIG. 6.25. The effect of 140 mEq/day of ammonium chloride by mouth on the urinary excretion of sodium, hydrogen and ammonium in a normal subject.

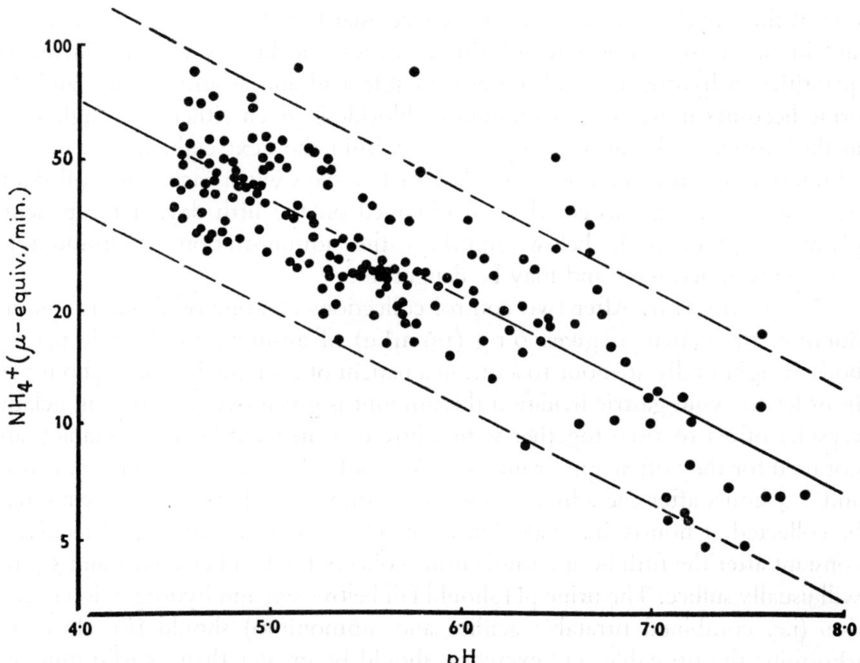

FIG. 6.26. Relation between the excretion of ammonium and urinary pH in normal subjects a few hours after the oral ingestion of a single dose of ammonium chloride ("short test"). The calculated regression line and 95 per cent range of observations are shown. (Wrong and Davies, 1959, *Quart. J. Med.*)

amount of ammonium excreted continues to rise after the pH has reached its minimum. This adaptive mechanism in chronic acidosis is not yet understood. It is not due to an increasing concentration of glutaminase in the tubule cells.

In normal circumstances the daily excretion of ammonium and free hydrogen ions is approximately the same (i.e. 20–30 mEq of each). When there is a need for an increased excretion of both (as in diabetic ketosis) the increase in ammonium greatly exceeds that of free hydrogen ions. Ammonium excretion may reach 400 mEq/day whereas the simultaneous excretion of free hydrogen ions will only be 70–100 mEq/day. These are very high excretion rates and are rarely seen except in prolonged diabetic ketosis. The response of a normal person to large quantities of ammonium chloride is illustrated in Fig. 6.25. It can be seen that after a delay of five days the ammonium excretion is about three times greater than that of free hydrogen ions.

Procedure Used to Estimate the Tubule's Ability to Excrete an Acid Urine and to Excrete Hydrogen Ions and Ammonia

The tubule's capacity to excrete hydrogen ions and ammonia is estimated by measuring its response to the oral administration of ammonium chloride. The ammonium chloride molecule is metabolised to urea and HCl. The addition of these hydrogen ions into the extracellular fluid tends to make it acidotic, and in order to compensate for this tendency the kidney excretes increased quantities of hydrogen ions both as titratable acid and as ammonium, and the urine becomes more acid. Ammonium chloride is given either as a single dose in the morning, the urine being studied within the next eight hours; or it is administered in divided doses each day for five days when each daily collection of urine is studied, particularly that obtained on the fifth day. If the patients plasma bicarbonate is below 20 mEq/l the administration of ammonium chloride is unnecessary and may be dangerous.

THE SHORT TEST. After two control collections of urine of about 1–2 hours duration the patient is given 0·1 g (1·9 mEq) of ammonium chloride per kg body weight orally at about 10 a.m.; in a patient of average size this is about 7 g. In order to avoid gastric irritation this amount is given over an hour, in gelatin capsules of 0·5 to 1·0 g together with a litre of water (enteric coated tablets are not used for they often appear intact in the stools). Venous blood is taken before and 2–4 hours after the administration of ammonium chloride. The urine may be collected at hourly intervals, but as the changes are maximal and relatively constant after the fifth hour a single urine collection taken between 3 and 5 p.m. will usually suffice. The urine pH should fall below 5·3, and hydrogen ion excretion (i.e. combined titratable acidity and ammonium) should rise above 60 μEq/min; the titratable acid excretion should be greater than 25 μEq/min and ammonium excretion greater than 35 μEq/min.

THE LONG TEST. Following two to three days control observations 7·5 g (140 mEq) of ammonium chloride is given by mouth in divided doses each day for five days. The maximum titratable acidity is reached in three to four days, whereas ammonium excretion takes four to five days to reach its peak. The chloride ions of the ammonium chloride are also eliminated through the kidney; at first these are excreted with almost equal quantities of sodium, but after two to three days the initial increase in sodium excretion subsides (Fig. 6.25). At the end of four to five days the urine pH should have fallen below 5·0 and the daily combined excretion of ammonium and titrable acid should rise above control values by about 120 mEq/day. If the renal response is normal, plasma bicarbonate and chloride concentrations should not alter by more than 6 mEq/l.

The ability to reduce the pH of the urine is always impaired in renal tubular acidosis (p. 237) and potassium deficiency (p. 218), it is sometimes impaired in hypercalcuria, while it appears superficially normal in the chronic renal failure which accompanies loss of nephrons (p. 180). The ability to excrete titratable acid normally is depressed in renal tubular acidosis; potassium deficiency, hypercalcuria and chronic renal failure. As ammonium excretion is related to the pH of the urine the value obtained in these tests must be considered in relation to the pH of the urine. The normal relationship is illustrated in Fig. 6.26. It can only be claimed that the capacity to excrete ammonium is depressed if it is lower than a normal person's capabilities at the same urine pH. According to these criteria ammonia excretion is depressed in chronic renal failure and in some cases of hypercalcuria, it is normal in most cases of renal tubular acidosis and some cases of potassium deficiency; and it is raised in most cases of potassium deficiency and some cases of renal tubular acidosis.

CHLORIDE EXCRETION

It has already been pointed out that the activity of the sodium pump in transporting sodium ions out of the lumen of the tubule causes an electrical potential gradient between the cell and the lumen; the lumen being negatively charged and the cell positively. It is probable that this is sufficient to account for the reabsorption of chloride from the tubule lumen which accompanies sodium reabsorption, the chloride ion diffusing passively down the potential gradient from the lumen into the tubule cell. Under exceptional experimental conditions, however, it can be shown that active processes for the reabsorption of chloride also exist. The importance of these active mechanisms in the differential absorption of chloride ions, as opposed to bicarbonate ions, which occurs in those conditions where there is a reciprocal change in the plasma concentration of these two ions, is not known.

POTASSIUM EXCRETION

Potassium is the principal intracellular cation. It should be remembered that in this respect the cells of the tubule are the same as other cells.

It has been shown both by direct tubular puncture and by indirect experiments, that the potassium that is filtered at the glomerulus is nearly all reabsorbed in the proximal tubule, and that the amount which eventually appears in the urine is secreted in the distal tubule. As with sodium, therefore, glomerular filtration rate is unrelated to potassium excretion; a point of the greatest importance to patients suffering from most forms of chronic renal disease and in whom glomerular filtration rate is severely impaired.

Diffusion of potassium from the tubule cell into the tubule lumen is passive. It is dependent in part of the cell's ability to maintain the potassium concentration gradient between the lumen and the cell but more importantly on the electronegativity of the tubule lumen, which is a consequence of active sodium reabsorption. There is no evidence that the potassium that is secreted is in any way exchanged for sodium that is reabsorbed. For instance during the intravenous infusion of sodium sulphate the impermeant negatively charged sulphate ions in the glomerular filtrate are not reabsorbed. A small amount of sodium reabsorption therefore causes the electronegativity of the tubule lumen to become very great. This then increases back diffusion of sodium from the cell into the lumen so that effective sodium reabsorption from the lumen is small Nevertheless there is a simultaneous maximal secretion rate of potassium ions from the cells to the tubule lumen. There is also evidence that the diffusion of potassium into the lumen proceeds at such a rate that the same potassium concentration gradient is achieved however high the rate of flow of the tubule fluid. In other words the more fluid delivered into the distal tubule the greater the urinary excretion of potassium, even if distal tubule sodium reabsorption remains unchanged. There is also evidence that the net movement of potassium into the tubule lumen is dependent on the permeability of the cell membrane on the luminal side of the cell and on the presence of a potassium pump which moves potassium back from the lumen into the cell. Though there is a certain reciprocity between potassium and hydrogen ion secretion there is again no evidence that there is a direct "pump-related" competition between potassium and hydrogen secretion It is more probable that the apparent reciprocity is due to changes in intracellular potassium and hydrogen ion concentration. For instance when Pco_2 rises there is a rise in intracellular hydrogen ion concentration and a fall in the intracellular potassium concentration. These changes are accompanied by a rise in urinary hydrogen secretion and a fall in potassium excretion.

Procedure Used to Test the Tubules Ability to Control Potassium Excretion

Unlike sodium, where the serum concentration tends to remain unchanged or *fall* with sodium retention, serum potassium *rises* with potassium retention. This makes the testing of the kidney's ability to deal with an increased potassium load a potentially dangerous procedure, and it is therefore never attempted. Urinary excretion is the main route of potassium elimination, and if the serum potassium is found to be persistently raised it is clear that there is a tubular defect of potassium excretion.

To show that there is a potassium deficit and that it is due to excess urinary loss is more difficult. Except when serum potassium is below 3 mEq/l a low concentration is uncertain evidence of potassium deficiency; though it is more likely if there is a concomitant rise in serum bicarbonate. If potassium depletion is suspected or evident, and there is no obvious diminished intake, or leak from the intestinal tract, it is almost certain that it is due to abnormal loss in the urine. This is confirmed by measuring the oral intake of potassium and its output in the urine.

The patient is placed on a normal diet containing 80–100 mEq of potassium per day and the daily urinary potassium excretion is measured for a control period, during which it should be 10–20 mEq less than the intake (this amount is eliminated in the faeces). If the urinary excretion is greater than the intake, particularly when the plasma potassium concentration is low, there is unequivocal evidence of a urinary leak of potassium. The following relationship between the lower concentrations of plasma potassium and the urinary excretion of potassium, when the patient is eating a normal ward diet, is a reliable substitute for a balance study. When there is a renal leak of potassium and the plasma concentration of potassium has fallen to 3 mEq/l or lower, the urinary excretion of potassium is greater than 20 mEq/24 hours; whereas if the potassium deficiency is due to some other cause (such as diarrhoea) the urinary excretion of potassium at these low plasma potassium concentrations will be less than 20 mEq/24 hours. This distinction will usually persist even when potassium deficiency has caused severe renal functional impairment. After some years, however, the potassium deficiency itself may affect the kidney's ability to retain potassium.

If the findings on a normal diet are within normal limits and yet a urinary leak of potassium seems very likely, the patient is placed on a low potassium diet, since in some instances the tubular abnormality may only become apparent when the potassium intake is reduced. On a diet containing 25–30 mEq/day of potassium the urinary excretion of potassium should fall to 25–30 mEq/day within four to seven days.

Potassium excretion may be excessive in hyperaldosteronism, and Cushing's disease, following the use of diuretics, and in certain tubular disorders, particularly those associated with renal tubular acidosis. In all of these there may be hypokalaemia. Potassium excretion may be abnormally low in hypoaldosternism (Addison's disease), acute renal failure or in terminal chronic renal failure when there may be hyperkalaemia.

CALCIUM EXCRETION

Calcium reabsorption from the glomerular filtrate normally occurs in the proximal tubule. When the serum calcium rises, however, and there is an increased amount of calcium filtered, evidence of calcium reabsorption can also be obtained in the distal and collecting tubules. Parathyroid hormone increases calcium absorption from the distal tubule, it has no effect on the proximal tubule. The initial functional disturbances associated with hypercalcuria are an impairment in the ability to concentrate and to acidify the urine.

Urinary calcium excretion rises and falls with the concentration of filtrable plasma calcium and to a minor extent with changes in glomerular filtration rate. Parathyroid hormone *decreases* calcium clearance, increases calcium absorption from the bowel, and liberates calcium from bone; these mechanisms tend to raise the plasma calcium, but the net effect is an increase in calcium excretion. It is doubtful if a high urinary excretion of calcium is ever due to a primary disturbance of tubular function. It is usually due either to a raised plasma calcium or increased parathyroid hormone activity such as a parathyroid tumour, when the hypercalcuria may itself cause severe renal structural and functional disturbances (p. 224). When there is severe depression of filtration rate hypercalcaemia may not be associated with hypercalcuria, but it may appear as renal failure improves.

Procedure Used to Determine the Presence of Hypercalcuria

Hypercalcuria is difficult to define. A few years ago there were reports that 90 per cent of normal subjects studied in England excreted less than 300 mg of calcium per day. It was therefore considered that a urinary excretion of more than 300 mg per day was greater than normal. Recently, however, there have been claims that the proportion of normal subjects who excrete more than 300 mg per day is rising; perhaps as a result of the Milk Marketing Board's advertising. Now therefore the upper limit of normal calcium excretion is probably nearer 400 mg per day

More precisely hypercalcuria can be defined as the daily excretion of more than 200 mg of calcium when the diet contains less than 150 mg. A simple way to perform such a balance study is to place the patient on a rice diet. The rice is cooked in distilled water,★ but salt can be added in normal amounts, and jams, sugar and fruit are allowed; drinking water must also be distilled. Such a diet contains about 90–130 mg of calcium a day. The urine calcium excretion is estimated on the fourth day when it should contain less than 200 mg. In children the upper level of urinary calcium excretion is 7 mg/kg/24 hours, the usual rate is about 3–4 mg/kg/24 hours.

MAGNESIUM EXCRETION

The average daily intake of magnesium is approximately 250 mg with a urinary excretion of 100 mg per day. The filtration of magnesium at the glomerulus and its reabsorption from the tubule parallel that of calcium. In the same way the control of urinary magnesium excretion appears to be almost iden-

★ London tap water contains 10 mg/100 ml of calcium.

tical to that of calcium in that it is raised by a rise in the concentration of circulating parathormone, etc. It is probable that calcium and magnesium share a common intratubular transport mechanism. Nevertheless magnesium metabolism is less disturbed than calcium metabolism in renal disease. Paradoxically in acute renal failure, though the urinary excretion of both calcium and magnesium cease there is a fall in plasma calcium and a rise in plasma magnesium. In chronic renal failure plasma magnesium remains normal even when the glomerular filtration rate falls below 5 ml/min. Very rarely a renal lesion may cause an excessive loss of magnesium and cause magnesium deficiency.

Procedure Used to Detect a Renal Leak of Magnesium

There is no standardised way to do this. Nevertheless it is usually not difficult to establish that a renal leak of magnesium is taking place for with rare exceptions it only occurs in patients with advanced renal disease. If such a patient has a low plasma magnesium and there is no other obvious cause for magnesium deficiency then it is overwhelmingly likely that the deficiency is due to excess urinary excretion. This can be confirmed by finding that though the plasma magnesium is low the urinary excretion of magnesium is not reduced.

PHOSPHATE EXCRETION

There is no evidence that phosphate is secreted by the tubule. Phosphate excretion therefore depends on a balance between filtration and reabsorption. In normal circumstances all the phosphate in the plasma is filtrable. Tubular reabsorption is mainly controlled by the concentrations of circulating parathyroid hormone, calcitonin and thyroid hormone. Phosphate reabsorption (like bicarbonate and sodium reabsorption) is also related to glomerular filtration rate, in such a way that changes in filtration rate produce little change in phosphate excretion. In other words the greater the amount of phosphate filtered the greater is the amount absorbed. On the other hand, changes in plasma phosphate concentration and extracellular fluid volume opposite produce changes in phosphate secretion. A rise in plasma phosphate is associated with an increased phosphate clearance. This is immensely important for the diurnal swing of plasma phosphate is very pronounced and is maximal in the morning; a time which is often chosen to do studies on renal function. The effect of changes in extracellular fluid volume on phosphate clearance has to be kept in mind when trying to measure the tubules maximal capacity to reasorb phosphate (Tm PO_4).

Procedure Used to Detect the Presence of an Abnormal
Handling of Phosphate by the Kidney

The only reliable and reproducible method is to estimate the maximal capacity of the tubules to reabsorb phosphate (Tm PO_4, p. 91). This is achieved by raising the plasma phosphate concentration by a steady intravenous infusion of about 200 ml of buffered phosphate over three hours until the plasma phosphate rises to a level greater than 5 mg/100 ml. Conditions both before and during this test have to be rigorously controlled; a high phosphate diet before the test must be avoided; because of the diurnal rhythm of phosphate the test should always be done at the same time of day; as glucose is absorbed along the same pathways as phosphate the patient should be fasting; other substances such as PAH which may compete for tubular transport mechanisms should be

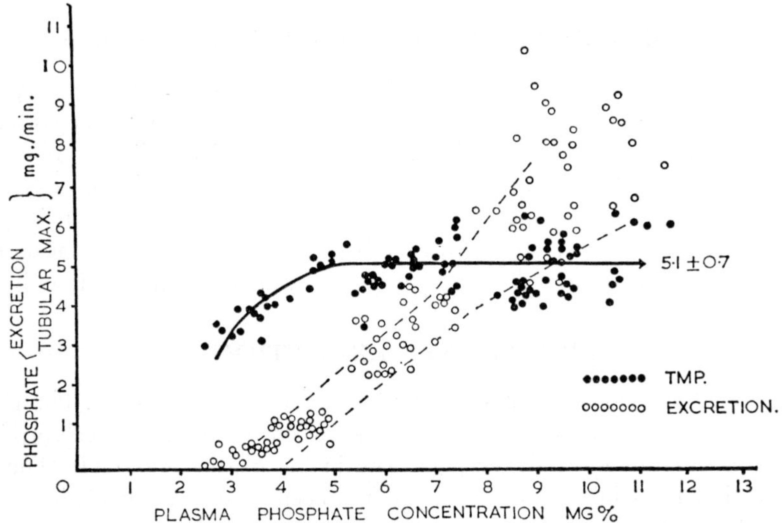

Fig. 6.27. Single estimation of Tm PO_4 and phosphate excretion corrected for filtration rate, plotted against phosphate concentrations in normal subjects ("phosphate tubular max" phosphate reabsorbed). Phosphate reabsorption reaches a maximum of about 5·0 mg/min and then levels out. The value at which it does so is the Tm PO_4, or maximum capacity of the tubule to reabsorb phosphate. In this figure the reabsorption and excretion have been adjusted to a glomerular filtration rate of 131 ml/min; it is now more usual to relate these to 1 litre of filtrate (see text). (Anderson and Parsons, 1963, Clin. Sci.)

avoided; and the test should not be prolonged for otherwise it may induce endocrine changes which will alter the result. And when all these precautions have been taken the normal range is still so wide that it may not be exceeded even in proven primary hyperparathyroidism. Fig. 6.27 shows the results in normal subjects. The maximal capacity to reabsorb phosphate (Tm PO_4) is 38 ± 5 mg/l of glomerular filtrate. It is necessary to relate the maximal rate of phosphate reabsorption to a fixed volume of glomerular filtrate because changes in filtration rate are accompanied by automatic and parallel changes in phosphate reabsorption. Parathyroid hormone diminishes phosphate reabsorption by inhibiting phosphate reabsorption in the distal tubule. Thyroid hormone increases phosphate reabsorption. Phosphate reabsorption is also reduced in severe renal failure and certain primary disturbances of the tubules. When patients are grouped according to their Tm PO$_4$ per litre of glomerular filtrate, the groups correspond to their diseases. It is then possible to discriminate groups of patients with hyper- and hypoparathyroidism, thyrotoxicosis, and over production of growth hormone, from healthy persons. Tm PO$_4$ unrelated to filtration rate does not discriminate patients. There is a close correlation between Tm PO$_4$ per litre of glomerular filtration rate and the fasting plasma phosphate so that when the capacity to reabsorb is diminished the plasma phosphate falls, while the plasma phosphate rises when reabsorption increases.

Tm PO$_4$ per litre of glomerular filtration rate (Tm PO$_4$/l GFR) is a time consuming performance subject to many technical pitfalls. It has been found however that in the fasting state it is possible to predict Tm PO$_4$/l GFR from

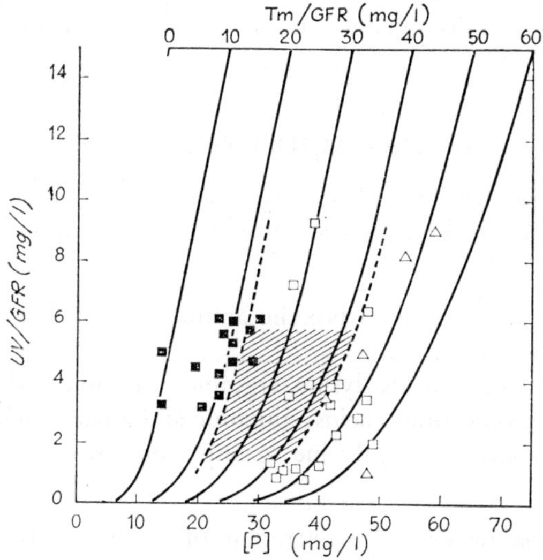

Fig. 6.28. The relation between U$_{PO_4}$V/GFR and plasma phosphate in groups of patients with ■ hyperparathyroidism; △ hypoparathyroidism; □ thyrotoxicosis. The shaded area indicates the 95% range of Tm PO$_4$/GFR (22–42 mg/l) and U$_{PO_4}$V/GFR (14–57 mg/l) in normal persons. (Bijvoet, Morgan and Fourman, 1969, *Clin. Chim. Acta.*)

the relation of urinary phosphate excretion (U$_{PO_4}$× V/GFR) to the plasma phosphate. This is shown in Fig. 6.28. A prediction made in this way is even simpler to make than it at first appears for U$_{PO_4}$× V/GFR is

$$\text{U}_{PO_4} \times \text{V} \bigg/ \frac{\text{U creatinine} \times \text{V}}{\text{P creatinine}}$$

which becomes

$$\frac{\text{U}_{PO_4} \times \text{P creatinine}}{\text{U creatinine}}.$$

Thus a prediction of Tm PO$_4$/l GFR can be made from a measurement of the concentration of phosphate and creatinine in the plasma and in an untimed (as V has been eliminated) but simultaneous sample of urine. The error of the prediction is too large to be of value in single determinations, but the prediction is much improved by repeat determinations. Moreover the use of the prediction makes it practicable to make successive observations when following the clinical progress of a patient.

Other methods used to detect the presence of an abnormal handling of phosphate by the kidneys include estimates of the clearance of phosphate alone, or the phosphate to creatinine clearance ratio. The first is valueless and the second is only of value if the duration of the clearance period is 24 hours, the dietary intake of phosphate is constant from day to day and the plasma phosphate sample is always taken 4–5 hours after the last meal (e.g. at midday). As the phosphate to creatinine clearance ratio rises as the plasma phosphate concentration increases the results obtained must therefore be compared with those obtained over a wide range of plasma phosphate concentrations in normal subjects.

AMINO ACID EXCRETION

Amino acids are filtered, and actively reabsorbed in the proximal tubule by four main transport mechanisms, each of which deals with one of the following groups of amino acids:

1. The monoamino-monocarboxylic amino acids such as alamine, valine, trytophan and cysteine.
2. The dibasic amino acids: lysine, arginine, ornithine and cystine.
3. The dicarboxylic amino acids: glutamic and aspartic acids.
4. The imino-acid and glycine group: proline, hydroxyproline and glycine.

Amino-aciduria or excessive excretion of amino acids is classified into "overflow" or "renal" types. Overflow amino-aciduria is due to disorders of metabolism in which the circulating concentration of certain amino acids rises. The amount of these amino acids which is then filtered exceeds the tubules' capacity for reabsorption and the quantity which is not reabsorbed "overflows" into the urine. The inability to deaminate amino acids in severe liver failure causes an overflow of all groups of amino acids, while phenylketonuria which is due to an impaired ability to metabolise phenylanaline is an example of a single amino acid overflow amino-aciduria.

In renal amino-aciduria the primary defect is either an absence or deficiency or either group 1 or 2 active transport mechanisms. This can arise either as a hereditary anomaly of amino acid transport without other evidence of abnormal tubular function, e.g. cystinuria; or as one of several tubular abnormalities all of them caused by damage to the proximal tubules. Such damage may develop acutely as in cadmium and uranium poisoning or more chronically with copper in Wilson's disease, or galactose in infantile galactosaemia.

URIC ACID EXCRETION

Ninety-eight per cent of the filtered uric acid is reabsorbed by the proximal tubule, while 80 per cent of the uric acid in the urine is secreted by the distal tubule. The daily excretion of uric acid is 0·5 to 1·0 g. The amount depends to a large extent on the content of cell nuclei in the diet for uric acid is derived from purine bases liberated in the degradation of both ingested, and endogenous nucleoproteins.

The concentrations of uric acid found in the urine are such that the uric acid is in a supersaturated state. The liability to precipitation is obviously greatest when the urine is acid. The solubility of total uric acid, i.e. free uric acid and urates in urine is only 8 mg/100 ml at pH 5·0, 22 mg/100 ml at pH 6·0, and 158 mg/100 ml at pH 7·0. In addition precipitation of sodium urate in the urine and in the medulla is probably enhanced by the high concentrations of sodium in the medulla and urine when concentrated urine is being formed.

Procedures Used to Test the Ability of the Tubules to Secrete Uric Acid; and to Detect the Presence of an Increased Urate Production

Plasma uric acid may be raised because of a diminished tubular secretion of uric acid, an increased endogenous production of uric acid, or a high protein intake. In order to assess the capacity of the kidneys to excrete uric acid, large amounts of RNA are given per day to progressively raise plasma uric acid and urinary uric acid excretion. An impairment in the ability to secrete uric acid is evident from the slope of the rise in the urinary output of uric acid in relation to the change in plasma uric acid. A normal subject excretes much more uric acid at each plasma uric acid level than a person who has an impaired ability to excrete uric acid (Fig. 6.29). An excess endogenous production can be discerned by placing the patients on a purine free diet consisting of milk, bread, fats and eggs for seven days. Twenty-four hour urine collections are made on the last two days when the daily uric acid excretion should be less than 600 mg.

There are many conditions in which there is a selective impairment in the ability to excrete uric acid. Many of them are due to a raised concentration of plasma lactic acid which is a well established inhibitor of uric acid excretion, whereas in familial gout the impairment in the ability to secrete uric acid appears to be a primary tubular disturbance. In renal failure the ability to excrete uric acid remains normal until the glomerular filtration rate falls below 20 ml min (p. 380). An increased production of uric acid of unknown cause is sometimes the cause of recurrent gout. Often, however, an increase in production is due to an identifiable cause such as a high cellular turn-over as in leukaemia, or when a tumour is rapidly destroyed, e.g. radiotherapy to a large retroperitoneal lymphosarcomatous mass. Many patients with transient gout have a high intake of purines and alcohol. The combination may cause a brisk rise in plasma uric acid, for the increased production of uric acid from the breakdown of the purines is accompanied by a diminished capacity

D

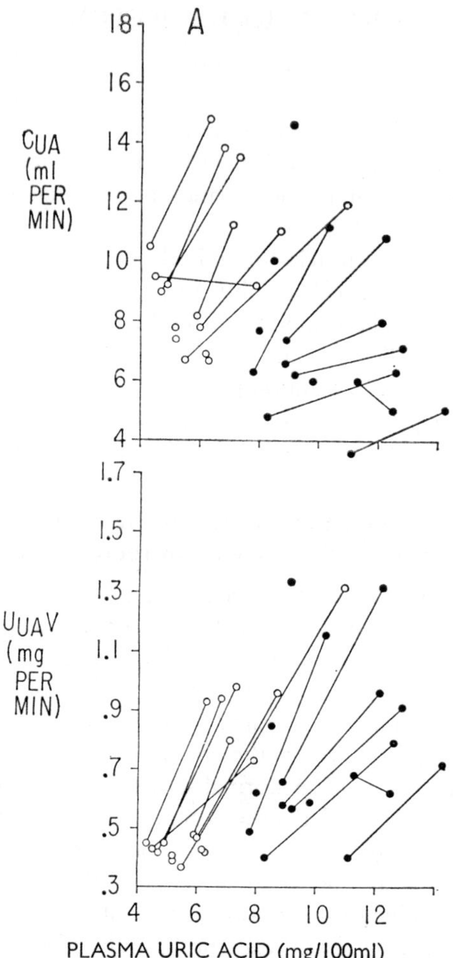

FIG. 6.29. The effect of the ingestion of large amounts of ribonucleic acid for three days on plasma urate concentration, the clearance of uric acid (C_{UA}), and the urinary excretion of uric acid ($U_{UA}V$) in patients with gout ● ; and in individuals without gout ○. The patients with gout have an impaired ability to excrete uric acid. (Nugent, MacDiarmid and Tyler, 1964, *Arch. Int. Med.*)

to excrete uric acid due to the increased lactic acid production caused by the alcohol intake. The position is aggravated if the alcoholic drink is beer for yeast has a high purine content.

MAXIMAL CAPACITY OF THE TUBULES TO TRANSPORT GLUCOSE AND PARA-AMINO HIPPURIC ACID

The capacity of the tubules to reabsorb or secrete certain substances may be limited, and a measure of this is obtained by estimating the maximal amount that the tubules can either secrete or reabsorb in one minute. This amount is referred to as the Tm of that substance (derived from the words "tubule" and "maximal"); it has a certain value particularly in relation to phosphate excretion.

Reabsorption Tm

The Tm of glucose (Tm$_g$) is a good example of a reabsorptive Tm. When blood glucose is within normal limits it is unusual for there to be glucose in the urine, since all the filtered glucose has been reabsorbed. To determine Tm$_g$ an intravenous infusion of glucose is given at a rate sufficient to raise the blood glucose substantially. Glycosuria occurs and the amount of glucose reabsorbed is calculated as follows:

$$\text{glucose filtered} - \text{glucose excreted} = \text{glucose reabsorbed}$$

or

$$\text{GFR} \times P_g - U_g \times V = T_g,$$

where GFR is glomerular filtration rate per minute, P_g is plasma glucose concentration, U_g the urine glucose concentration, V the rate of urine flow, and T_g the rate of glucose reabsorbed as mg per minute. The rate of glucose administration continues to be increased in a stepwise manner and the measurements are repeated; blood glucose and glycosuria increase steadily, but there comes a point beyond which the quantity of glucose reabsorbed remains constant; this is the Tm$_g$, and in normal man is 323 ± 64 mg/min.

The plasma glucose concentration at which glucose first appears in the urine is sometimes referred to as the renal threshold for glucose. This level is roughly correlated with Tm$_g$ but is a less constant value, for it is influenced by alterations in glomerular filtration rate. At the renal threshold for glucose the quantity of glucose being presented to the tubules by the glomerular filtrate is only just sufficient to exceed the tubule's ability to reabsorb all the glucose passing through; if plasma glucose remains unchanged but there is a fall in filtration rate, no glucose will appear in the urine and the renal threshold will have altered. But when estimating Tm$_g$ the blood glucose concentration is raised to such high values that, so long as a nephron has some filtration, the amount of glucose being presented to the tubule for reabsorption is far in excess of its maximum reabsorbing capacity; in this way alterations in glomerular filtration rate cannot influence the amount reabsorbed.

The main value of a Tm$_g$ is that it gives a quantitative expression of the total mass of functioning tubular cells. It is rarely estimated.

The Tm of bicarbonate and phosphate reabsorption have been discussed earlier (pp. 73, 85). The reabsorption of these ions is influenced by changes in the extracellular fluid volume. For instance it has been pointed out that there appears to be no limit to the tubule's capacity to reabsorb bicarbonate if the plasma bicarbonate is raised in such a way that the rise in the extracellular fluid volume is minimal. And it has also been demonstrated that even when the technique of raising the plasma bicarbonate includes a substantial expansion of the extracellular fluid volume of constant volume the Tm HCO_3 can still be altered by altering Pco_2.

The influence of extracellular fluid volume expansion on Tm PO_4 is not nearly so profound but can be easily demonstrated. Tm PO_4 is also influenced by parathyroid hormone. It is clear therefore that for Tm PO_4 and Tm HCO_3 to be of any value they must be measured during rigorously standardised conditions. In addition, unlike Tm_g which is uninfluenced by changes in glomerular filtration, tubular reabsorption of bicarbonate and phosphate varies directly with changes in glomerular filtration rate, so that for purposes of comparison Tm HCO_3 and Tm PO_4 have to be related to a standard glomerular filtration rate.

Secretion Tm

In this context a substance is considered to be secreted by the tubules only if the amount excreted in the urine is greater than that which has been filtered. This is, of course, a convenient but grossly arbitrary definition, for some substances which are actively secreted by the tubules (e.g. potassium) have a total urinary excretion which is usually less than that which has been filtered. To measure the true amount secreted, therefore, it would be necessary to know the amount which has been reabsorbed, and in ordinary circumstances this is not possible.

Those substances which have the greatest rate of tubular secretion according to the definition given above are those which are not normally present in body fluids, and include diodone, phenol red, penicillin and para-amino-hippuric acid (PAH). Because of its ease of estimation and its high rate of active secretion PAH is the substance which has been most often used to obtain a secretory Tm. The procedure is similar to that used for estimating glucose Tm. Intravenous PAH is administered at a rate sufficient to maintain plasma PAH level at about 20 mg per 100 ml at which level the tubules are being presented with PAH at a rate much greater than their ability to secrete it into the tubule lumen; Tm_{PAH} is then calculated as follows:

$$\text{PAH excreted} - \text{PAH filtered} = \text{PAH actively secreted,}$$

or

$$U_{PAH} \times V - GFR \times P_{PAH} = Tm_{PAH}.$$

In normal man Tm_{PAH} is 68 ± 11 mg/min. Again, it is rarely estimated. It is of great interest that the secretion Tm of PAH, in line with the reabsorption Tm of HCO_3 and PO_4, is also depressed by expansion of the extracellular fluid volume.

Limitations of Existing Renal Function Tests

There is as yet no test which will give information about the number of functioning nephrons. This is a serious disadvantage. The kidney's capacity to hypertrophy is very great and it has been repeatedly shown that the removal of

Interpretation of the Results of the Two Most Widely Used Tests of Renal Function, i.e. Glomerular Filtration Rate and the Ability to Concentrate

The information derived from these two tests alone allows a certain measure of subdivision of renal disorders

Glomerular function (filtration rate)	Tubular function (ability to concentrate)	Interpretation	Renal disorder
Decreased	Decreased	Number of functioning nephrons diminished or Both glomerular and tubular function impaired; number of functioning nephrons variable	Chronic glomerular nephritis, polycystic kidneys, etc., etc. 1. Severe urinary obstruction 2. Severe renal ischaemia, e.g. acute renal failure from loss of blood 3. Severe electrolyte abnormality, e.g. potassium deficiency and hypercalcaemia 4. Renal poisons, e.g. acute renal failure from the ingestion of mercury
Normal or slightly decreased	Decreased	Tubular function definitely impaired, glomerular function normal or impaired to a much smaller extent than tubular function	1. Urinary tract obstruction, either recent, moderate or unilateral 2. Chronic pyelonephritis in its early stages 3. Moderate electrolyte abnormality, e.g. potassium deficiency and hypercalcaemia 4. Inborn functional defect of renal tubules, e.g. Fanconi's syndrome 5. Compulsive polydipsia
Decreased	Normal	Glomerular function impaired, tubular function normal	1. Moderate acute renal ischaemia, e.g. haemorrhage insufficient to cause acute renal failure 2. Acute nephritis

one kidney produces little or no permanent change in overall function. Similarly there is much histological evidence that in those chronic renal diseases in which nephrons are destroyed, the surviving nephrons hypertrophy, and it must be assumed that the function of the surviving nephrons increase with their size. It is therefore theoretically possible for a renal disease to destroy about half the nephron population and yet produce little or no change in renal function, and it follows that an unchanging renal function is not proof that a disease is quiescent, e.g. in persistent pyelonephritis. Conversely, when renal function is persistently reduced to half its normal value it is almost certain that a great deal more than half of the original renal parenchyma must have been destroyed. These speculations would be unnecessary if, during life it were possible to obtain an estimate of the number of surviving nephrons.

BIBLIOGRAPHY

ABER, G. M., and BISHOP, J. M. (1965). "Serial changes in renal function, arterial gas tensions, and the acid–base state in patients with chronic bronchitis and oedema." *Clin. Sci.*, **28**, 511.

ANDERSON, J., and PARSONS, V. (1963). "The tubular maximal resorptive rate for inorganic phosphate in normal subjects." *Clin. Sci.*, **25**, 431.

BARKER, E. S. (1960). "Physiologic and clinical aspects of magnesium metabolism." *J. chron. Dis.*, **11**, 278 .

BIJVOET, O. L. M. (1969). "Relation of plasma phosphate concentration to renal tubular reabsorption of phosphate." *Clin. Sci.*, **37**, 23.

BIJVOET, O. L. M., MORGAN, D. B., and FOURMAN, P. (1969). "The assessment of phosphate reabsorption." *Clin. Chim. Acta*, **26**, 11.

CLAPP, J. R., and ROBINSON, R. R. (1966). "Osmolality of distal tubular fluid in the dog." *J. clin. Invest.*, **45**, 1847.

DENIS, G., PREUSS, H., and PITTS, R. (1964). "The pNH_3 of renal tubular cells." *J. clin. Invest.*, **43**, 571.

DUNN, M. J., and WALSER, M. (1966). "Magnesium depletion in normal man." *Metabolism*, **15**, 884.

EDWARDS, N. A., and HODGKINSON, A. (1965). "Phosphate metabolism in patients with renal calculi." *Clin. Sci.*, **29**, 93.

FRICK, A., RUMRICH, G., ULLRICH, K. J., and LASSITER, W. (1965). "Microperfusion study of calcium transport in the proximal tubule of the rat kidney." *Pflüger's Archives*, **286**, 109.

GIEBISCH, G., and MALNIC, G. (1970). "Some aspects of renal tubular hydrogen ion transport." *Proc. 4th Int. Congress of Nephrology*, 1969. Vol. 1, p. 181. Published by S. Karger.

GIEBISCH, G. (1969). "Functional organisation of proximal and distal tubular electrolyte transport." *Nephron*, **6**, No. 3, 260. (Potassium excretion.)

GOTTSCHALK, C. W. (1964). "Osmotic concentration and dilution of the urine." *Amer. J. Med.*, **36**, 670.

GUTMAN, A. B., YÜ, T. F., and BERGER, L. (1959). "Tubular secretion of urate in man." *J. clin. Invest.*, **38**, 1778.

KASSIRER, J. P., and SCHWARTZ, W. B. (1966). "The response of normal man to selective depletion of hydrochloric acid." *Amer. J. Med.*, **40**, 10.

KENNEDY, T. J. (1960). "The effect of carbon dioxide on the kidney." *Anesthesiology*, **21**, 704.

LEMANN, J., LENNON, E. J., GOODMAN, J. R., LITZOW, J. R., and RELMAN, A. S. (1965). "The nett balance of acid in subjects given large loads of acid and alkali." *J. clin. Invest.*, **44**, 507.

MANITIUS, A., and EPSTEIN, F. (1963). "Some observations on the influence of a magnesium deficient diet on rats with special reference to renal concentrating ability." *J. clin. Invest.*, **42**, 208.

MASSRY, S. G., COBURN, J. W., and KLEEMAN, C. R. (1969). "The influence of ECV expansion on renal phosphate handling in the dog." *J. Clin. Invest.*, **48**, 1237.

MILES, B. E., PATON, A., and DE WARDENER, H. E. (1954). "Maximum urine concentration." *Brit. med. J.*, **2**, 901.

MILNE, M. D. (1964). "Disorders of amino-acid transport." *Brit. med. J.*, **1**, 327.

MORGAN, T. (1970). "A microperfusion study of some factors controlling sodium absorption and glomerular filtration in the nephron of the rat." Supplement II to *Circulation Research*, **26** and **27**, II–245.

NORDIN, B. E. C., and SMITH, D. A. (1965). "Diagnostic procedures in disorders of calcium metabolism." J. & A. Churchill, London.

ORLOFF, J., and BURG, M. (1971). "Kidney." Annual Review of Physiology. **33**, 83. (Ammonia production.)

PAK POY, R. K., and WRONG, O. (1960). "The urinary pCO$_2$ in renal disease." *Clin. Sci.*, **19**, 631.

PITTS, R. F. (1964). "Renal production and excretion of ammonia." *Amer. J. Med.*, **36**, 686.

RAPOPORT, S., WEST, C. D., BRODSKY, W. A., and MACKLER, B. (1949). "Urinary flow and excretion of solutes during osmotic diuresis in hydropenic man." *Amer. J. Physiol.*, **156**, 433.

RECTOR, F. C., CLAPP, J. R., and HUDDESTON, M. (1962). "Evidence for active chloride reabsorption in the distal renal tubule of the rat." *J. clin. Invest.*, **41**, 101.

RECTOR, F. C., SELDIN, D. W., ROBERTS, A. D., and SMITH, J. S. (1960). "The role of plasma CO$_2$ tension and carbonic anhydrase activity in the renal reabsorption of bicarbonate." *J. clin. Invest.*, **39**, 1706.

RELMAN, A. S. (1968). "The acidosis of renal disease." *Amer. J. Med.*, **44**, 706.

ROYER, P., HABIB, R., and MATHIEU, H. (1963). "Problèmes actuels de Néphrologie infantile." Édition Médicales Flammarion, France, p. 26. (Bicarbonate secretion.)

SCHRIER, R. W., and DE WARDENER, H. E. (1971). "Tubular reabsorption of sodium ion: influence of factors other than aldosterone and glomerular filtration rate." *New Eng. J. Med.*, **285**, 1231.

SMITH, H. W., GOLDRING, W., and CHASIS, H. (1938). "The measurement of the tubular excretory mass, effective blood flow and filtration rate in the normal human kidney." *J. clin. Invest.*, **17**, 263.

STAMP, T. C. B., and STACEY, T. E. (1970). "Evaluation of therapeutic renal phosphorus threshold as an index of renal phosphorus handling." *Clin. Sci.*, **39**, 505.

SYMPOSIUM ON ACID-BASE HOMEOSTASIS. Guest Editor F. C. Rector. *Kidney International*, **1**, 273.

STANBURY, S. W. (1958). "Some aspects of disordered renal tubular function." (Phosphaturia.) *Advanc. intern. Med.*, **9**, 231.

STRUYVENBERG, A., DE GRAEFF, J., and LAMEYER, L. D. F. (1965). "The role of chloride in hypokalaemic alkalosis in the rat." *J. clin. Invest.*, **44**, 326.

VIEIRA, E. L., and MALNIC, G. (1968). *Amer. J. Physiol.*, **214**, 710.

VERNEY, E. B. (1946). "Absorption and excretion of water. The antidiuretic hormone." *Lancet*, **2**, 739 and 781.

WALKER, A. M., and HUDSON, C. L. (1937). "The reabsorption of glucose from the renal tubule in amphibia and the action of phlorizin upon it." *Amer. J. Physiol.*, **118**, 130.

WARDENER, DE H. E. (1956). "Vasopressin tannate in oil and the urine concentration test." *Lancet*, **1**, 1037.

WARDENER, DE H. E., and DEL GRECO, F. (1955). "The influence of solute excretion rate on the production of a hypotonic urine in man." *Clin. Sci.*, **14**, 715.

WARREN, Y., LUKE, R. G., KASHGARIAN, M., and LEVITIN, H. (1970). "Micropuncture studies of chloride and bicarbonate absorption in the proximal tubule of the rat in respiratory acidosis and in chloride depletion." *Clin. Sci.*, **38**, 375.

WHANG, R., and WELT, L. G. (1963). "Observations in experimental magnesium depletion." *J. clin. Invest.*, **42**, 305.

WOMERSLEY, R. A., and DARRAGH, J. H. (1955). "Potassium and sodium restriction in the normal human." *J. clin. Invest.*, **34**, 456.

WRONG, O., and DAVIES, H. E. F. (1959). "The excretion of acid in renal disease." *Quart. J. Med.*, N.S., **28**, 259.

7

Diurnal Rhythm

THE urinary excretion of water and most electrolytes is normally greater during the day than at night, a fortunate phenomenon which ensures that the night's repose shall be undisturbed. This pattern is not only due to the fact that fluid and food are usually ingested during the day; it will persist even if identical quantities of food and water are ingested at regular intervals throughout the 24 hours. As the evening approaches and during the night, the excretion of sodium, potassium, bicarbonate and chloride ions gradually diminishes, while the pH of the urine falls, and its concentration rises; the process is reversed in the morning (Fig. 7.1).

The mechanism responsible for this rhythm is unknown; it has been shown that there is a small nocturnal fall in glomerular filtration rate, but this cannot explain all the changes that occur; for instance, the excretion of phosphate *increases* at night and diminishes during the day. It is possible that the changes in water excretion, and particularly the changes in urine concentration, follow a diurnal alteration in antidiuretic hormone secretion. There is no doubt that an antidiuretic mechanism is present, for at night a large drink of water only produces a small increase in urine flow. The changes in electrolyte excretion are preceded, by a few hours, by similar fluctuations in steroid excretion. It is probable that this is only coincidental, for it fails to explain why the changes in sodium and potassium excretion should be parallel; it has also been reported that under certain conditions the excretion of steroid will rise gradually throughout the day and night, and yet the diurnal rhythm of electrolyte and water excretion continues uninterruptedly.

A normal diurnal rhythm persists during undernutrition, water deprivation, salt deprivation, the sustained action of pitressin and a temporary disturbance of sleep rhythm. For instance, a person going from east to west on a ship across the Atlantic will show a peak of electrolyte excretion one hour (ship time) earlier each day. But the clock "gains" an hour each day so that in fact the diurnal rhythm remains unchanged in relation to European time. Reversal or abolition of the diurnal rhythm occurs commonly in the four most frequent causes of generalised oedema, i.e. cardiac failure, liver failure, the nephrotic syndrome and malnutrition (e.g. anorexia nervosa). In these conditions the volume of urine passed at night may be equal to or exceed the daytime total (Fig. 7.2). It may also be reversed in chronic renal failure, malignant hypertension, renal artery stenosis, small bowel insufficiency (e.g. idiopathic steatorrhoea), Addison's disease, hyperaldosteronism, Cushing's Syndrome and follow-

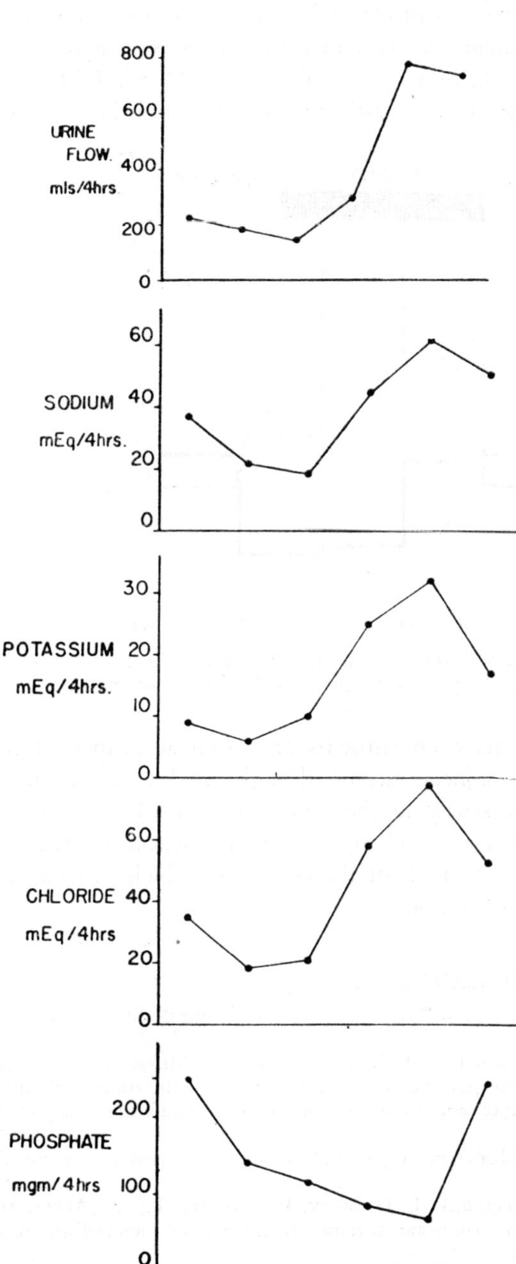

FIG. 7.1. Diurnal rhythm of urinary excretion of water, sodium, potassium, chloride and phosphate in a normal subject.

ing a head injury. In a normal person the diurnal rhythm can be abolished and occasionally reversed by the administration of cortisone.

A knowledge of a patient's pattern of electrolyte and water excretion may sometimes be of help in treatment. An oedematous person with a reversed rhythm, for instance, may only have a diuresis following the administration of a diuretic, if it is given in the evening, rather than in the morning.

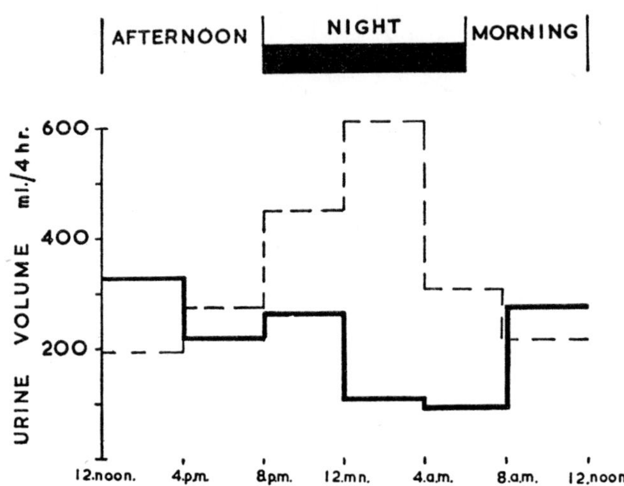

Fig. 7.2. Pathological reversal of the diurnal rhythm of urinary excretion of water (- - - -) compared with the normal rhythm (———) in a patient following a head injury.

The diurnal rhythms of urinary constituents are often accompanied by diurnal rhythms in their plasma concentrations, though synchronous changes in blood and urine are not necessarily in the same direction. This is of the utmost importance when trying to assess changes in renal function. Inattention to these rhythms was the cause of much of the confusion which surrounded earlier discussions on phosphate excretion.

BIBLIOGRAPHY

BORST, J. G. G., and DE VRIES, L. A. (1950). "The three types of 'natural' diuresis." *Lancet*, **2**, 1.

FINKENSTAEDT, J. T., DINGMAN, J. F., JENKINS, D., LAIDLAW, J. C., and MERRILL, J. P. (1954). "The effect of intravenous hydrocortisone and corticosterone on the diurnal rhythm in renal function, and electrolyte equilibria in normal and Addisonian subjects." *J. clin. Invest.*, **33**, 933.

FLEAR, C. T. G., COOKE, W. T., and QUINTON, A. (1959). "Water diuresis and steatorrhoea." *Clin. Sci.*, **18**, 137.

FOURMAN, P., REIFENSTEIN, E. C., KEPLER, E. J., DEMPSEY, E., BARTTER, F., and ALBRIGHT, F. (1952). "Effect of desoxycorticosterone acetate on electrolyte metabolism in a normal man." *Metabolism*, **1**, 242.

GOLDMAN, R. (1951). "Studies in diurnal variation of water and electrolyte excretion: nocturnal diuresis of water and sodium in congestive cardiac failure and cirrhosis of the liver." *J. clin. Invest.*, **30**, 1191.

KLEITMAN, N. (1949). "Biological rhythms and cycles." *Physiol. Rev.*, **29**, 1.
LEWIS, P. R., and LOBBAN, M. C. (1956). "Patterns of electrolyte excretion in human subjects during a prolonged period of life on a 22-hour day." *J. Physiol. (Lond.)*, **133**, 670.
PAPPER, S., and ROSENBAUM, J. D. (1952). "Diurnal variation in the diuretic response to ingested water." *J. clin. Invest.*, **31**, 401.
PAYNE, R. W., and DE WARDENER, H. E. (1958). "Reversal of urinary diurnal rhythm following head injury." *Lancet*, **1**, 1098.
ROSENBAUM, J. D., FERGUSON, B. C., DAVIS, R. K., and ROSSMEISL, E. C. (1952). "The influence of cortisone upon the diurnal rhythm of renal excretory function." *J. clin. Invest.*, **31**, 507.
STANBURY, S. W., and THOMSON, A. E. (1951). "Diurnal variations in electrolyte excretion." *Clin. Sci.*, **10**, 267.
THOMAS, J. P., COLES, G. A., and EL-SHABOURY, A. H. (1970). "Nocturia in patients on long term steroid therapy." *Clin. Sci.*, **38**, 415.
THOMAS, S. (1959). "Effects of change in posture on the diurnal renal excretory rhythm." *J. Physiol.*, **148**, 489.
WESSON, L. G. (1964). "Electrolyte excretion in relation to diurnal cycles of renal function." *Medicine*, **43**, 547.
WESSON, L. G., and LAULER, D. P. (1961). "Diurnal cycle of glomerular filtration rate and sodium and chloride excretion during response to altered salt and water balance in man." *J. clin. Invest.*, **40**, 1967.

8

Renal Function in Relation to Age

Renal function in the foetus

The outstanding fact is that foetal urine is hypotonic to its own plasma.

Renal function in infancy

In contrast to adults the intake of food and the rate of growth are more important than the kidney in keeping the biochemical environment of the infant stable. In addition, though the infant's kidney is perfectly adequate for normal purposes it is less adaptable than that of an adult in an emergency. The normal daily rhythms of urinary excretion are not present at birth. They only gradually become established over a period of years, though some difference between "day" and "night" excretory rates manifest themselves at an early stage. Failure to develop a normal diurnal rhythm may occasionally be the cause of nocturnal enuresis after infancy.

Glomerula filtration rate, calculated on a surface area basis, is proportionately less than in an adult and yet the concentration of urea in the blood is lower. This is due to the relatively larger quantities of nitrogen that are being retained at this time of life, and in normal circumstances the lower glomerular filtration rate is perfectly adequate to dispose of the small amount of waste products of protein catabolism. The hazards of this situation are evident when the child becomes ill and ceases to store nitrogen. A sharp increase in protein catabolism is then liable to produce a rapid rise in blood urea and, if protein administration is continued the blood urea may rise rapidly though there has been no alteration in the glomerular filtration rate.

Tubular function. The ability to dilute and concentrate the urine to adult levels does not take place until approximately the fourteenth day and the third month respectively. The ability to excrete a water load does not reach adult proportions until the end of the first month. The inability to concentrate the urine is due initially to (i) an inability to respond to ADH because the renal medulla has not developed sufficiently, and (ii) the small amounts of urea passing down the tubule. After a few weeks the kidney has matured sufficiently to enable it to respond to ADH but the ability to concentrate remains low because of the small amounts of urea that are sequested in the medulla. At this point, however, if an infant is given suitable quantities of urea by mouth the ability to concentrate rises to adult levels within a few hours, the increase in osmolality being equal to the increased concentration of urea in the urine.

100

The control of sodium excretion is even less elastic than that of water and an excess infusion of normal saline may produce a hypertonic oedema because of the greater difficulty in getting rid of sodium. In infants 5 to 7 months of age retention of sodium occurs when the intake is greater than 50 mEq/day. Alternatively, urinary sodium excretion may continue though there is a negative balance of sodium from diarrhoea or vomiting. Consequently, during the first few months an inadequate intake of water or an attack of diarrhoea may lead to severe dehydration; or an excessive administration of water may cause over-hydration.

The other tubular functions which have been found to be relatively less efficient than in an adult are the ability to excrete a highly acid urine, and both Tm_{PAH} and Tm_g. All functions become comparable to those of an adult by the end of the first year. Ammonia excretion, however, is within normal limits in the first few days.

Titratable acid excretion is remarkably low for the first year of life. This is due in part to a poor ability to secrete hydrogen ions against a gradient and also to the low phosphate content of the urine. The low urinary phosphate content is due to the infant's retention of phosphate for the formation of bone and muscle. If phosphate is administered titratable acid excretion rises and the usually low plasma bicarbonate values rise to adult levels. In addition the infant's renal threshold for bicarbonate is 21·5 to 22·5 mEq/l which is much lower than the 24 to 26 mEq/l found in the adult. It appears therefore that the infant's normal state of mild metabolic acidosis is secondary to a combination of inadequate kidneys and insufficient urinary buffer. This explains the infant's liability to develop severe acidosis if given large quantities of dietary protein.

Proteinuria and glycosuria occur in about a quarter of normal premature infants, and infants up to the third day, when the urine then becomes free of protein and glucose.

Renal function during senescence

After the age of 30 there is a gradual reduction in renal functional capacity. The functions which have been studied include glomerular filtration, renal blood flow, secretion Tm, urea clearance, and the ability to concentrate.

By the age of 90 each of these functions has decreased to approximately half its value at the age of 30. It is important to note however that though the creatinine clearance may be halved, the plasma creatinine is normal. This is because the production of creatinine by the reduced muscle mass of the elderly is smaller than normal. It must not be assumed, therefore, if the plasma creatinine of an elderly person is normal, then his glomerular filtration rate is the same as that of a younger person with the same plasma creatinine. This is extremely relevant when administering digitalis and certain antibiotics which, if the dose is not adjusted to the degressed glomerular filtration rate, may accumulate and cause toxic symptoms. Histological appearances show that there is a gradual loss of nephrons so that it is highly probable that every function is involved.

It is certainly very noticeable that elderly patients are not able to concentrate their urine to the same extent as adolescents.

BIBLIOGRAPHY

ALEXANDER, P., and NIXON, D. A. (1961). "The foetal kidney." *Brit. med. Bull.*, **17**, 112.

BOSS, J. M. H., DLOUKA, H., KRAUS, M., and KRECEK, J. (1964). "The structure of the kidney in relation to age and diet in white rats during the weaning period." *J. Physiol.*, **168**, 196.

CUTLER, R. E., and ORME, B. M. (1969). *J. Amer. med. Ass.*, **209**, 539.

EDELMAN, C. M., BARNETT, H. L., and TROUPKOU, V. (1960). "Renal concentrating mechanisms in newborn infants. Effects of dietary protein and water content, role of urea, and responsiveness to antidiuretic hormone." *J. clin. Invest.*, **39**, 1062.

EDELMAN, C. M., SORIANO, J. R., BOICHIS, H., GRUSKIN, A. B., and ACOSTA, M. I. (1967). "Renal bicarbonate reabsorption and hydrogen ion excretion in normal infants." *J. Clin. Invest.*, **46**, 1309.

KRECEK, J., and HELLER, J. (1962). "Neurohypophysis and the regulation of water and electrolyte metabolism in infants and mammals." *Proc. Internat. Union of Phys. Sci.*, *22nd Congress*, **I**, 53

MCCANCE, R. A., and HATEMI, N. (1961). "Control of acid-base stability in the newly born." *Lancet*, **I**, 293.

MCCANCE, R. A., and WIDDOWSON, E. M. (1956). "Metabolism and renal function in the first two days of life." "Modern Views on the Secretion of Urine", p. 217. J. & A. Churchill Ltd., London.

MILLER, J. H., and SHOCK, N. W. (1953) "Age differences in the renal response to antidiuretic hormone." *J. Gerontol.*, **8**, 446.

RHODES, P. G., HAMMEL, C. L., and BERMAN, L. B. (1962). "Urinary constituents of the new born infant." *J. Paediat.*, **60**, 18.

SAKAI, T., LEUMANN, E. P., and HOLLIDAY, M. A. (1969). "Single injection clearance in children." *Pediatrics*, **44**, 905.

SHOCK, N. W. (1946). "Kidney function tests in aged males." *Geriatrics*, **I**, 232.

SHOCK, N. W., and DAVIES, D. F. (1950). "Age changes in glomerular filtration rate, effective renal plasma flow, and tubular excretory capacity in adult males." *J. clin. Invest.*, **29**, 496.

SPITZER, A. (1971). "Renal physiology impact of recent developments on clinical nephrology." *Pediatrics clinic of North America*, **18**, 377.

VERNIER, R. L., and BIRCH-ANDERSON, A. (1962). "Studies of the human foetal kidney." *J. Paediat.*, **60**, 754.

WATKIN, M., and SHOCK, M. H. (1955). *J. Clin. Invest.*, **34**, 969.

9

The Renal Circulation

At rest about one-fifth of the cardiac output flows through the kidney, though the oxygen consumption of the kidney does not amount to more than 8–10 per cent of the oxygen consumption of the whole body. The normal renal blood flow is approximately 1,100 ml/min. It is a greater irrigation per unit weight of tissue than any other organ. This extraordinary phenomenon is confined to the cortex; the medulla only receives 6 per cent of the total renal blood flow and has an irrigation which is comparable to that of other tissues. The reason for this high cortical perfusion is not understood for, though experimentally a substantial and sustained reduction in renal blood flow is always associated with some fall in glomerular filtration rate, renal function in all other measurable respects may remain perfectly normal. In the following discussion it is to be remembered that changes in renal blood flow are generally accompanied by similar changes in the glomerular filtration rate, though frequently the degree of change may be different.

Some Factors which Cause a Reduction in Renal Blood Flow

The normal renal blood flow is very great, consequently if a change does occur, the flow is nearly always reduced. The upright posture, undernutrition, exercise, pain, heat, adrenaline and advancing years are some of the physiological factors associated with such a reduction. The pathological causes are discussed below.

Circulatory insufficiency

Clinically the most frequent cause of a fall in renal blood flow is circulatory insufficiency. Contraction of the blood volume and cardiac failure both cause renal vasoconstriction and a fall in renal blood flow, whether or not there is a concomitant decrease in blood pressure.

Contraction of the blood volume may be secondary to traumatic, surgical or spontaneous bleeding, acute haemolysis, severe diarrhoea and vomiting, barbiturate poisoning, burns, or negative protein balance. Sudden changes in blood volume produce the most marked changes in the renal circulation, but there is a delay between the time of the haemorrhage and the onset of renal vasoconstriction. A haemorrhage which is severe enough to induce peripheral vasoconstriction, with pallor and coldness of the hands, feet and face, may not cause a fall in renal blood flow within the next one to two hours. If, however, the blood volume remains reduced for four to seven hours there is severe renal vasoconstriction, which may be sufficient to cause necrosis of the renal cortex. The cause of this vasoconstriction is nervous and humoral. Therapeutically the delay is sometimes an advantage, for early transfusion may prevent the onset of severe renal ischaemia; but conversely once ischaemia has developed, transfusion is only associated with a slow recovery; the ischaemia continuing for several hours though the blood volume is normal.

Cardiac failure induces renal vasoconstriction both when the cardiac output is low (when the fall in renal blood flow is proportionately greater than the fall in cardiac output) and when the output is high as in cor pulmonale and thyrotoxicosis. In the latter the cardiac output may be doubled and yet the renal blood flow may fall to 20 per cent of its normal value. The cause of this vasoconstriction is uncertain, but the inability of a high spinal anaesthetic to alter the renal blood flow in established cardiac failure suggests that it may be humoral. This is supported by the finding that some increase in renal blood flow occurs following the administration of the adrenaline antagonist dibenamine. Large increases in renal venous pressure have been found to produce transient reductions in renal blood flow. But this is not the cause of the fall in renal blood flow in cardiac failure, for the renal venous pressures usually encountered are not in this high range, and in chronic heart failure the venous pressure and renal blood flow may vary independently.

A teleological explanation for the renal vasoconstriction which occurs with circulatory distress is that it maintains the arterial pressure and switches the available cardiac output to organs which are less able than the kidney to function with a reduced blood flow.

Acute uterine catastrophies

There is a close association between the incidence of abortion, accidental haemorrhage, and eclampsia on the one hand and severe renal ischaemia on the other. Abortion used to be the most frequent cause of acute renal failure.

In many of these conditions haemorrhage must be partly responsible for the renal ischaemia, but it is probable that other mechanisms are also involved. The intravascular laying down of fibrin in the glomerular capillaries in accidental haemorrhage is one mechanism, and endothelial capillary swelling in eclampsia is another. In experimental animals an acute rise in intra-uterine pressure causes a marked fall in renal blood flow; if such a mechanism is present in man it may be an important contributory factor in the causation of renal ischaemia in some of the conditions mentioned above (e.g. concealed accidental haemorrhage).

Electrolyte and endocrine abnormalities

Most forms of electrolyte abnormalities cause a reduction in renal blood flow. With simple water depletion, or with combined salt and water depletion, this reduction is caused by the contraction of the blood volume. But with water intoxication due to salt loss, or excess water intake, the mechanism is obscure. Potassium deficiency and hypercalcaemia also cause a fall in renal blood flow. Initially these circulatory changes are quickly and completely reversible; if, however, they are prolonged and are associated with the development of structural changes, recovery will be incomplete.

The renal blood flow is also reduced in hyper- and hypo-adrenalism, hypopituitarism and myxoedema.

Vasoconstrictors other than those produced by the endocrine glands

These consist mainly of exogenous substances and include a variety of cytotoxic poisons such as carbon tetrachloride, corrosive sublimate (mercuric chloride), propylene glycol, etc. Frequently tubular necrosis follows, both from direct action of the poison on the cells and from intense renal ischaemia (p. 159).

Some infections such as Weil's disease and scrub typhus are also associated with severe reductions in renal blood flow.

Disorders of the renal vasculature

Atheroma of the large intrarenal arteries may occasionally lead to wedge-shaped loss of renal parenchyma and a substantial fall in renal blood flow; while hypertension (particularly the malignant form), polyarteritis nodosa, eclampsia, diabetes and amyloidosis frequently produce such obliterative changes in the arterioles and glomerular capillaries that severe fatal renal ischaemia may result. Changes in the renal vessels in diffuse lupus erythematosus and scleroderma may also lead to renal failure. The acute glomerular capillaritis of acute nephritis does not usually affect the renal blood flow, but there are occasional instances of severe renal ischaemia.

Gradual destruction of the renal parenchyma as a cause of a decrease in renal blood flow

Loss of nephrons is at first compensated for by an increased flow of blood through the remaining hypertrophied nephrons, e.g. the changes which occur following unilateral nephrectomy. Eventually, however, with further loss of nephrons the renal blood flow inevitably diminishes. Among the conditions which have not yet been considered and which produce a gradual destruction of the renal parenchyma there are: persistent glomerular nephritis, pyelonephritis, polycystic disease, congenital tubular disorders, renal tuberculosis and urinary tract obstruction.

Some Factors which Cause Renal Hyperaemia

These include cold, large protein intake, hyperpyrexia, sudden increase in blood volume, emotion, aminophylline derivatives, methedrine, magnesium sulphate, polycythaemia, pregnancy, and growth hormone. In general such increases in renal blood flow are of no clinical importance, though occasionally aminophylline is used to raise the renal blood flow and glomerular filtration rate when trying to obtain an adequate diuresis with diuretics.

Adjustment of the Renal Circulation to Changes in Haematocrit

In the normal kidney the fall in haematocrit which occurs in anaemia is associated with a substantial decrease in renal blood flow, a small reduction in plasma flow and an almost unchanged glomerular filtration rate; when the

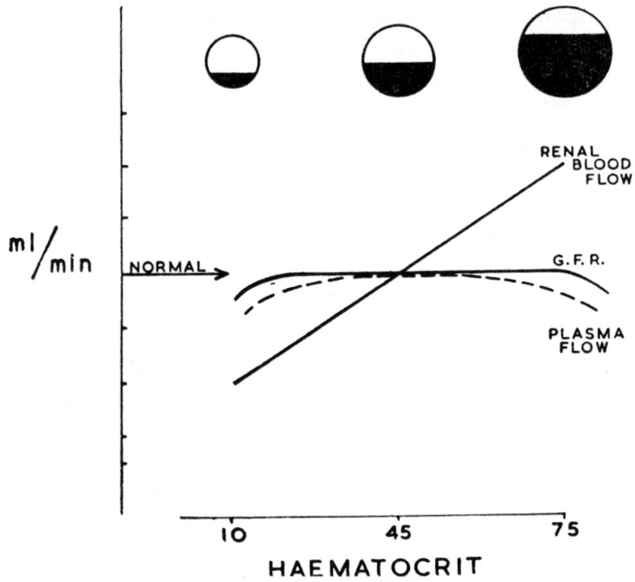

FIG. 9.1. Schema of the changes in renal blood flow, plasma flow and glomerular filtration rate which occur in the normal kidney in response to changes in haematocrit. The three circles illustrate what is presumably taking place in the renal vessels, i.e. the renal plasma flow remains constant because the diameter of the renal vessles varies directly with the changing fraction of red cells.

haematocrit falls below approximately 20, however, the renal ischaemia becomes much more pronounced and there is a marked reduction in plasma flow and glomerular filtration (Fig. 9.1). These changes are more pronounced when the anaemia causes salt and water retention ("cardiac failure").

Conversely the rise in haematocrit which occurs in polycythaemia is associated with a substantial *increase* in renal blood flow, but again there is only a small reduction in plasma flow and an almost unchanged rate of glomerular filtration; at haematocrits above approximately 75, however, both the renal plasma flow and glomerular filtration rate tend to be sharply depressed.

These changes suggest that the kidney is mainly concerned with the maintenance of a constant renal plasma flow and glomerular filtration, and not with the total renal blood flow. The mechanisms responsible for these adjustments are not known, but they appear to be local in origin and unrelated to changes in cardiac output.

Clinically the important point is that such adjustments may take some days to complete, and that in diseased kidneys take place even more slowly or not at all. The result is that a perfectly justifiable transfusion for anaemia in chronic renal failure may be followed by a rapid deterioration in renal function. The explanation is as follows. It has been pointed out earlier that a reduction in glomerular filtration rate to 50 per cent of normal produces little absolute change in the blood concentrations of waste products, but with further reductions in filtration rate these concentrations rise steeply. If, therefore, owing to renal parenchymal destruction the glomerular filtration rate is low, it is clear that a further small decrease in filtration will produce a large increase in blood concentrations of waste products. Such a decrease in filtration may follow the rise in haematocrit which accompanies a transfusion; it is due to the failure of the renal vessels to dilate sufficiently quickly to accommodate the rising fraction of red cells; the renal plasma flow and filtration rate are automatically reduced and the patient may die of acute anuria. If it is considered necessary to treat the chronic anaemia of chronic renal failure with transfusions, it is best to give small amounts of packed cells and not to try and raise the P.C.V. above 25. It is best to give packed red cells in order to minimise the risk of causing heart failure which is the other hazard of transfusing patients with renal failure. An estimate of glomerular function should be obtained between each transfusion.

Adjustment of the Renal Circulation to Changes in Arterial Pressure

The rate of blood flow is related to the arterial pressure and the resistance of the vessels, i.e. $F = P/R$ where F = blood flow, P = arterial pressure and R = vascular resistance. Alterations in resistance are produced almost entirely by changes in the calibre of the vessels, i.e. by vasoconstriction and vasodilatation. Such changes usually occur as part of a general alteration in total peripheral resistance, e.g. hypertension and haemorrhage are both associated with an increase in total peripheral resistance and, in each, renal vasoconstriction contributes to the increase. Occasionally, however, changes in renal resistance may occur which do not stem from some central demand for circulatory adjustment. For instance, there are the changes in renal vascular resistance which accompany changes in haematocrit (see above), and the following changes which accompany alterations in arterial pressure.

It is well established that the kidney has an independent mechanism which alters the calibre of the renal vessels in response to changes in arterial pressure. This relationship between the rate of renal blood flow and the arterial pressure is most easily demonstrated in the isolated perfused dog's kidney, and is illustrated in Fig. 9.2. It can be seen that over a pressure range of about 0 to 90 mmHg the blood flow rises with the pressure; from 90 to 200 mmHg the flow remains relatively unaltered; and after 200 mmHg the flow rises once again. The alterations in vascular lumen occur in the arteries on the afferent side of the glomerulus, for the glomerular filtration rate parallels the changes in the renal blood flow. The changes in the diameter of the arterial lumen are due to the innate property of the smooth muscle in the arterial walls to respond to a stretching force by a contraction, and a diminution of tension by a relaxation; a property which can be demonstrated in many sites in the body including the arteries of other organs and the umbilical artery. It is probable, for instance, that

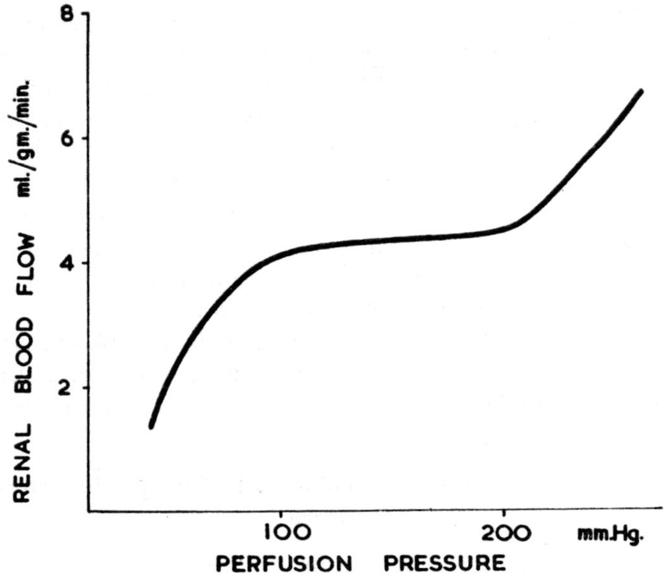

FIG. 9.2. Renal circulatory autoregulation. The relationship between the perfusion pressure (i.e. renal artery pressure) and the renal blood flow in a dog's kidney, showing the relative constancy of the blood flow when the perfusion pressure is between 100 and 200 mmHg.

this phenomenon is responsible for the dilatation of an artery that occurs distal to the site of an obstruction. The constancy of the renal blood flow during alterations in blood pressure is known as renal circulatory autoregulation.

Recently a hypothesis has been put forward that renal circulatory autoregulation is due to a different mechanism from that which is responsible for circulating autoregulation in other vascular beds. It is proposed that changes in perfusion pressure cause an initial change in renal blood flow and glomerular filtration rate which causes a change in the sodium concentration delivered to the macula densa of the distal tubule, that this in turn induces a change in the rate of renin production by the granular cells in that part of the afferent arteriole near to the macula densa and that this causes the afferent arteriole to change the size of its lumen in the direction which will correct this sequence. There are many objections to this hypothesis. Perhaps one of the most potent is that it cannot explain the rapid oscillations of renal blood flow which take place in the first few seconds after the renal perfusion pressure is suddenly altered (Fig. 9.3).

Indirect evidence for the presence of a similar stabilising mechanism in the renal vasculature of man has been obtained on several occasions, though the exact range over which it occurs is not known. It must almost certainly be

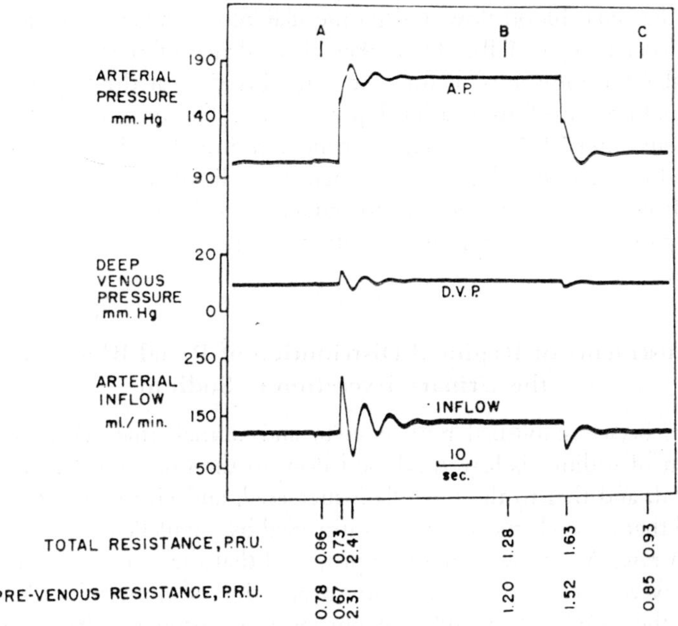

FIG. 9.3. Circulatory autoregulation. The effect on renal arterial blood flow to an isolated kidney of increasing the arterial pressure. There are several rapid oscillations of blood flow before the renal blood flow stabilises at a level slightly greater than before the rise in pressure. Such oscillations could not be a function of a biochemical reflex from the distal tubule to the afferent arteriole. See text. (Waugh, 1964, Suppl. I to *Circulation Research*.)

over a lower range than in the dog, for the mean blood pressure in man is lower than that in the dog. There is some evidence that renal circulatory autoregulation in man is present down to a mean arterial pressure of about 60 mmHg. Such observations are difficult to obtain, for in most circumstances changes in arterial pressure produce a central demand for compensatory alterations in the peripheral resistance which have priority over purely local circulatory reflexes; the latter are best observed following small changes in arterial pressure produced by changes in cardiac output.

Teleologically this intrinsic pressure-flow relationship is difficult to understand. One suggestion is that it protects the glomerular filtration rate from the normal fluctuations in pressure, so that the tubules are presented with a continuous steady quantity of materials. As many of the factors which influence tubular function are slow to change the extent of their activity, a stability of this nature may be of value.

Clinically there are two aspects of this local pressure-flow relationship which are of interest. The first is purely speculative; does this mechanism, which responds to a rise in arterial pressure by vasoconstriction ever become so disordered in disease that it causes excessive vasoconstriction at normal blood pressures? The other is more practical and is related to the treatment of hypertensive patients with hypotensive drugs. When renal function is substantially normal the renal blood flow and glomerular filtration rate remain unchanged as the blood pressure falls. But if there is evidence of renal damage (reduced glomerular filtration, etc.) before the administration of the hypotensive agent the normal pressure-flow relationship may either fail, or only become manifest after a long interval. In these circumstances glomerular filtration rate will fall, the blood urea rise steeply, and the patient may die of acute upon chronic renal failure. It is always wise therefore to induce a fall in blood pressure gradually in such patients, and to repeat estimations of glomerular function at frequent intervals.

Adjustments of Regional Distribution of Renal Blood Flow and the Urinary Excretion of Sodium

It has been established both in man and animals that when the urinary excretion of sodium is low the blood flow to the outer cortex of the kidney is reduced, and that to the medulla is increased, and vice versa. It was, at first, assumed that these changes were accompanied by parallel changes in glomerular filtration rate. And it was therefore proposed that the cause of the low urinary sodium excretion was due to a greater proportion of glomerular filtrate passing through the deep juxta medullary nephrons. It was proposed that these nephrons reabsorbed sodium more avidly because they have long loops of Henle. None of these assumptions seem to be warranted. It has been found that redistribution of filtrate does not occur with changes in urinary sodium excretion. And it has been pointed out that though the juxta medullary nephrons do have longer loops of Henle they also have a much higher rate of filtration. Thus any overall redistribution, if it did occur, might not have any effect on sodium reabsorption. It is possible therefore that the redistribution of blood flow that occurs with changes in sodium excretion may be the consequence, rather than the cause, of the changes in sodium excretion. This conclusion is re-enforced by the observation that the rise in urinary sodium excretion produced by frusemide and ethacrynic acid are also associated with a redistribution of regional blood flow.

Shunts

There is no convincing evidence that true shunting of blood ever takes place in the kidney. Nevertheless, there are two renal circulatory phenomena which have sometimes had the word shunt applied to them. One is the kidney's capacity for intense vasoconstriction, and the other is the way in which it separates plasma from red cells.

"Shunting" of whole blood

It has been claimed that in some circumstances, the cortex may become ischaemic because the blood which should have travelled to the cortex is shunted through the medulla. This conclusion was first reached from observations made on experimental animals subjected to the following stimuli: prolonged application of tourniquets to the hind limbs, bleeding, stimulation of the sciatic nerves and the administration of certain substances such as adrenaline, in large quantities. During and immediately after stimulation the renal circulation was studied by means of angiographs, injections of methylene blue, and histological sections. These techniques give an indication of the *distribution* of blood within the kidney at any one time, but are not measures of the *rate* of blood flow in any one place. It was found that the stimuli were associated with the following change in the distribution of blood; the cortex contained less and the medulla more, that is, the cortex on section was pale and the medulla was dark. Mainly from this evidence it was suggested that the ischaemia of the cortex was due to the hyperaemia of the medulla; the blood intended for the cortex having been by-passed, diverted, or shunted through the medulla.

There is much evidence however, that this assumption was unwarranted. It has been pointed out that to demonstrate that ischaemia is due to the opening of a shunt it is necessary to show that the decrease in flow in the ischaemic area is of the same order as the increase in flow in the shunt, i.e. if a large diversion of the normal cortical blood flow takes place it should be possible to demonstrate cortical ischaemia without significant reduction in renal blood flow. But when renal blood flow is measured, the cortex becomes pale and the medulla dark only when the total renal blood flow is greatly reduced. It is clear therefore, that the ischaemic pallor of the cortex cannot be due only to an increase in medullary flow, whether or not a small increase does occur. That such an increase is unlikely has been demonstrated with temperature measuring needles simultaneously recording from medulla and cortex; for when the total renal blood flow is markedly reduced by nor-adrenaline, adrenaline and stimulation of the renal nerves, the changes in temperature which take place (and which presumably reflect changes in blood flow) are the same in the two sites. It has even been suggested that when there is pallor of the cortex and congestionof the medulla it is probable that there is no blood flowing through the medulla, for it has been found that indian ink injected intravenously may sometimes fail to appear in the medulla.

The importance of the observations which led to the renal shunt hypothesis is that they showed that in certain circumstances the cortex of the kidney has a disconcerting tendency to shut off its blood supply almost completely. It is probable that in most instances of intense renal vasconstriction the blood flow through the cortex virtually ceases while medullary blood flow continues at a very reduced rate.

"Shunting" of plasma from red cells

The haematocrit of the blood in the renal cortex is about 50 per cent of that in the large blood vessels, and in the medulla it is only 30 per cent. This high proportion of plasma in the cortex is partly due to (i) its predominantly capillary bore circulation, for there is a tendency in small vessels for red cells to travel quickly down the centre in a narrow stream, while plasma passes more slowly in a wide peripheral cuff; and (ii) there is some evidence that some plasma probably lies in the interstitial space.

The even higher proportion of plasma in the medulla indicates that the blood flow through the medulla is mainly plasma. The most reasonable hypothesis for this phenomenon is that the plasma is "stripped" from the red cells at the point where the afferent arterioles supplying the juxtamedullary glomeruli leave the interlobular arteries. It has been shown on models that when blood flows through a tube whose branches come off at right angles (as they do from the interlobular arteries) the sleeve of plasma in the central tube passes selectively into the branches with little admixture of red cells. The functional importance of this manoeuvre is obscure. It is possible that it contributes to a low intra-medullary pO_2 (see below).

Significance of the Counter-current Circulation in the Medulla

It has been pointed out (p. 8) that the blood supply to the medulla flows through long looped vessels (the vasa recta) which, though they are relatively wide, have walls of capillary thickness throughout their entire course. And that the blood within them is obliged to flow in a counter-current fashion, first down towards the tip of the papilla and then upwards to the corticomedullary junction. As the walls of the vasa recta are of capillary thickness the blood they contain is in nearly all respects in equilibrium with medullary interstitial fluid, and therefore with the fluid flowing through the thin capillary like descending limbs of Henle. In addition it is very likely that at all times the fluid in the collecting ducts must also be in equilibrium with the pO_2 and Pco_2 of the medullary interstitial fluid, and there is evidence that under the influence of ADH the fluid in the collecting ducts is also in equilibrium with respect to its osmolality, urea concentration and probably hydrogen ion concentration.

The importance to the medullary interstitial fluid of a counter-current flow in the vasa recta is two-fold. (i) It magnifies the *rise* in concentration which follows the transfer of any solute or gas from the tubules into the medullary interstitial fluid. (ii) It magnifies the *fall* in concentration of any solute or gas which is removed from the medullary interstitial fluid. Both are clinically important.

An example of the first consequence of the counter-current circulation was detailed on pp. 51, 53 where it was shown how it contributes to the high medullary concentrations of sodium chloride and urea, which in turn make it possible for the urine to become hypertonic. It is probable that it is also responsible for the high P_{CO_2} of alkaline urine and the low pH of acid urine. The high osmolality of the medulla is one reason why the medulla is so susceptible to infection, it inhibits the action of complement and the mobilisation and phagocytic properties of polymorphonuclear leucocytes. The most clear-cut example of the second consequence is the fact that the pO_2 of urine is lower than that of renal venous blood. This is because the initially high pO_2 of the arterial blood in the descending limb of the vasa recta is in equilibrium with the low pO_2 of the venous blood in the ascending limb; it follows that the pO_2 of the supposedly arterial blood reaching the tip of the papilla, and which is in equilibrium with the urine emerging from the collecting tubule, is lower than normal arterial blood. Clinically, it is possible that this regional hypoxia is a factor in the characteristic localisation of renal tuberculosis, and in the aetiology of necrotising papillitis.

BIBLIOGRAPHY

BARGER, A. C. (1966). "Renal hemodynamic factors in congestive heart failure." *Ann. N.Y. Acad. Sci.*, **139**, 276. (Regional redistribution of blood flows.)

BRADLEY, S. E., and BRADLEY, G. P. (1947). "Renal function during chronic anaemia in man." *Blood*, **2**, 192.

EICHNAR, L. W., FARBER, S. J., BERGER, A., EARLE, D., RADER, B., PELLEGRINO, E., ALBERT, R. E., ALEXANDER, J. D., TAUBE, H., and YOUNGWORTH, S. (1953). "Cardio-vascular dynamics in heart failure." *Circulation*, **7**, 674.

EMERY, E. W., GOWENLOCK, A. H., RIDDELL, A. G., and BLACK, D. A. K. (1959). "Intrarenal variations in haematocrit." *Clin. Sci.*, **18**, 205.

EPSTEIN, F. H., POST, R. S., and MacDOWELL, M. E. (1953). "The effect of an A–V fistula on renal haemodynamics and electrolyte excretion." *J. clin. Invest.*, **32**, 233.

FISHMAN, A. P., MAXWELL, M. H., CROWDER, C. H., and MORALES, P. (1951). "Kidney function in cor pulmonale." *Circulation*, **3**, 703.

KIIL, F. (1971). Blood flow and oxygen utilization by the kidney. "Kidney Hormones". Edited by J. W. Fisher. Academic Press, London and New York, 1.

LADEFOGED, J., and MUNK, O. (1971). Distribution of blood flow in the kidney. "Kidney Hormones." Edited by J. W. Fisher. Academic Press, London and New York, 31.

LAUSON, H. D., BRADLEY, S. E., and COURNAND, A. (1944). "Renal circulation in shock." *J. clin. Invest.*, **23**, 381.

LILINEFIELD, L. S., LASSEN, N. A., and ROSE, J. C. (1958). "The diverse distribution of red cells and albumin within anatomic regions of the kidney." *Amer. J. Med.*, **25**, 126.

PHILLIP, R. A., DOLE, V. P., HAMILTON, P. B., EMERSON, K., ARCHIBALD, R. M., and VAN SLYKE, D. D. (1946). "Effects of acute haemorrhagic and traumatic shock on renal function of dogs." *Amer. J. Physiol.*, **145**, 314.

RENNIE, D. W., REEVES, R. B., and PAPPENHEIMER, J. R. (1958). "Oxygen pressure in urine and its relation to intrarenal blood flow." *Amer. J. Physiol.*, **195**, 120.

SCHER, A. M. (1951). "Focal blood flow measurement in cortex and medulla of kidney." *Amer. J. Physiol.*, **167**, 539.

THURAU, K., SCHNERMANN, J., NAGEL, W., HORSTER, M., and WAHL, M. (1967). Composition of tubular fluid in the macula densa segment as a factor regulating the function of the juxtaglomerular apparatus. "Circulation Research", Vol. 20 and 21, Suppl. II. 79. (Autoregulation.)

SELKURT, E. E., and HALPERS, M. J. (1963). "The influence of haemorrhagic shock on renal hemodynamics and osmolar clearance." *Amer. J. Physiol.*, **205**, 147.

SEMPLE, S. J. G. and DE WARDENER, H. E. (1959). "The effect of increased renal venous pressure on circulatory autoregulation of isolated dog kidneys." *Circulat. Res.*, **7**, 643.

SYMPOSIUM on "Autoregulation of Blood Flow". (1964). *Circulation Res.*, **15**, suppl. 1.

THURAU, K. (1964). "Renal hemodynamics." *Amer. J. Med.*, **36**, 698.

THURAU, K., and WOBER, E. (1962). "On the localisation of autoregulative resistance changes in the kidneys. Micropuncture measurements of the pressure in the tubules and peritubular capillaries of the rat kidney in changes of arterial pressure." *Pflügers Arch. ges. Physiol.*, **274**, 553.

TRUETA, J., BARCLAY, A. E., DANIEL, P. M., FRANKLIN, K. J., and PRITCHARD, M. M. L. (1947). "Studies of the Renal Circulation." Blackwell Scientific Pubs., Oxford.

WARDENER DE, H. E., McSWINEY, R. R., and MILES, B. E. (1951). "Renal haemodynamics in primary polycythaemia." *Lancet*, **2**, 204.

10

The Kidney and Erythropoiesis

ANAEMIA is a constant feature of renal failure and mainly due to depressed erythropoiesis. Fig. 10.1 illustrates the average fall in haemoglobin plotted against the rise in blood urea in patients with chronic renal failure. On the other hand, it is well-established that about 10 per cent of patients with carcinoma

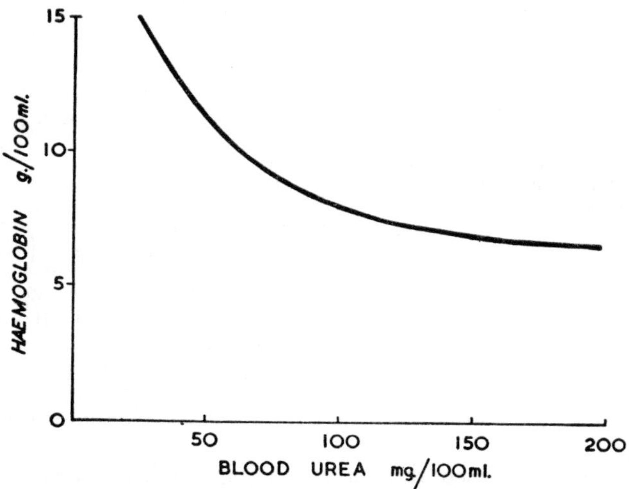

FIG. 10.1. Schema of the mean relationship between the haemoglobin concentration and the blood urea; individual plots show a considerable scatter.

of the kidney have polycythaemia and that on occasion a reversible polycythaemia accompanies a hydronephrosis or polycystic kidneys. Some patients in the early stages of glomerular nephritis before the onset of renal failure may also have polycythaemia with enlarged red cell masses. Clinically therefore, it appears that loss of renal tissue is usually associated with a decrease in red cell formation, and an increase in renal tissue sometimes associated with an increased red cell formation. The connection between hydronephrosis, polycystic kidneys and glomerular nephritis with erythropoiesis is obscure. It is probable that the stimulus is relative renal hypoxia from ischaemia.

The kidneys produce a substance called renal erythropoietic factor, which, when incubated with plasma, produces an erythropoietic stimulating factor or erythropoietin which directly stimulates the bone marrow. As one stimulus for the production of renal erythropoietic factor is renal ischaemia the analogy with renin and angiotensin is very close. It has been demonstrated however that renal erythropoietic factor is not the same substance as renin.

The rate of production of erythropoietin depends on the presence of a certain quantity of renal parenchyma regardless of its excretory efficiency. This has been shown by comparing one group of animals in which one kidney has been irradiated and the other has been removed, with another group in which one kidney has been irradiated but the other has been left in place with the cut end of its ureter stitched in the peritoneal space. The blood urea rose equally in both groups. The animals with an irradiated contracted kidney and no other renal substance became anaemic. Those with a similarly diseased kidney but in whom

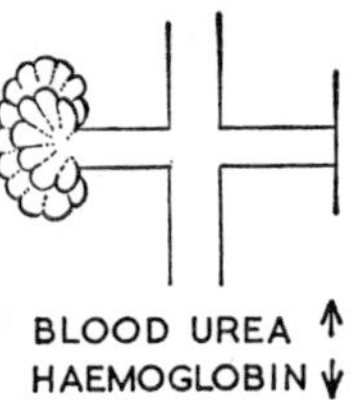

Fig. 10.2. Illustration of an experiment demonstrating that the fall in haemoglobin in renal failure is not due to the accumulation of "waste products". Right kidney irradiated. (Osnes, 1959, *Brit. med. J.*)

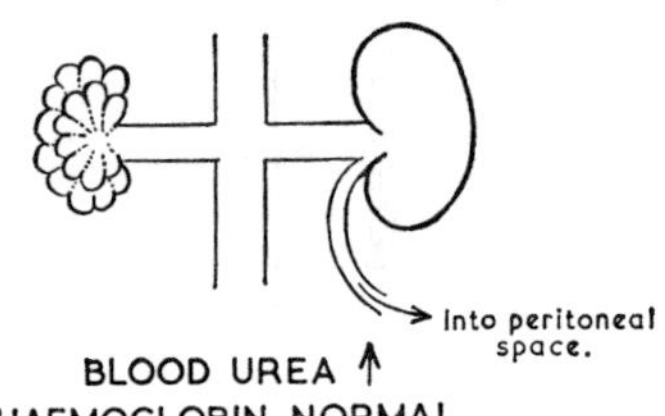

the other kidney was present though excreting its urine into the peritoneal space did not become anaemic (Fig. 10.2). It has been shown that patients after bilateral nephrectomy usually have no erythropoietin in their circulating blood. Nevertheless a haemorrhage may induce a brisk rise in erythropoietin level indicating that the kidney is not the only site which produces erythropoietin. On the other hand, in patients with chronic renal failure, changes in erythropoiesis can be produced by bleeding and transfusion in the absence of detectable erythropoietin levels in the blood indicating that there are hormonal agents responsible for erythropoiesis other than erythropoietin. In man it would appear that the anaemia of chronic renal failure is due mainly to certain biochemical changes associated with advancing ureamia which directly inhibit erythropoiesis. It has been shown for instance that erythropoiesis increases after dialysis and after lowering the blood urea with a low protein diet, regardless of the presence of detectable erythropoietin in the blood.

Renal polycythaemia should be suspected in a patient whose polycythaemia is associated with a normal arterial saturation but with no increase in white cells or platelets and no enlargement of the spleen. If, in addition, there is an episode of haematuria the diagnosis becomes increasingly likely. Occasionally there is a tendency to think that the haematuria has been caused by the polycythaemia when, in fact, it is due to the renal lesion responsible for the polycythaemia. About 1 per cent of all patients with an initial diagnosis of polycythaemia vera are subsequently found to have renal polycythaemia. A few of these have a palpable spleen, which is misleading. Polycythaemia also occurs in some patients following transplantation when it is probably due to the vascular damage in the transplanted kidney caused by immunological rejection.

BIBLIOGRAPHY

FORSSELL, J. (1958). "Nephrogenous polycythaemia." *Acta med. scand.*, **161**, 169.

HOFFMAN, G. C. (1971). "Erythropoietin after transplantation." *Idem.*, p. 431.

JONES, N. F., PAYNE, R. W., HYDE, R. D., and PRICE, T. M. L. (1960). "Renal polycythaemia." *Lancet*, **1**, 299.

NAETES, J. P. (1960). "The rôle of the kidney in erythropoiesis." *J. clin. Invest.*, **39**, 102.

NAETES, J. P., and WITTEK, W. (1968). "Erythropoiesis in anephric man." *Lancet*, **1**, 941.

NATHAN, D. G., BECK, L. H., HAMPERS, C. L., and BUTTON, L. (1971). Hematopoiesis in renal failure. "Kidney Hormones." Edited by J. W. Fisher. Academic Press, London and New York, 411.

NATHAN, D. G., SCHUPAK, E., STOHLMAN, F., and MERRILL, J. P. (1964). "Erythropoiesis in anephric man." *J. clin. Invest.*, **43**, 2158.

OSNES, S. (1959). "Experimental study of an erythropoietic principle produced in the kidney." *Brit. med. J.*, **2**, 650.

RAMBACH, W. A., KURTIDES, E., ALT, H. L., and DEL GRECO, F. (1963). "Azotaemic anemia and the effect of hemodialysis." *Trans. Amer. Soc. Artific. Int. Organs*, **9**, 57.

11

The Kidney and Hypertension

THERE are seven important points to note when considering the relationship between the kidney and hypertension:

(1) Anephric man and animals develop severe hypertension when they are overloaded with salt and water.

(2) Animal experiments into the nature of hypertension have been concerned mainly with the rise in arterial pressure which takes place when the main trunk of one or both renal arteries are occluded.

(3) Partial occlusion of a main renal artery in man causes hypertension.

(4) Renal disease in man is often associated with hypertension.

(5) Hypertension in man causes occlusive lesions of the renal arterial tree, particularly the smaller arteries and arterioles, and it also causes disturbances of renal function.

(6) The evidence is becoming vanishingly small that persistent hypertension following partial occlusion of a renal artery is often related to the renin–angiotensin system.

(7) There is as yet no evidence that essential hypertension in man is due to renal dysfunction.

EXPERIMENTAL HYPERTENSION

Renoprival hypertension

As the name implies this form of hypertension follows bilateral nephrectomy. It was first performed in animals which subsequently developed hypertension. Many explanations were put forward amongst which there was one that proposed that the rise in blood pressure might be due to retention of salt and water (Fig. 11.1).

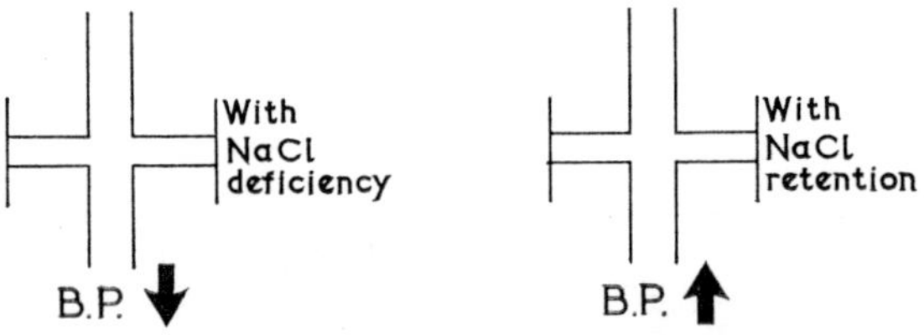

FIG. 11.1. Renoprival hypertension. The blood pressure depends on the retention of sodium chloride.

Renal hypertension

It has been firmly established in experimental animals that partial occlusion of the renal artery is followed by hypertension. In some animals both renal arteries must be occluded whereas in the rat it is sufficient to occlude only one renal artery (Fig. 11.2). Hypertension does not appear to be due to renal ischaemia, for it can be induced by an occlusion which does not interfere with renal blood flow. An unchanged renal blood flow despite partial occlusion of the renal artery, may at first seem paradoxical, but it is probably maintained by renal circulatory autoregulation, the phenomenon discussed in the previous section (p. oo). There is also evidence that hypertension may follow a partial occlusion of the renal artery even if the occlusion is adjusted so that the mean renal arterial pressure distal to the point of occlusion remains unchanged.

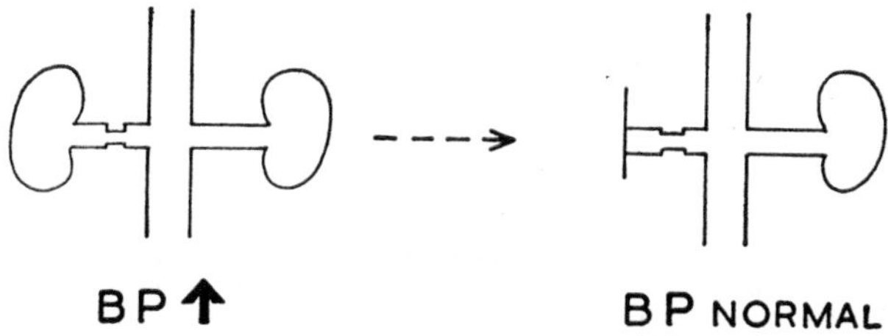

Fig. 11.2. Renal hypertension.

The stimulus is the reduction in pulse pressure. Renal artery occlusion causes the juxta glomerular apparatus to release renin into the general circulation which reacts with plasma angiotensinogen to form a vasoconstrictor angiotensin. Until recently it has been assumed that the initial rise in blood pressure that accompanied these changes were due to the observed rise in plasma angiotensin. Nevertheless it was less certain what caused the hypertension to persist, for after a few weeks the plasma angiotensin returns to normal. Lately, however, it has been shown that effective immunisation of rabbits against endogenous angiotensin does not prevent the development of persistent hypertension when a renal artery is partially occluded. This experiment makes it difficult to believe that angiotensin is very important in the aetiology of hypertension following partial renal artery occlusion. On the other hand it is not clear what does cause the blood pressure to rise in experimental renal artery occlusion. It has been claimed that salt and water retention does not occur. It is just possible however that this conclusion is erroneous and that the hypertension is indeed due to the salt and water retention consequent upon lowering the peritubular venous capillary pressure (p. 64).

Vicious circle renal hypertension

This form of hypertension is intimately connected with renal hypertension and occurs in the following circumstances. If renal hypertension is induced in the rat by occluding only one renal artery, the subsequent removal of the occlusion, or of the "occluded" kidney, may or may not be followed by a return of the blood pressure to normal. The deciding factor is the extent of hypertensive vascular damage present in the untouched kidney (Fig. 11.3). It has been suggested therefore that perhaps the mechanism is the same as in renal hypertension; the occlusion being produced by hypertensive vascular changes

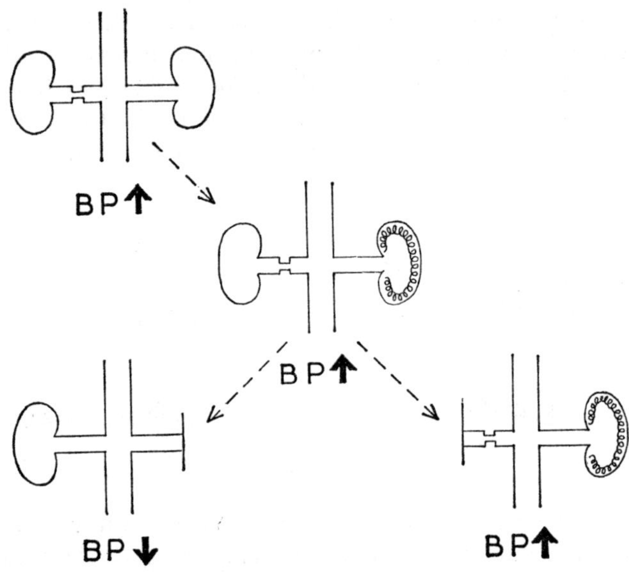

FIG. 11.3. Vicious circle hypertension.

throughout the periphery of the renal arterial bed. If such a self-perpetuating hypertensive mechanism occurs in man it is clearly of the utmost therapeutic importance. But again it is not clear which particular mechanisms cause the blood pressure to rise.

Experimental hypertension and perirenal compression

If one kidney is surrounded by some hard unyielding substance such as colloidon, the blood pressure rises rapidly and the animal dies of malignant hypertension within a few days. The mechanism which causes this rise in blood pressure is totally obscure. It is not related to a decrease in pulse pressure for the diminished distensibility of the kidney in these conditions causes a pronounced increase in intrarenal pulse pressure.

Experimental hypertension and adrenal function

Angiotensin stimulates the adrenal cortex to secrete aldosterone. Partial occlusion of the renal artery is therefore associated with a raised concentration of circulating aldosterone, some degree of sodium retention, and a urinary leak of potassium. It is interesting that when sodium and water retention is induced by an excess of aldosterone secondary to a prolonged experimental infusion of angiotensin the concentration of plasma sodium *falls* whereas an experimental infusion of aldosterone, and an aldosterone secreting tumour, cause a *rise* in plasma sodium. There is some evidence which suggests that this difference is because angiotensin stimulates anti-diuretic hormone secretion, whereas aldosterone does not. This phenomenon explains why the plasma renin concentration of patients with hypertension is inversely related to the plasma sodium concentration (Fig. 11.4).

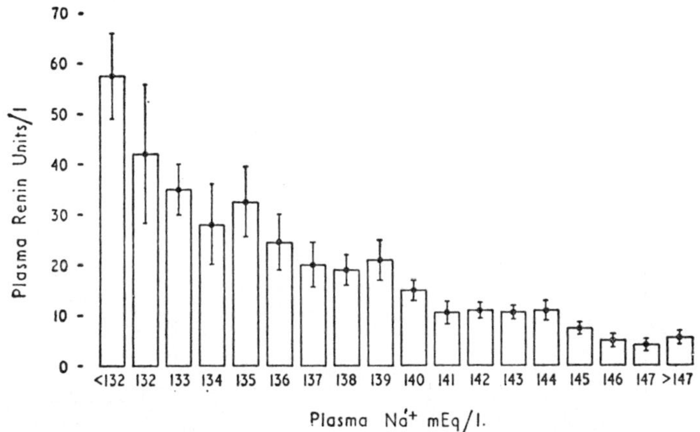

FIG. 11.4. Relationship between plasma renin and sodium concentrations in 253 patients with hypertension. (Brown *et al.*, 1965, *Brit. med. J.*)

Correlation Between Experimental and Clinical Findings

Statistically it is evident that in man renal disease is associated with hypertension; it is not unreasonable therefore, to suspect that some, if not all, the renal mechanisms which have been shown to produce hypertension in animals may eventually be proved to have their clinical counterpart. Some parallels can already be drawn.

Renoprival Hypertension

The most important recent advance in understanding those mechanisms responsible for hypertension in man has come from treating patients suffering from terminal renal failure with maintenance haemodialysis. *It has been found that in anephric patients the blood pressure is directly related to the total exchangeable sodium* (Fig. 11.5). An increase in exchangeable sodium causes a rise in blood pressure while removal of sodium and water by ultrafiltration during haemodialysis lowers the blood pressure. It has also been found that the blood pressure of the great majority of patients in terminal renal failure, before they are placed

E

on maintenance haemodialysis, is very susceptible to alteration of sodium and water balance. There is therefore conclusive evidence that salt and water retention can cause the blood pressure to rise. And it is probable that salt and water retention is an important factor in the aetiology of hypertension in chronic renal failure.

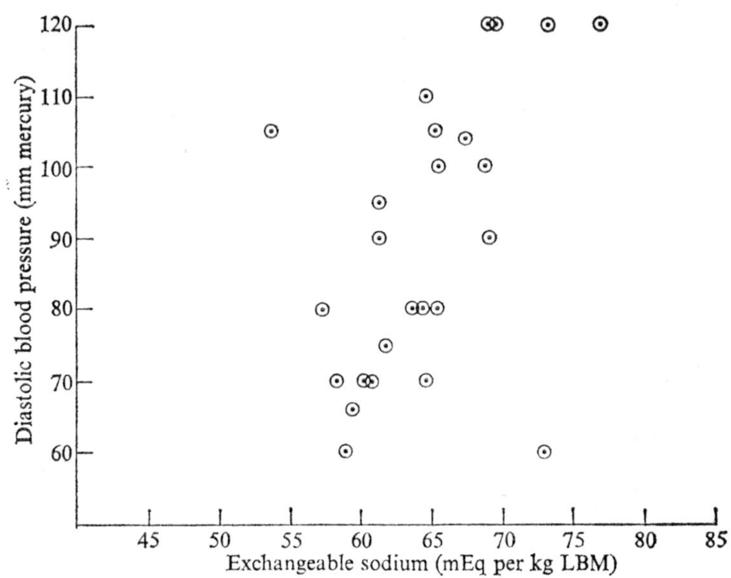

FIG. 11.5. The relation between exchangeable sodium and the diastolic blood pressure in anephric subjects. (Wilkinson, Scott, Udall, Kerr and Swiney, 1970, *Quarterly Journal of Medicine*.)

Alterations in pulse pressure

Following haemorrhage, or acute reductions of the extracellular volume by vomiting and diarrhoea, the pulse pressure diminishes whether or not there is a fall in mean arterial pressure; in these circumstances the renin mechanism is stimulated and the maintenance of the blood pressure in such an acute situation may in part be controlled by an increased quantity of circulating angiotensin.

A reduced pulse pressure to the renal arterial tree also occurs in coarctation of the aorta. In this condition, though there is no evidence that the renin mechanism is hyperactive or that the rate of renal blood flow is abnormal, it is nevertheless probable that the hypertension is renal in origin and that the stimulus to the kidney is the diminished pulse pressure. Unfortunately the best evidence that the hypertension of coarctation of the aorta is renal is again experimental. It has been shown that artificial "coarctation" of the aorta in an animal only induces hypertension when there is a kidney below the "coarctation", and that the hypertension can be abolished by transplanting the kidney into the neck.

Chronic anaemia provides a good example that a reduced renal blood flow is an unlikely cause of hypertension, for the renal blood flow may be decreased considerably, yet a raised arterial pressure is most unusual; the pulse pressure in anaemia, however, is much increased.

Renal hypertension

Hypertension due to partial occlusion of one or both renal arteries, or overall occlusion of the renal arterial tree, are clinical counterparts to the animal experiments. With renal artery stenosis there is often persistent increase

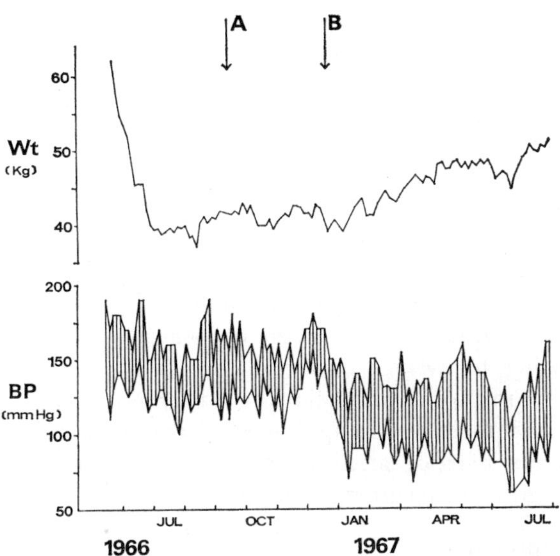

Fig. 11.6. The effect of bilateral nephrectomy (B) on uncontrollable hypertension in a patient on maintenance haemodialysis with a very high plasma renin. There is an immediate fall in blood pressure which is maintained though there is a rise in weight. At point (A) the patient had an attack of acute infectious hepatitis. (Brown, Curtis, Lever, Robertson, de Wardener and Wing, 1969, *Nephron.*)

in plasma renin and angiotensin. This gives rise to a severe secondary hyper-aldosteronism which may be so pronounced that the most prominent clinical feature may not be the rise in blood pressure, but the thirst and polyuria caused by the negative potassium balance due to the renal loss of potassium. A most striking example of overall occlusion of the renal arterial tree giving rise to a high renin output and secondary aldosteronism is malignant hypertension when the rate of aldosterone secretion is often greater than in primary aldosteronism. It is not clear how much the rise in blood pressure in these two clinical situations is due to the vasoconstrictor action of the angiotensin, or to the salt and water retention and increase in extracellular volume caused by the fall in the peritubular venous capillary pressure around the tubules, and the raised plasma aldosterone concentration.

There is no doubt, however, that occasionally a high plasma renin and angiotensin can cause severe hypertension by themselves in the absence of an increase in extracellular blood volume. This phenomenon is seen in a few patients with terminal renal failure on maintenance haemodialysis whose blood pressure is impossible to control however much salt and water are removed from them. After a bilateral nephrectomy, however, the blood pressure falls in spite of a simultaneous rise in exchangeable sodium and water to normal (Fig. 11.6). Occasionally severe vascular changes with extensive destruction of the renal parenchyma may be associated with a *normal* or *low* blood pressure. This is seen sometimes in young persons dying with small contracted kidneys, or at any age in renal amyloidosis. Such patients are invariably sodium losers excreting large volumes of urine.

Vicious circle hypertension

The mechanism responsible for this form of hypertension probably aggravates every case of hypertension in man, but it is only possible to demonstrate its presence in patients suffering from hypertension and unilateral renal disease. In most of these, removal of the diseased kidney does not lower the blood pressure, and it is probable that this is because the hypertension has produced irreversible renal vascular changes in the opposite kidney. This interpretation is quite convincing, for when a unilateral lesion is of short duration the blood pressure often returns to normal following a nephrectomy.

It is clear that if there is a strong suggestion that vicious circle hypertension occurs in unilateral renal disease, it is probable that the same mechanism perpetuates and aggravates hypertension in bilateral renal disease.

Perirenal compression

Occasionally a perirenal haematoma following an injury may cause hypertension. The arterial pressure rises within a few weeks of the accident but it can be lowered by removing the organising clot.

HYPERTENSIVE VASCULAR DISEASE IN MAN

Structural Changes

Hypertension, however caused, eventually leads to changes in renal structure and function; the structural changes are sometimes known as nephrosclerosis. Initially these mainly occur in the vessels, but, as the lesions progress, there are secondary ischaemic changes in the nephrons. The vascular changes may be either acute or chronic. The acute changes are found in association with malignant hypertension; they consist of gross thickening of the intima of the smaller arteries, and focal necrosis of arterioles. The chronic lesions are found mainly in association with non-malignant hypertension, they consist mainly of a less marked thickening of the whole wall of the smaller arteries.

Acute changes

The most important change is a thickening of the intima of the comparatively large intralobular arteries so that their lumens become extremely small. In younger patients this is due to a cellular hyperplasia in which there is no collagen or elastic fibres. In older patients it is due to an increased quantity of fibro-elastic tissue similar to that found in much smaller quantities in non-malignant hypertension. There is little doubt that this subintimal proliferation is due directly to the rise in blood pressure. Teleologically it is reasonable that the normal mechanism whereby the rise in blood pressure induces a renal functional vasoconstriction (p. 107) should be reinforced by a structural narrowing, but the exuberance of this support is sometimes lethal.

The other acute vascular change consists of localised areas of necrosis of the whole thickness and circumference of an arteriole. These necrotic lesions contain large amounts of fibrin so that the change is often called fibrinoid necrosis.

Subintimal proliferation occludes the smaller arteries. At first this produces only a thickening of glomerular capillary walls but subsequently the glomeruli atrophy and are replaced by collagen. Arteriolar necrosis may be associated with focal areas of acute necrosis in the glomeruli which can be recognised as collections of structureless eosin-staining material containing disintegrating nuclei and narrow capillary lumens.

There is a strong suggestion that the principal factor which determines whether the lesions accompanying the rise in blood pressure are acute or chronic is a difference in the state of the vessels and not the height of the pressure. The nature of this difference is unknown. Acute changes are more likely if the rate of rise in blood pressure is rapid or if the hypertension is initially caused by a renal disease such as glomerular nephritis or pyelonephritis.

Chronic changes

The chronic vascular changes which are found characteristically in prolonged hypertension may also be found in patients with normal blood pressure. There is a generalised narrowing of the arterioles and intralobular arteries with fibro-elastic tissue and the deposition of an eosinophilic structureless material. Gradually complete occlusion of the lumen may occur and a patchy ischaemia of increasing severity develops. This process may, of course, develop in previously normal kidneys, and may occasionally be severe enough to cause renal failure; but it also complicates most longstanding cases of renal disease, when it then contributes to, and accelerates, the kidney's eventual destruction. In the larger arteries these chronic vascular lesions eventually cause focal wedge-shaped areas of degeneration situated between relatively normal renal tissue. In the affected areas the glomeruli tend to be crowded together. The glomerular tufts show a diffuse thickening with collagen accompanied by a similar thickening of the glomerular capsule; eventually the collagenised tuft and capsule become fused, the capillary lumens are obliterated and the glomerulus is replaced by fibrous tissues. At first, the tubules between these glomeruli lose their lumens, but the cells show little change so that the glomeruli appear to be packed in solid wedges of relatively normal cells. Later the cells atrophy and there is fibrous tissue replacement. When these vascular changes are far advanced there may be no normal tissue left and it may then be impossible, histologically, to distinguish them from the end stages of such renal diseases as glomerular nephritis or chronic interstitial nephritis, in which vascular changes are only a complication.

Functional Changes

The only consistent abnormality is in the handling of sodium chloride. Though patients with a high blood pressure are in normal salt balance they have a remarkable tendency suddenly to excrete abnormally large quantities of salt in response to certain stimuli, e.g. an osmotic diuresis induced by manni-

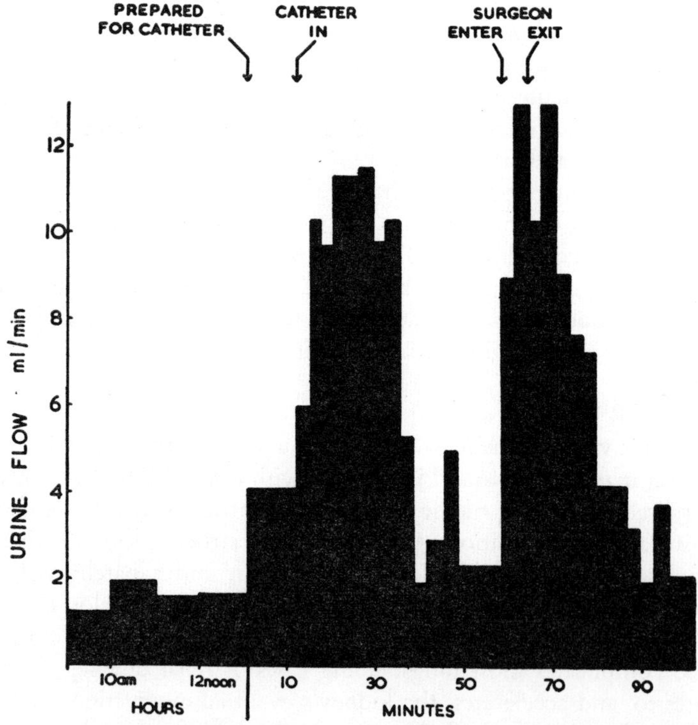

FIG. 11.7. The effect on urine flow of (1) catheterising the bladder and (2) a brief interview with a surgeon, in a patient suffering from hypertension. The sudden increase in urine flow were associated with a sudden increase in sodium excretion. Miles and de Wardener, 1953, *Lancet*.)

tol, an intravenous administration of angiotensin or saline, and certain emotional situations (Fig. 11.7). The mechanism responsible for this phenomenon in man has been investigated most thoroughly following an intravenous administration of saline. The result suggests that the sudden rise in urinary sodium excretion is due directly to the raised hydrostatic pressure in the capillaries of the kidney. It is certainly well established that in animal experiments an acute rise in hydro-

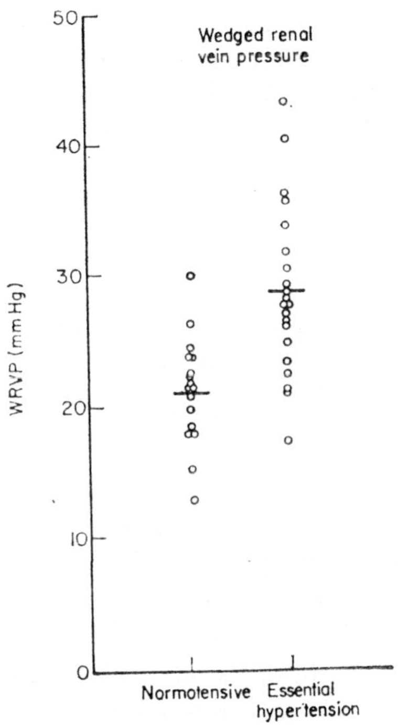

FIG. 11.8. The wedged renal venous pressure in normal man and in patients with essential hypertension. (Lowenstein, Berenbaum, Chasis and Baldwin, 1970, *Clinical Science.*)

static pressure in the peritubular venous capillaries diminishes sodium reabsorption and thus raises urinary sodium excretion. In man it has been found that the peritubular capillary pressure of patients suffering from hypertension is always slightly greater than in normal subjects. During the intravenous administration of saline however this difference becomes suddenly very much greater (Fig. 11.8). Presumably the presence of the saline in the blood permits a greater proportion of the arterial pressure in the afferent arteriole to be transmitted through to the peritubular venous capillaries, either because the viscosity of the blood is lowered or because of renal vasodilation.

In the earliest stages of essential hypertension, before there is any marked change in renal blood flow or glomerular filtration rate, it is sometimes possible to demonstrate an impaired ability to dilute or alkalinise the urine. In addition many patients with hypertension have an impaired ability to excrete uric acid which causes a rise in serum uric acid. This phenomenon is associated with a higher incidence of cerebrovascular and ischaemic heart disease. None of these abnormalities of tubular function has been explained.

Otherwise essential hypertension initially causes little disturbance in renal function; renal blood flow measurements show renal vasoconstriction with a normal rate of flow, while complex and speculative calculations suggest that the efferent glomerular arteriole constricts to a greater extent than the afferent, and that this is one of the reasons why glomerular filtration rate also remains unchanged. Renal biopsies at this time show no abnormality of structure. Gradually renal blood flow and glomerular filtration decrease, the latter always to a lesser extent than the former; small amounts of protein appear in the urine and there is some diminution of the ability to concentrate; at this stage renal biopsies show hypertensive vascular changes with scattered local changes in the glomeruli. Unless malignant hypertension supervenes it is unusual for these changes to become sufficiently extensive to cause symptomatic renal failure. With malignant hypertension proteinuria increases and the urine contains many red cells and granular casts; tubular capacity to concentrate is lost; renal blood flow and glomerular filtration rate fall precipitously, and renal failure rapidly develops. The extent of the proteinuria is greatest in those who rapidly develop renal failure, and daily excretion rates above 5 g/day may occur together with a nephrotic syndrome. (Very occasionally however malignant hypertension may be associated with a urine that is free of protein.) If the blood pressure can be lowered without immediately aggravating the renal failure most of the acute structural and functional changes disappear.

Extracellular Fluid Volume, Renin and Aldosterone in Essential Hypertension

About 80 per cent of patients with non-malignant essential hypertension have an extracellular fluid space which is slightly smaller than normal, with a normal plasma renin which rises normally upon depleting the extracellular fluid volume with a salt free diet. The other 20 per cent of patients have a normal extracellular fluid volume with a normal or low plasma renin which does not rise upon depleting the extracellular fluid volume. Aldosterone secretion rates are normal in both groups, but because of the liver's depressed ability to destroy aldosterone in hypertension (cause unknown) plasma aldosterone is greater than normal in both groups, the larger group having the higher concentration. It appears therefore that in the majority of patients with hypertension, there is evidence of a mild partially compensated urinary leak of sodium, and that this compensation does not take place via the angiotensin aldosterone mechanism. In the other 20 per cent the tendency for the hypertension to cause a urinary leak of sodium is completely submerged by an unknown sodium retaining mechanism which inhibits the renin aldosterone mechanism. There is some evidence that this sodium retention is due to the presence of an unusual steroid. The arterial pressure in this smaller group is easily controlled with spironolactone.

UNILATERAL RENAL DISEASE ASSOCIATED WITH HYPERTENSION

The importance of this group of patients is that in a few the hypertension may be due to the renal lesion, and that nephrectomy, or correction of an obstruction or by-pass of a renal arterial occlusion may cure the hypertension. On the other hand, only approximately 0·25 per cent of all patients with a raised diastolic pressure are found to have a unilateral renal lesion which surgery can benefit. It is also important to note that demonstrable partial occlusion of the renal artery may not be associated with hypertension; or that if partial occlusion of the renal artery is associated with hypertension, occlusion may not be its cause. Occlusion of the renal arterial tree may be either in the main renal artery or its main segmental branches before they enter the parenchyma of the kidney, or in the smaller arteries within the renal parenchyma. The lesions in the main artery and its branches include atheromatous plaques, "fibromuscular hyperplasia", aneurysm and embolisms, and external compression from a tumour. Unilateral parenchymatous renal lesions include chronic childhood pyelonephritis, irradiation of the kidney and tuberculosis of the kidney.

Clinical features

On the whole there is little to distinguish these patients from the other 99·75 per cent of patients suffering from hypertension. There may be a recent history of abdominal trauma, emboli or thrombi in other sites, or of pain in the flank or loin. The diastolic pressure may have been noted to rise rapidly and the patient may complain of thirst and polyuria. Stenosis of the renal artery is sometimes associated with a systolic murmur which is heard best posteriorly over the affected artery. There is also a slender statistical connection between occlusive disease of the renal arteries, a negative family history of hypertension, an onset of hypertension under 30 years or after 55 years of age, and the presence of proteinuria.

Renal structure

The characteristic appearance in the parenchyma is best seen in occlusion of the main renal artery or its branches. The tubules become small with narrow lumens and shrunken cuboidal cells. The glomeruli remain relatively unchanged but are crowded together because of the tubular atrophy. On the other hand, the arterioles are normal, in striking contrast to the arterioles from the opposite kidney which is being perfused with a raised arterial pressure.

E§

Renal function

Experimentally partial occlusion of a renal artery perfusing functioning renal parenchyma causes a variable fall in renal plasma flow and glomerular filtration rate. The most characteristic change, however, is a great increase in tubular reabsorption of sodium in the proximal tubule. This is due to the lowering of the peritubular venous capillary pressure. The increase in sodium reabsorption causes a marked increase in water reabsorption from the proximal tubule. This has two consequences, it reduces the utine flow and raises the concentration of those substances in the tubule lumen which are not reabsorbed, i.e. creatinine, inulin, PAH or Hypaque. A kidney being perfused by a partially occluded renal artery therefore will produce urine at a slow rate which nevertheless contains a lower concentration of sodium than that from the opposite kidney but a higher concentration of creatinine, inulin or PAH. Clearly, the pattern is only discernible if the process is unilateral or at least more pronounced on one side than the other. If this phenomenon can be demonstrated it is highly probable that a considerable proportion of functioning proximal tubules are being perfused at a low pressure. It is then justifiable to imply that a similar proportion of functioning juxta-glomerular apparati are also being perfused at a low pressure and to conclude therefore that at least part of the hypertension is probably due to partial occlusion of the renal arteries. The opposite also holds. The unequivocal demonstration of a unilateral renal abnormality or renal artery stenosis in the absence of this characteristic functional pattern implies that either the occlusion to the renal arteries is not sufficient to lower the perfusion pressure, or that the low perfusion pressure is not affecting functioning proximal tubules and therefore functioning juxta-glomerular apparati.

Diagnosis

The methods available include an intravenous pyelogram (I.V.P.), aortography, individual renal functional studies, renal biopsy, isotope renogram, and renal vein renin concentration. The intensity with which these techniques are used depend on how suggestive are the clinical features, the age of the patient, and what is considered it might be appropriate to do if occlusive renal arterial disease were found.

I.V.P. It is imperative that an intravenous pyelogram be performed on any patient in whom one or more of the clinical features described above is present. An I.V.P. in such a patient must be performed with a rapid infusion of contrast medium and the taking of films at 15 sec, 1, 2 and 3 min after the injection, in addition to the other films taken at 5, 10 and 20 min. Ureteric compression must not be used during the first few minutes. If there is unilateral occlusion of the renal arterial tree the contrast medium appears first in the pelvis and ureter of the unaffected kidney, and in the first few minutes the contrast medium on the affected side is *less dense* than on the "normal" side. This is due to the slow urine flow and reduced glomerular filtration rate of the affected kidney.

Ten to 20 min later, however, the picture is reversed. Because of the increased sodium and water reabsorption which accompanies the vascular occlusion the contrast medium on the affected side is now *denser* than on the normal side. At this time it is possible to compare the lengths of the two kidneys; a difference greater than 1·5 cm is abnormal and nearly always accompanies partial occlusion of the renal artery.

These characteristic findings can sometimes be made more distinct by performing the pyelogram during a water or a urea-saline diuresis. If the I.V.P. is normal and the clinical features not particularly suggestive of occlusive arterial disease no further test need be carried out.

AORTOGRAM. It is doubtful if this should ever be performed unless there is very strong clinical suspicion of a renal vascular cause for the hypertension or the intravenous pyelogram suggests that it is a likely possibility.

INDIVIDUAL RENAL FUNCTIONAL STUDIES. Ureteric catheters are introduced via a cystoscope into each ureter and urine collected from each kidney during the intravenous administration of urea, saline and vasopressin. The characteristic finding is that the affected kidney has a urine flow 50 per cent less than on the other side, with at least a 20 per cent increase in creatinine concentration and a 20 per cent reduction in sodium concentration.

This test need only be performed when (*a*) the I.V.P. and aortogram suggest that there is occlusion of the renal arterial tree but the pattern of change in the I.V.P. does not define the characteristic functional abnormality sufficiently well, and (*b*) if there is some doubt about the functional capacity of the opposite kidney. Individual renal studies are difficult to perform in a reliable way and can give rise to painful complications. They should be avoided as much as possible.

RENAL BIOPSY. If this test is used a sample should be obtained from both sides. The two biopsies must be performed on separate days. It is the contrast in the histological findings between the two sides which is diagnostic.

ISOTOPE RENOGRAM. The popularity of this test in the diagnosis of occlusive vascular disease is due more to its convenience than to its reliability.

RENIN CONCENTRATION IN THE RENAL VEIN. Blood is obtained from both renal veins. Occlusive renal arterial disease is reported to be associated with raised concentration of renin in the venous blood from the affected side. One account claimed that if the renin concentration ratio between the two sides is 1·5 or more unilateral surgical interference is likely to lower the blood pressure.

Treatment

Overall the influence of operation on blood pressure and survival is disappointing. This is probably due to the difficulty in obtaining accurate renin estimations. If the patient is young and the disease is unilateral it is justifiable to attempt either to correct or by-pass the occlusion or to perform a nephrectomy. Nephrectomy is the more satisfying procedure in terms of both immediate and long term mortality. In the majority of instances, however, the patients are middle-aged or elderly and the cause of the occlusion is atheroma. If the hypertension can be controlled satisfactorily with hypotensive drugs the patient should not be subjected to an operation. Treatment with spironolactone alone may be sufficient.

BIBLIOGRAPHY

AMES, R. P., BORKOWSKI, A. J., SICINSKI, A. M., and LARAGH, J. L. (1965). "Prolonged infusions of angiotensin II and norepinephrine, blood pressure, electrolyte balance, and aldosterone and cortisol secretion in normal man and in cirrhosis with ascites." *J. clin. Invest.*, **44**, 1171.

BEILIN, L. J., WADE, D. N., HONOUR, A. J., and COLE, T. J. (1970). "Vascular hyperactivity with sodium loading and with desoxycorticosterone induced hypertension." *Clin. Sci.*, **39**, 793.

BRECKENBRIDGE, A. (1966). "Hypertension and hyperuricaemia." *Lancet*, **1**, 15.

BRECKENRIDGE, A., DOLLERY, C. T., and PARRY, E. H. O. (1970). "Prognosis of treated hypertension." *Quart. J. med.*, **39**, 411.

BROWN, J. J., CHUNIN, R. H., FERISS, B., FRASER, R., LEVER, A. F., and ROBERTSON, J. I. S. (1970) "Effets d'un traitement prolongé par la spironolactone sur les electrolyte plasmatiques et la pression sanguine des malades atteints d'hyperaldosteronisme 'primaire'." *Actualités Néphrologiques*, 132.

BROWN, J. J., CURTIS, J. R., LEVER, A. F., ROBERTSON, J. I. S., DE WARDENER, H. E., and WING, A. J. (1969). "Plasma renin concentration and the control of blood pressure in patients on maintenance haemodialysis." *Nephron*, **6**, 329.

BYROM, F. B. (1954). "The pathogenesis of hypertensive encephalopathy and its relation to the malignant phase of hypertension. Experimental evidence from the hypertensive rat." *Lancet*, **2**, 201.

BYROM, F. B., and WILSON, C. (1941). "The vicious circle in chronic Bright's disease. Experimental evidence from the hypertensive rat." *Quart. J. Med.*, N.S. **10**, 65.

CORREA, R. J., STEWART, B. H., and BOBLITT, D. E. (1962). "Intravenous pyelography as a screening test in renal hypertension." *Amer. J. Roentgenol.*, **88**, 1135.

FLOYER, M. A., (1957). "Role of the kidney in experimental hypertension." *Brit. med. Bull.*, **13**, 29.

FOURNIER, A., SEFAR, M., FENDLER, J. P., MEYER, P., and MILLIEZ, P. (1970). *Actualités Néphrologiques*, 86.

GARDNER, D. L., and MATTHEWS, M. A. (1969). "Ultrastructure of the wall of small arteries in early experimental rat hypertension." *J. Path.*, **97**, 51.

GENEST, C. C., and NOWACZYNSKI, W. (1970). "Aldosterone and electrolyte balance in human hypertension." *J. Roy. Coll. Phycns. Lond.*, **5**, 77.

GROLLMAN, A., and GROLLMAN, E. F. (1962). "The teratogenic induction of hypertension." *J. clin. Invest.*, **41**, 710.

HARRIS, J. J., CRANE, M. G., and JOHNS, V. I. (1967). "Plasma renin activity in hypertension." *Ann. Intern. Med.*, **66**, 1036.

HAWTHORNE, E. W., PERRY, S. L. C., and POGUE, W. G. (1953). "Development of experimental renal hypertension in the dog following reduction of renal artery pulse pressure without reducing mean pressure." *Amer. J. Physiol.*, **174**, 393.

JERUMS, G., and DOYLE, A. E. (1969). "Renal sodium handling as responsiveness of plasma renin levels in hypertension." *Clin. Sci.*, **37**, 79.

KAUFMAN, J. J., LUPV, A. N., and MAXWELL, M. H. (1969). "Renovascular hypertension. Clinical characteristics, diagnosis and treatment." *Cardiovascular Clinics*, **1**, 80.

KINCAID, O. W. (1964). "Progress in Angiography." Charles C. Thomas, Springfield, Ill., p. 280.

KLEINKNECHT, D., and MAXWELL, M. H. (1970). *Actualités Néphrologiques*, 63.

KOHLSTAEDT, K. G., and PAGE, I. H. (1940). "Liberation of renin by perfusion of kidneys following reduction of pulse pressure." *J. exp. Med.*, **72**, 201.

LEDINGHAM, J. M. (1971). "Blood pressure regulation in renal failure." *J. Roy. Coll. Phycns. Lond.*, **5**, 103.

LOUIS, W. J., RENZINI, V., MACDONALD, G. L., BOYD, G. W., and PEART, W. S. (1970). "Renal clip hypertension in rabbits immunised against angiotensin II." *Lancet*, **1**, 333.

LUKE, R. G., KENNEDY, A. C., BRIGGS, J. D., STRUTHERS, N. W., WATT, J. K., SHORT, D. W., and STIRLINS, W. B. (1968). "Results of surgery in hypertension due to renal artery stenosis." *Brit. Med. J.*, **1**, 76.

McCORMACK, L. J., BÉLAND, J. E., SCHNECKLOTH, R. E., and CORCORAN, A. C. (1958). "Effects of antihypertensive treatment on the evolution of the renal lesions in malignant nephrosclerosis." *Amer. J. Path.*, **34**, 1011.

MENDOWITZ, M. (1969). The biology of hypertension. "The Biological Basis of Medicine." Academic Press, London and New York, 142.

PAGE, I. H., and McCUBBIN, J. W. (1968). "Renal Hypertension." Year Book Medical Publishers.

PEART, W. S. (1965). "The renin-angiotensin system." *Pharmacol. Revs.*, **17**, 143.

ROBERTSON, P. W., KLIDJIAN, A., HULL, D. H., and HILTON, D. D. (1962). "The assessment and treatment of hypertension." *Lancet*, **2**, 567.

SCOTT, H. W., and BAHNSON, H. T. (1951). "Evidence for renal factor in hypertension of experimental coarctation of aorta." *Surgery*, **30**, 206.

SIMMONS, J. L., and MICHELAKIS, A. M. (1971). "Renovascular hypertension. The diagnostic value of renal vein renin ratios." *J. Urol.*, **104**, 497.

STAMEY, T. A. (1963). "Renovascular Hypertension." Baillière, Tindall and Cox.

TALBOTT, J. H., CASTLEMAN, B., SMITHWICK, R. H., MELVILLE, R. S., and PECORA, L. J. (1943). "Renal biopsy studies correlated with renal clearance observations in hypertensive patients treated by radical sympathectomy." *J. clin. Invest.*, **22**, 387.

VANDER, A. J. (1967). "Control of renin release." *Physiological Reviews*, **47**, 359.

WILKINSON, R., SCOTT, D. F., ULDALL, P. R., KERR, D. N. S., and SWINEY, J. (1970). "Plasma renin and exchangeable sodium in the hypertension of chronic renal failure." *Quart. J. Med.*, **155**, 377.

WILLIAMS, T. F. (1963). "Renal cortical necrosis, renal infarction, and hypertension due to renal vascular disease." Diseases of the Kidney by Strauss M. B., and Welt, L. G. J. & A. Churchill, London, p. 526.

12

The Kidney's Control of Urinary Sodium Excretion in Disease

Normal Control of the Volume and Concentration of Body Fluids

WATER is added to body fluids principally by oral intake, but there is also a small contribution of 200–300 ml a day which is an end product of metabolism. Water is lost via the skin, lungs and kidneys; loss from the gut is negligible unless there is vomiting, diarrhoea or a fistula. The intake of water is controlled by thirst, while its output is adjusted by the kidneys; the amount of water lost from the skin and respiratory tract is mainly dependent on atmospheric conditions and is thus beyond the body's internal authority.

Thirst

The sensation of thirst appears to originate in the hypothalamus; it is influenced by a wide variety of factors, the two most important being the osmolality of the extracellular fluid, and the blood volume. The first can easily be demonstrated by administering hypertonic saline, and the second by performing a substantial venesection. It is probable that the thirst centre is directly stimulated by changes in osmolality, but it is not known how it is aware of changes in blood volume.

Renal control of extracellular fluid tonicity

The control of water output by the kidney is intimately connected with the control of sodium chloride excretion, both varying with the need to keep the tonicity of body fluids and the blood volume within normal limits. It is probable that the osmolality of the intra- and extracellular fluids is the same, so that it is possible for the kidney to maintain tonicity of body fluids simply by adjusting the osmolality of the extracellular fluid. Theoretically this could be achieved by altering the urinary excretion of either water or salt, but in practice it is done mainly by altering the excretion of water. The neurohypophysis responds to changes in plasma osmolality by rapid alterations in the rate at which the antidiuretic hormone (ADH) is secreted into the circulation, and ADH in turn controls the concentration of the urine and therefore, the volume of urine that is excreted. For instance, a drink of water lowers plasma osmolality; this inhibits ADH production by the neurohypophysis and within 20–30 min the urine

134

becomes hypotonic, whereas with fluid deprivation and a rise in plasma osmolality the mechanism is reversed.

Renal control of extracellular fluid and blood volume

Changes in blood volume induce alterations in both sodium and water excretion. It is clear that if the tonicity of body fluids is to remain constant the ratio of salt to water released or retained must be in isotonic proportions. This synchronisation of the different mechanisms which control salt and water excretion can be demonstrated by bleeding a normal subject, when there is a prompt and simultaneous *decrease* in both salt and water excretion; or, conversely, by administering blood or a "plasma expander" such as albumin when there is a simultaneous *increase* in salt and water excretion.

The efferent mechanism responsible for changes in water excretion consists mainly in altering the rate of secretion of antidiuretic hormone (ADH); those mechanisms responsible for the changes in salt excretion are more obscure. There is now considerable evidence that changes in sodium excretion which originate from a change in blood volume are due almost entirely to changes in tubular reabsorption of sodium. When blood volume changes are rapid, the mechanisms responsible for this diminished tubular reabsorption include changes in peritubular venous capillary pressure, and changes in the circulating concentration of an unidentified hormone. When blood volume changes are more prolonged, changes in the circulating concentration of aldosterone become important.

The afferent stimulus produced by a change in blood volume is generally considered to be a change in pulse pressure in vascular compartments from the walls of which afferent impulses travel centrally. The carotid baroreceptors have been shown to be such a site for the control of aldosterone secretion. It is not known where the afferent stimuli originate which control ADH secretion.

CHANGES IN URINARY SODIUM EXCRETION IN SOME DISEASES ASSOCIATED WITH GENERALISED OEDEMA

Generalised oedema is due to retention of salt and water by the kidneys. This occurs in acute glomerular nephritis, cardiac failure, malnutrition, the nephrotic syndrome and chronic liver failure.

Acute glomerular nephritis

The cause of the sodium retention and oedema in this condition is not known for certain. It is not due to heart failure for there is no evidence that the heart is failing as a pump. There is usually some degree of hypoproteinaemia and the fall in glomerular filtration rate is greater than the fall in renal blood flow. There is therefore a fall in filtration fraction and plasma protein osmotic pressure in the peri-tubular capillaries, which would tend to decrease sodium reabsorption and thus increase urinary excretion of sodium. Renal biopsy however shows that the glomerular tufts tend to be obliterated by cellular proliferation. It is possible therefore that the cause of the increased reabsorption of sodium is a diminished hydrostatic pressure in the peri-tubular capillaries.

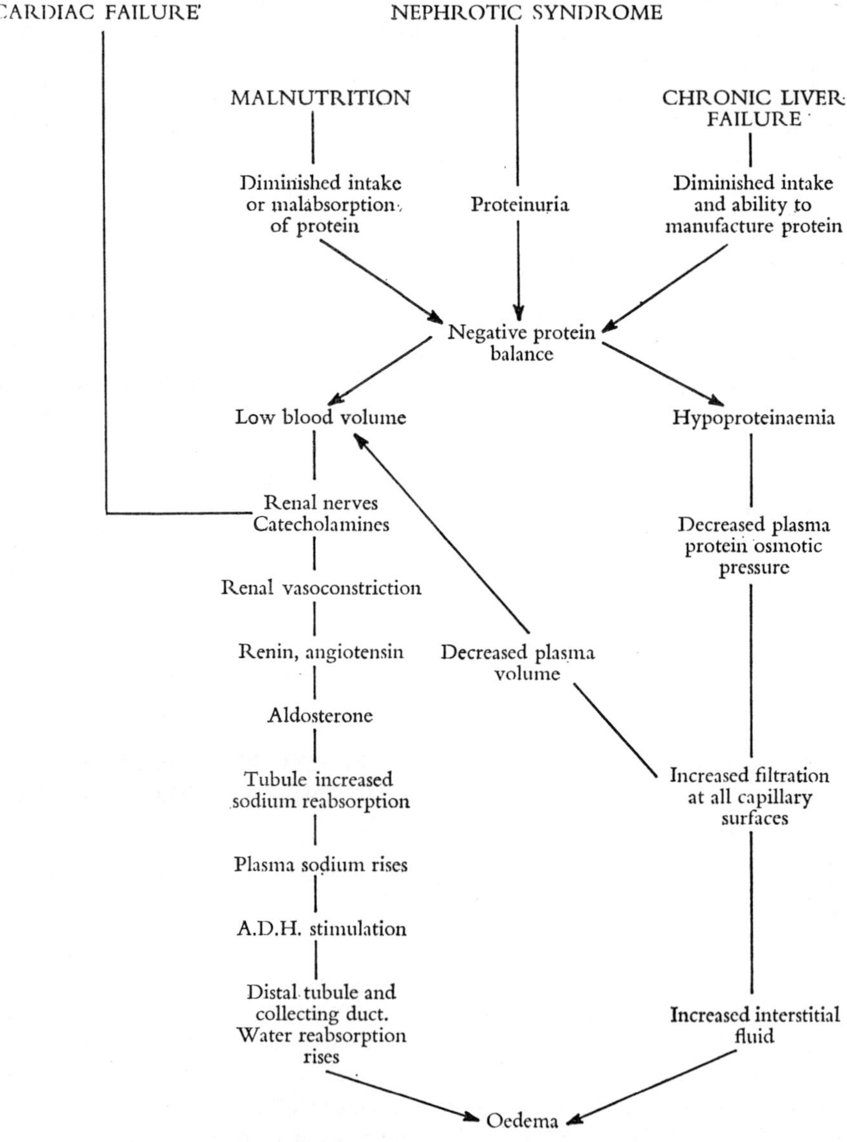

Fig. 12.1. The aetiology and some of the mechanisms responsible for generalised oedema.

Cardiac failure

In heart failure there is intense renal vasoconstriction which lowers the hydrostatic pressure in the peritubular venous capillaries, and there is also a raised filtration fraction which raises the peritubular oncotic pressure. Both of these changes are known to increase tubular reabsorption of sodium and depress urinary sodium excretion. The renal vasoconstriction is due to the high circulating concentration of catecholamines and renal nerve stimulation, both of which may also have direct stimulting effects on tubular sodium reabsorption. The renal vasoconstriction may also cause a release of renin and an increased secretion of aldosterone (Fig. 12.1). It should be noted however that oedema from cardiac failure can still form after bilateral adrenalectomy.

Nephrotic syndrome, malnutrition and chronic liver failure

The diminished urinary excretion of sodium in these conditions is associated with a high secretion rate of aldosterone and a reduced blood volume due to the negative nitrogen balance. The probable sequence of events is illustrated in Fig. 12.1. It is to be noted that the principal mechanism is increased sodium reabsorption due to secondary aldosteronism. But there is a considerable amount of evidence which demonstrates that excess aldosterone alone does not cause oedema. The most important evidence is that in normal man the continuous infusion of aldosterone only causes sodium retention for about 3–10 days. And it is a well established observation that oedema does not occur in primary aldosteronism from an aldosterone producing adrenal tumour (see below). In both of these examples the aldosterone causes an initial slight increase in total exchangeable sodium, extracellular fluid volume and plasma volume which in turn causes a compensatory decrease in sodium reabsorption from the proximal tubules. This swamps the increased sodium reabsorption in the distal tubules caused by the aldosterone. This compensatory mechanism is known as the aldosterone escape phenomenon (see below). It is clear therefore that an increased aldosterone secretion rate can only cause oedema if the aldosterone escape phenomenon does not prevent it from doing so. The absence of the aldosterone escape phenomenon in the nephrotic syndrome, malnutrition and chronic liver failure may be due to the fact that the plasma volume is low and does not rise above normal when aldosterone increases sodium reabsorption.

CHANGES IN SODIUM EXCRETION IN SOME DISEASES NOT ASSOCIATED WITH OEDEMA

The various disturbances of urinary sodium excretion in bengin essential hypertension have been outlined in the previous chapter. Those that occur in primary and secondary hyperaldosteronism (without oedema) and in chronic renal failure are discussed here.

Primary hyperaldosteronism and hyperadrenalism

In these two conditions sodium reabsorption in the distal tubule is being stimulated and yet generalised oedema does not occur. This is presumably due to the aldosterone "escape" phenomenon. The individual steps of this phenomenon may be the following. The aldosterone's sodium retaining effect on the distal tubule increases the extracellular fluid volume. But an increase in extracellular fluid and blood volume causes an increase in the circulating concentration of the unknown natriuretic hormone (p. 65) which controls urinary sodium excretion. This inhibits sodium reabsorption in several sites along the nephron including particularly the proximal tubule. Less sodium reabsorbed in the proximal tubule causes more sodium to reach the distal tubule. In the presence of aldosterone this causes an even greater reabsorption of sodium and secretion of potassium in the distal tubule. Thus the compensatory decrease in proximal tubule reabsorption by the unknown hormone not only tends to prevent the rise in the extracellular fluid volume becoming evident as oedema but it also stimulates an increase in urinary potassium excretion. Eventually overall sodium balance is achieved. Equilibrium is presumably achieved when the rise in the circulating concentration of the unknown hormone is such that the proximal tubule releases sufficient sodium to swamp the distal tubule's increased sodium reabsorption. The aldosterone escape phenomenon is not related to a change in arterial pressure.

Secondary aldosteronism without clinical oedema

The two most prominent examples of this syndrome are malignant hypertension and renal artery stenosis. A detailed account of those mechanisms which probably maintain sodium balance in renal artery stenosis (Fig. 12.2) is probably applicable to what takes place in malignant hypertension for in both, the renal arterial tree is partially occluded. The persistent diminution in vascular hydrostatic pressure in the peri-tubular capillaries of the kidney with the stenosed renal artery causes a persistent increase in sodium and water reabsorption in that kidney. This tends to increase the extracellular fluid volume. In addition the fall in pressure in the afferent arterioles of the kidney with the stenosed renal artery causes a release of renin from the juxtaglomerular apparatus, the formation of angiotensin and a rise in the circulating concentration of aldosterone. The aldosterone increases sodium reabsorption from the distal tubules of both kidneys. This also tends to increase the volume of the extracellular space. An increase in extracellular fluid and plasma volume, however, causes an increase in the circulating concentration of the unknown natruiretic hormone (see above). This hormone probably has its greatest effect on the proximal tubule of the normal kidney where it inhibits sodium reabsorption. As in primary aldosteronism therefore there is thus an increased delivery of sodium into the distal tubule of the normal kidney. This in turn increases potassium excretion from the normal kidney which leads to hypokalaemia. Equilibrium occurs when the diminution in sodium reabsorption in the proximal tubule of the normal kidney is sufficient to counteract the increased sodium reabsorption along the whole of the nephrons in the kidney with the stenosed renal artery, and along the distal tubules of the normal kidney. A remarkable homeostatic manoeuvre. The rise in arterial pressure which accompanies a renal artery stenosis sufficiently severe to cause secondary aldosteronism may also contribute slightly to the compensatory increase in sodium excretion from the normal kidney. But this

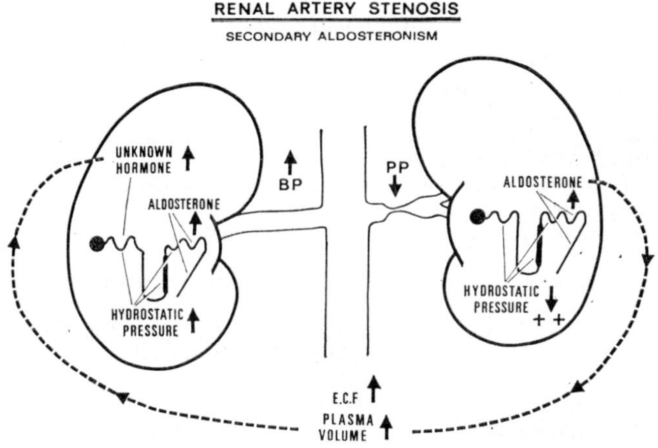

FIG. 12.2. Renal artery stenosis and urinary sodium excretion.

effect is of little importance, for patients with hypertension due to renal artery stenosis do not become oedematous when the blood pressure is reduced with hypotensive drugs.

Chronic renal failure

In chronic renal failure the intake of sodium is usually normal and the patients are usually in salt balance. Therefore as the number of nephrons diminishes sodium excretion per nephron must increase. Or in other words, in chronic renal failure there is a fall in the proportion of filtered sodium that is reabsorbed from each remaining nephron. The mechanisms responsible for this nice adjustment are not known. It occurs in spite of normal or raised aldosterone secretion rates. It is possible that the diminished reabsorption is due to the accumulation of some waste product which has a toxic effect on sodium reabsorption. On the other hand there is much evidence that it may be due to the release of a similar, or the same, unknown natruiretic hormone which controls urinary sodium excretion in response to changes in the extracellular fluid volume in normal animals.

In spite of this alteration in tubular sodium reabsorption to compensate for the falling filtration rates it is not uncommon for patients terminally to develop either a tendency to loose sodium or to retain sodium. Sometimes a patient may slide from one tendency to the other unexpectedly (p. 183). It is of the utmost importance to be aware of this possibility for obviously the treatment of the two conditions is dramatically opposed. A tendency to retain sodium is associated with hypertension, while a tendency to lose sodium with either a normal or a low arterial pressure. The first is treated with diuretics and the second with sodium supplements. Selective tubular disturbances of sodium reabsorption of unknown cause are discussed on p. 231.

BIBLIOGRAPHY

ANDERSSON, B. (1957). "Polydipsia, antidiuresis and milk ejection caused by hypothalamic stimulation. The Neurohypophysis." *Proc. 8th Symposium Colston Res. Soc.*, p. 131. Butterworths Scientific Pubs., London.

BARTTER, F. C. (1956). "The role of aldosterone in normal homeostasis and in certain disease states." *Metabolism*, **55**, 369.

BRICKER, N. S. (1967). Editorial. "The control of sodium excretion with normal and reduced nephron populations." *Amer. J. Med.*, **43**, 313.

BROD, J., and FEJFAR, Z. (1950). "The origin of oedema in heart failure." *Quart. J. Med.*, **19**, 187.

COPE, C. L., and PEARSON, J. (1963). "Aldosterone secretion in severe renal failure." *Clin. Sci.*, **25**, 331.

DUNCAN, L. E., LIDDLE, G. W., and BARTTER, F. C. (1956). "The effect of changes in body sodium on extracellular fluid volume and aldosterone and sodium excretion by normal and edematous men." *J. clin. Invest.*, **35**, 1299.

GUZ, A., NOBLE, M. I. M., TRENCHARD, D., CLARKSON, E. M., and DE WARDENER, H. E (1966). "The significance of a raised venous pressure during sodium and water retention." *Clin. Sci.*, **30**, 295.

HAYSLETT, J. P., BOYD, J. E., and EPSTEIN, F. H. (1969). "Aldosterone product ion in chronic renal failure (33685)." *Proc. Soc. exp. Biol. (N.Y.)* **130**, 912.

HAYSLETT, J. P., KASHGARIAN, M., and EPSTEIN, F. H. (1969). "Mechanism of change in excretion per nephron when renal mass is reduced." *J. clin. Invest.*, **48**, 1002.

LARAGH, J. H. (1960). "Aldosterone in fluid and electrolyte disorders: hyper- and hypo-aldosteronism." *J. chron. Dis.*, **11**, 292.

LARAGH, J. H., ULICK, S., JANUSZEWICZ, V., DEMING, Q. B., KELLY, W. J., and LIEBERMAN, S. (1960). "Aldosterone secretion in primary aldosteronism and malignant hypertension." *J. clin. Invest.*, **39**, 1091.

LOMBARDO, T. A., EISENBERG, S., OLIVER, B. B., VIAR, W. N., EDELMAN, E. E., and HARRISON, T. R. (1951). "Effects of bleeding on electrolyte excretion and on glomerular filtration." *Circulation*, **3**, 260.

NELSON, D. H., and AUGUST, J. T. (1959). "Failure of aldosterone to maintain sodium retention in normal subjects and Addisonian patients." *J. clin. Invest.*, **37**, 919.

ORRINGER, E. P., WEISS, F. R., and PREUSS, H. G. (1971). "Azotaemic inhibition of organic anion transport mechanisms and characteristics." *Clin. Sci.*, **40**, 159.

PETERS, J. P. (1951). "Sodium, water and oedema." *J. Mt. Sinai Hosp.*, **17**, 159.

SCHRIER, R. W., and DE WARDENER, H. E. (1971). "Tubular reabsorption of sodium ion: influence of factors other than aldosterone and glomerular filtration rate." *New Eng. J. Med.*, **285**, 1231.

SMITH, H. W. (1957). "Salt and water volume receptors." *Amer. J. Med.*, **23**, 623.

STAMEY, T. A. (1963). "Renovascular Hypertension." Williams and Wilkins, Baltimore.

VERNEY, E. B. (1946). "Absorption and excretion of water. The antidiuretic hormone." *Lancet*, **2**, 739 and 781.

WELT, L. G., and ORLOFF, J. (1951). "The effects of an increase in plasma volume on the metabolism and the excretion of water and electrolytes by normal subjects." *J. clin. Invest.*, **30**, 751.

13

The Nephrotic Syndrome

A NEPHROTIC* syndrome is a clinical state in which there is a combination of oedema, proteinuria and hypoproteinaemia, irrespective of aetiology or any other clinical features. This definition stresses the occasional clinical similarities of many unrelated diseases, for the nephrotic syndrome may occur in any of the following conditions: glomerular nephritis, anaphylactoid purpura, disseminated lupus, polyarteritis nodosa, malaria, amyloid disease, diabetes, renal vein thrombosis, cardiac failure, the administration of certain drugs such as troxidone (Tridione) and mercurial compounds (teething powders), it may also occur as a congenital condition.

STRUCTURAL CHANGES

The changes depend upon the aetiology of the nephrotic syndrome. Biopsy studies with the light microscope have shown that the nephrotic syndrome can occur without any changes in the glomerulus. Observations with the electron microscope, however, have shown that even in those biopsies in which there are no changes to be seen with the light microscope there are unequivocal alterations in the cytoplasmic extensions of the epithelial cells which lie on the basement membrane.

The tubule changes vary widely; they are most marked in the proximal tubules. Some are dilated and lined with flattened pale cells with poorly staining nuclei, while others appear to be occluded by large swollen tubule cells containing vacuoles and much fatty material. Often there are no changes apparent on light microscopy.

---

* The term "nephrosis" is gradually becoming extinct. Clinicians have continually disagreed on an exact clinical definition, and pathologists have used the word in a morphological sense to describe any "degenerative" condition of the kidney which they found difficult to classify. Jean Oliver's well-known broadside against the use of the word "nephrosis" begins ". . . that etymologically absurd and conceptually obfuscatory term nephrosis". He continues: "This curious barbarism was introduced by the clinician Friedrich Muller, apparently because to his ear 'osis' had the proper antithetical ring to 'itis' and so seemed appropriate as a sort of counter-term to nephritis. The suffix 'osis' had at the time an accepted meaning, 'to be full of', as in lipoidosis or carcinomatosis, so that by all the custom and usage of medical nomenclature nephrosis means 'full of kidney'. On this etymologically nonsensical basis an elaborate superstructure of vague and varied conceptual meaning has developed. . . ."

At the moment "a nephrotic syndrome" has an accepted and precise clinical definition. For this reason the term "nephrotic syndrome" has been used here, but perhaps in time it will be described by a more rational substitute such as "proteinuric hypoproteinaemia". "Protein losing kidney" has also been used.

FUNCTIONAL CHANGES

In addition to oedema, proteinuria and hypoproteinaemia, the blood lipids are usually raised and the serum calcium reduced. There may also be changes in renal function.

OEDEMA is due to the contraction of the blood volume (p. 136) and to a lesser extent the diminished plasma protein osmotic pressure; and both stem from a decreased quantity of circulating plasma proteins. Sometimes, however, it is possible to observe a plasma albumin concentration of less than 1 g/100 ml in young patients who have little or no oedema. Such patients' kidneys are clearly not retaining sodium and their blood volume is normal. The absence of oedema illustrates nicely the trivial importance of the plasma protein osmotic pressure on the formation of oedema. Presumably in such patients the increased capillary filtration which must accompany the fall in plasma protein osmotic pressure is compensated for, either by some peripheral vascular adjustment which causes a fall in hydrostatic capillary pressure, or the lymphatic system rapidly drains away the increased formation of interstitial fluid.

PLASMA VOLUME. When the patient is in a steady oedematous state the plasma volume and blood volume are usually within the lower levels of the normal range. At first this appears to contradict the hypothesis that the oedema is due to an increased sodium reabsorption due to a diminished blood volume. Nevertheless if the oedema is forcibly evacuated with diuretics the blood volume then falls to below normal. It then becomes obvious that the normal value which was obtained when the patient was oedematous was only normal because of the expansion of the extracellular fluid volume. The blood volume in the nephrotic syndrome shows another interesting phenomenon. It is that upon standing the blood volume may shrink in an exaggerated manner. Reductions of up to 1,000 ml having been recorded. It is possible therefore that for a large part of the day the blood volume of a patient with a nephrotic syndrome is well below those low-normal values which are measured with the patient lying in bed. It is not surprising that such patients tend to suffer from postural hypotension and faint easily.

Protein Metabolism

HYPOPROTEINAEMIA is due to a fall in the albumin fraction, and albumin concentrations below 1 g per 100 ml are sometimes seen. The concentrations of the globulins, however, are liable to increase (except for the smaller globulins) so that if total proteins only are estimated the severity of the decrease in albumin concentration may be disguised. Nevertheless, because globulin molecules are larger and heavier than those of albumin the plasma protein osmotic pressure falls. There is a rough correlation between the appearance of oedema and the plasma albumin concentration, the dividing line being about 2·5–3·0 g per 100 ml.

As the plasma proteins are qualitatively normal the protein disturbance is simply one of negative balance; this is also shown by the marked diminution in muscle protein, which is manifest as muscle wasting. The possible mechanisms for the negative protein balance are: (i) loss of protein in the urine; (ii) increased protein breakdown; and (iii) decreased protein synthesis. There is certainly proteinuria. Total excretion rate of albumin and globulins is usually above 5 g/day, and is often as much as 10–15 g/day. In addition there is a urinary loss of amino acids, the nitrogen content of which averages about half the total amount of nitrogen lost as protein. The problem is thus narrowed down to whether the proteinuria is the only cause of the negative protein balance or whether there is, in addition, increased protein breakdown, or decreased protein synthesis.

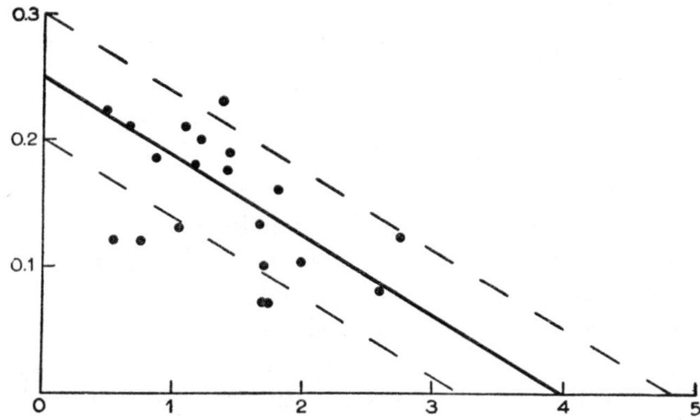

Fig. 13.1. Relation between reduced serum albumin concentration (abscissae g/100 ml) and daily albumin losses in urine (ordinates g/kg body weight). (Squire, Blainey and Hardwicke, 1957, *Brit. med. Bull.*)

A normal subject synthesises about 0·2 g/kg/day of albumin. And it is interesting that the maximum capacity to synthesise albumin is only double this amount, to approximately 26 g/day/70 kg man. A low concentration of plasma albumin increases the synthesis, and reduces the catabolism of albumin. In patients with the nephrotic syndrome it has been found that usually there is a rise in albumin synthesis up to a maximum of twice the normal rate. Sometimes albumin synthesis does not increase and very occasionally it may be depressed. Albumin breakdown may also vary but in some patients it is increased. Faecal loss of albumin is not raised. The rate of total gamma globulin synthesis increases up to sixfold so that in spite of heavy urinary loss of globulins, total plasma globulin is often normal. The plasma concentration of some of the smaller globulins, which leak easily into the urine is low, while the plasma concentration of the larger globulins is increased. The most oedematous patients often have a high urinary excretion of protein, together with an increased breakdown and a diminished synthesis of albumin. The relation between urinary excretion of protein and plasma albumin concentration is shown in Fig. 13.1.

The consequences of the loss of globulins are not clear, but globulins are known to be associated with the activity of certain enzymes and vitamins, and the carriage of some tracer metals. The loss of gamma globulins may be a factor in the well-known liability of the nephrotic patient to infection; it is also the probable explanation why immunisation procedures for poliomyelitis, influenza, tetanus or diphtheria often do not produce satisfactory levels of antibody. There is a diminution of all globulin fractions except a_2 globulin, which is markedly increased.

PROTEINURIA. The cause of the proteinuria is also in doubt. The possibilities are either an increased glomerular capillary permeability or a decreased capacity of the tubules to reabsorb protein. The evidence suggests that though occasionally there is impaired reabsorption, usually proteinuria is due to increased glomerular permeability. Assuming this to be correct, it follows that the increased quantity of protein which leaks into the tubule probably provokes the tubular protein reabsorbing mechanisms to increased activity, and it is generally thought that it is this increased quantity of protein continuously passing through the tubular cells which causes the structural changes in the tubules. Proximal tubule fluid in the dog contains an average of 5 mg/100 ml of albumin. Assuming the same concentration in man, and a total 24-hour glomerular filtration rate of 180 litres, there is normally a tubular reabsorption of less than 10 g per day of protein. But when the permeability of the glomerulus increases, tubular reabsorption of protein also increases. As the passage of the albumin through the tubule cell almost certainly involves some fragmentation of the molecule it is clear that an increased tubular reabsorption of albumin may be one important cause of an increase in overall protein breakdown. This is probably one reason for the recurrent finding of hypoproteinaemia in a patient with a relatively low urinary loss of protein, i.e. less than 5 g/day. If an immunological technique for the estimation of the albumin in the urine is available, it is possible to dispense with the frustration inherent in trying to collect all the urine passed in a 24-hour period in order to get an index of the extent of the proteinuria. Instead, the albumin to creatinine ratio of a random sample of urine is estimated. In healthy subjects the ratio is well below 1 whereas in patients with the nephrotic syndrome it is well above 1. This boundary is sometimes used to delineate the point at which a relapse or a remission has occurred. With this technique the progress of the proteinuria is easily and accurately followed with a sensitivity which is difficult to achieve in any other way.

The proteins that appear in the urine are qualitatively the same as those in the circulating blood and in oedema fluid, but the proportions are different. Albumin, having a smaller molecule, is excreted in relatively much greater amounts than globulin, though small globulins account for 30–40 per cent of the proteinuria.

Proteinuria usually exceeds 5 g/day and characteristically fluctuates widely from day to day, being particularly sensitive to posture and exercise; daily excretions of up to 60 g/day are sometimes seen but the usual rate is 10–15 g/day; it is largely independent of the rate of urine flow. The daily urine volume obviously depends on whether oedema is forming, remaining unchanged or being evacuated. Glycosuria is also found, and microscopy shows the presence of fatty casts and doubly refractible lipid bodies.

SELECTIVE PERMEABILITY. The quantity of protein that is excreted, if expressed in terms of its clearance (i.e. the amount of protein excreted per minute divided by its plasma concentration) correlates well with its molecular weight; the smaller the molecular weight, the greater the clearance. In some patients the clearance of large molecular proteins, when compared to the simultaneous clearance of small molecular proteins is greater than in others. Those in whom the clearance of large molecular proteins is high have been defined as having a non-selective proteinuria. The semantics are unfortunate, for clearly the proteinuria cannot select anything. Selective permeability of the kidneys is a more comprehensible way to express the phenomenon.

Selective permeability is measured by comparing the clearance of a large molecule with that of a small one. One way of doing this is to compare the clearances of IgG (CIgG) and albumin (Calb) measuring both these substances with immunological techniques. Thus

$$\frac{CIgG}{Calb} = \frac{UIgG \times V}{PIgG} \Big/ \frac{Ualb \times V}{Palb}$$

where C = clearance, U = urine, P = plasma, and V = urine flow, and this formula resolves so that V is eliminated and

$$\frac{CIgG}{Calb} = \frac{UIgG}{PIgG} \Big/ \frac{Ualb}{Palb} \times 100$$

This is most convenient (see p. 87) for a timed collection of urine is not necessary, and selective permeability can then be estimated on any random sample of urine. The ratio CIgG/Calb is the selective permeability and if this is multiplied by 100 it can be expressed as a percentage. In practice the following sub-divisions are useful. Highly selective permeability lies below 15 per cent, moderate selective permeability between 15 and 30 per cent, and poorly selective permeability is greater than 30 per cent.

The quantitative pattern of the proteinuria, i.e. the selective permeability of the kidneys, must derive from the disease process in the kidney. It is hardly surprising, therefore, to find that there is some correlation between the selective permeability of the kidneys and the biopsy findings. As might be expected patients whose kidneys have insignificant histological changes tend to have highly selective permeability and those in whom there are unequivocal histological abnormalities usually have non-selective permeability. The selectivity of the permeability is unrelated to the total amount of protein excreted per day, it remains unchanged during wide fluctuations in protein excretion, and it does not change as the disease progresses. It is interesting that selective permeability remains unchanged even in those patients in whom the proteinuria is reduced by administration of steroids. This suggests that the proteinuria is not due to a simple enlargement of the pores in the basement membrane for if that were the case a diminution of proteinuria would be accompanied by a shrinkage of these pores and a progressive return of selective permeability towards normal.

Plasma electrolytes

With low concentrations of plasma albumin the total serum calcium is reduced and the concentration of ionised calcium also tends to be lower than normal. Children may develop tetany. The reason for the reduction in ionised calcium is unknown; it is probably due to diminished calcium absorption. Most patients also have some degree of potassium deficiency, though usually this is not sufficiently severe to cause symptoms. This deficiency is due to an increased urinary loss of potassium secondary to the increased aldosterone secretion, and to a diminished dietary intake of potassium because of anorexia. Potassium deficiency is liable to become severe during treatment with resins, diuretics or steroids (see below).

HYPERLIPAEMIA. Total plasma fat, cholesterol, tri-glycerides, and phospholiquids are all raised in the nephrotic syndrome. Plasma free fatty acids concentration remains normal. The concentration of total fat in the plasma may reach 2,000 mg/100 ml with cholesterol concentrations of 1,000 mg/100 ml. These rises are inversely related to the change in plasma albumin concentration, so that a rise in plasma albumin to normal is usually associated with a reciprocal fall in plasma cholesterol whether the rise in plasma albumin is due to a spontaneous remission, treatment with prednisone or the onset of chronic renal failure. Occasionally, however, the plasma cholesterol level may remain elevated for some months after the concentration of plasma albumin has returned to normal. The cause of these rises in the fatty constituents of the plasma is not clear.

Lipiduria

The normal daily urinary excretion of fats is less than 10 mg. In the nephrotic syndrome it may rise to 1,000 mg. It appears to be mainly due to the hyperlipaemia. The crystallisation of cholesterol esters gives rise to the classical birefringent urinary crystals.

Renal function

All degrees of renal functional efficiency or impairment are seen with the nephrotic syndrome. Some patients, particularly children, have a raised renal blood flow and glomerular filtration rate, while others have varying degrees of renal failure. Because of the negative nitrogen balance the concentration of urea in the blood may be much lower than is expected from the rate of glomerular filtration; this can be very misleading if renal function is being judged only by estimations of the blood urea. On the other hand, it is important to remember that some patients have particularly high creatinine to inulin clearance ratios, and that in such patients a creatinine clearance may be more than double the true glomerular filtration rate. In those patients who have a supernormal filtration rate, very low concentrations of blood urea (10–15 mg per 100 ml) are seen. If the deterioration of renal function is gradual, proteinuria sometimes diminishes and the oedema recedes. This is presumably because the rate of protein excretion is proportional to the filtration rate, and if this falls sufficiently the negative protein balance ceases. More often, however, as renal failure advances proteinuria and oedema remain unchanged.

Clinical Picture

The incidence of the nephrotic syndrome in relation to age and sex depends largely on its aetiology. The cases can be divided into those in whom the renal lesion is primary and those in whom it is only a feature in a more generalised disease. The primary lesions are more common in children and men under the age of 60; whereas when the lesion is a feature in a generalised disease the patients are mainly adults and the disease is equally distributed between the sexes.

Whatever the cause of the nephrotic syndrome the onset of *oedema* is usually gradual and fluctuating. At first there is occasional swelling of the ankles in the evening, or of the face in the morning. There may be transient attacks of more obvious oedema which rapidly disappears.

Eventually, after an interval of weeks or months, oedema persists and recovery from each exacerbation is less complete. When the condition is advanced the accumulation of fluid appears to be controlled only by the skin's limited ability to stretch. The legs and arms are unsightly lobulated balloons, shiny and pale; the abdomen protrudes both with oedema of the subcutaneous tissues and ascites; the face is spherical, bloated and disfigured particularly by circumorbital oedema, the eyes becoming pink pustular horizontal slits between distended eyelids. Pleural effusions are present, and oedema of the scrotum or vulva may produce huge swellings. The oedema is always soft and pits easily with little pressure.

As the oedema appears there is an increasing feeling of lethargy and weakness; and when there are pleural effusions there is dyspnoea. Headache is common and, for reasons which are not understood, patients with the nephrotic syndrome frequently have recurrent "colds" which, though they rarely mature beyond a sore throat and transient nasal obstruction, are often associated with an acute exacerbation of oedema and proteinuria. Bacterial infections also occur frequently and affect principally the skin, the lungs and the peritoneum. When ascites is present there may be sudden attacks of abdominal pain simulating bacterial peritonitis, but laparotomy shows only a few strands of fibrin and sterile fluid; the pain settles gradually after operation. Anorexia and diarrhoea frequently occur and, although oedema of the stomach and intestinal mucosa may be partly responsible for both, it is clear that the anorexia is also due to the state of advanced malnutrition. The latter is probably also the cause of (i) the lowered basal metabolic rate, for the thyroid gland function has been found to be normal, and (ii) the occasional presence of anaemia in the absence of renal failure.

The combination of anorexia, increased secretion of aldosterone, treatment with adrenal steroids, and the use of diuretics may sometimes cause severe potassium deficiency with depression of glomerular filtration rate and functional disturbances of the tubule (p. 218).

Diagnosis

The fact that a patient is suffering from a nephrotic syndrome is easy to observe; its cause is usually more difficult to ascertain. It is suspected from the attendant circumstances and some help can be obtained from renal biopsy. Sometimes the correct diagnosis is only obtained in retrospect or at autopsy.

Prognosis

The course of the nephrotic syndrome largely depends on its cause; it varies from complete recovery to death from renal failure; it may last only a few weeks or, with remissions and relapses, up to 20 years. In general, the prognosis is better in women than it is in men, and in the young rather than the elderly. Remissions of oedema may occur at any time and may last several months, with persistent proteinuria as the only continuing evidence of disease. Sometimes such a remission may appear complete, with no protein in the urine and yet relapse takes place several years later. Renal failure, hypertensive cardiac failure with malignant hypertension and intercurrent infections are the usual causes of death. There may be periods of transient hypertension and microscopical haematuria, but these signs, unless they are persistent or severe, do not necessarily imply advancing destruction of the renal parenchyma. Conversely, gradual structural obliteration often takes place without proteinuria diminishing. Renal biopsy may establish the diagnosis. It is of some limited value in prognosis. For instance if the glomeruli appear normal the prognosis is excellent whereas if there are many crescents death occurs within a year.

Treatment

The many varieties of treatment of the nephrotic syndrome are illustrated in Fig. 13.2. The conditions which give rise to the syndrome are listed at the top and the sequence of disturbed physiology which follows is shown below; the aim of the treatment can be looked upon as cutting across a chain of events at different levels.

Treatment of the initiating condition

This is rarely successful. Cessation of troxidone administration, or the surgical removal of a septic focus, which is giving rise to renal amyloidosis, are

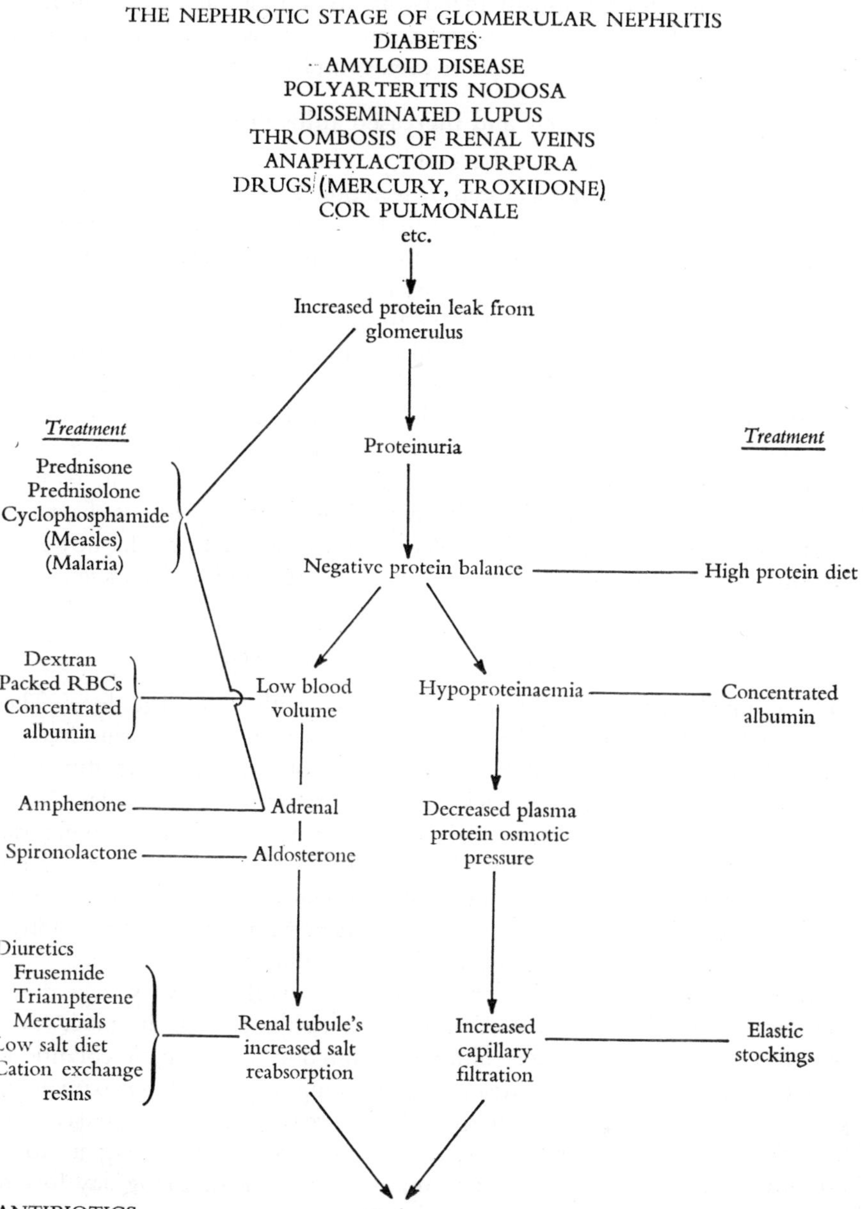

Fig. 13.2. Diseases in which the nephrotic syndrome develops; its pathological physiology and treatment.

two exceptions. Unfortunately, the cause of the nephrotic syndrome is seldom amenable to treatment, and usually therapy has to be aimed at a lower or more symptomatic level. Such symptomatic treatment, however, is occasionally followed by a long-lasting remission or even complete recovery.

Treatment of the proteinuria and increased aldosterone secretion

The administration of adrenal steroids to some patients causes a rapid diminution in proteinuria and aldosterone secretion, and there is a large diuresis and loss of oedema. Presumably the diminution in proteinuria is due to some alteration in glomerular permeability, and the decrease in aldosterone secretion to inhibition of adrenal function. The following account of the use of prednisone is mainly applicable to patients suffering from a nephrotic syndrome due to glomerular nephritis. It is now established that the only form of the nephrotic syndrome in this disease which will respond to prednisone is that in which the renal biopsy shows that the glomeruli are normal on light microscopy (see later). But it must be pointed out that in this group of patients the natural incidence of fairly rapid spontaneous remissions is about 65 per cent. Nevertheless it may be worthwhile, in children particularly, to try to cut short the dangers of hypovolaemia, protein depletion and oedema. In adults however the complications of prednisone therapy tend to outweigh its advantages.

ADRENAL STEROID THERAPY IN CHILDREN

It is claimed that the best response is obtained with very large doses. The aim is not only to get rid of the oedema but also to make the urine free of protein. At the onset the child is put to bed for one week. No treatment is given for this period unless a coincident infection has to be controlled. Very occasionally, within that time, there is a spontaneous diuresis and proteinuria may disappear or diminish greatly. If proteinuria is then less than 1 g/day no treatment is required but careful supervision should continue, for severe proteinuria usually recurs within two years. Treatment with steroid is divided into two stages: (i) treatment of the first attack, (ii) treatment of the relapse.

Treatment of the first attack is planned to last 4–8 weeks. As very large doses of steroids are administered it is advisable to keep the child in hospital. Care should be taken, however, to keep him away from others with septic conditions such as eczema and tonsillitis. At first prednisone 2 mg/kg per day (approximately) is given up to a maximum of 100 mg/day. This dose is continued for 10 days and then gradually reduced over the next 4–8 weeks. In a child weighing 30–40 lb the following course can be given: 60 mg/day for 10 days, 40 mg/day for 10 days, 20 mg/day for 10 days and 10 mg/day for 30 days (Fig. 13.3). The possible side effects include hypertension, oedema, cardiac failure, a rising blood urea, infection, potassium depletion, or mental changes. These are rare, but nevertheless the blood pressure, weight, and jugular venous pressure should be observed each day and periodic electrolyte estimations should be made. It is also evident that the contraindications to steroid therapy are cardiac failure, severe hypertension and advanced renal failure; dyspnoea from large pleural effusions is another contraindication. Even when treatment is eventually successful there may be little change in the first seven days except for fluid retention. There is then a gradually increasing diuresis and a marked fall in proteinuria (Fig. 13.3); in the most successful cases there is also a rise in glomerular filtration rate.

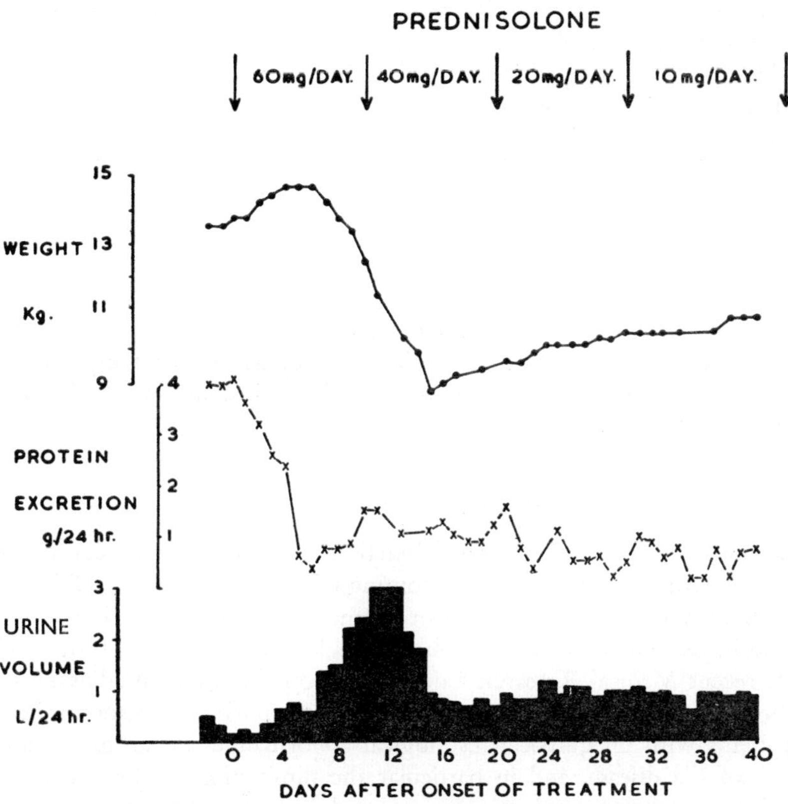

FIG. 13.3. Treatment of the nephrotic syndrome with prolonged courses of adrenal steroid in a child. Note the loss of weight *during* the administration of very large amounts of prednisolone, and the early decrease in proteinuria.

In 90 per cent of patients with normal glomeruli on renal biopsy the administration of prednisone will produce a remission. If there has been no response to this course it is probable that the evaluation of the renal biopsy was wrong, and that it does contain some glomerular abnormalities which have been missed. This usually becomes obvious later on a subsequent biopsy. If there has been no response to an eight week course of prednisone it is best to discontinue its use.

At the end of the initial course of treatment, injections of 10–20 units of corticotrophin are sometimes given once or twice weekly to stimulate adrenal activity in order to counteract the inhibiting effect of the prednisone. Prophylactic oral antibiotics (penicillin V) are given throughout the period of heavy dosage together with potassium supplements (potassium chloride 1–3 g/day), a small amount of calcium and vitamin D, and as much protein as the child will eat; no added salt is allowed. If there is a diuresis it is usually followed by an increase in weight and a phenomenal increase in appetite.

Treatment of a relapse. Fifty to 80 per cent of those in whom the first course of prednisone produced a remission will have a relapse subsequently. This may occur within days or after several years. If the relapses are so frequent that steroids cannot be stopped it may be possible to control the disease with the continuous administrations of a small dose daily, or on alternate days (e.g. 5 mg). If the amount of steroids which has to be given becomes unacceptable to the patient, parent or the doctor the administration of cyclophosphamide should be considered (see below). Supplements of calcium and potassium are always given during the administration of prednisone.

The fact that nephrotic children frequently have a remission of oedema following an accidental attack of measles has occasionally led to their being exposed to infection deliberately. The results are probably due to an increased endogenous secretion of adrenal steroids but they do not seem any better than after the administration of exogenous adrenal steroids; and measles is certainly far less pleasant for the child.

Adrenal steroids in adults

In adults deterioration of renal function, and hypertensive side effects of prednisone administration are more common than in children. In addition, large doses may cause acute perforation or haemorrhage from a peptic ulcer, acute psychosis, reactivation of an old tuberculous lesion, or coronary thrombosis.

A recent Medical Research Council trial on the use of prednisone in the nephrotic syndrome in adults due to glomerular nephritis, has demonstrated that in patients with unequivocal histological abnormalities in the glomeruli, the course of the disease, and in particular the diminution in the extent of the proteinuria, is the same whether or not prednisone 20–30 mg per day is given for at least two months. The only advantage of prednisone administration is in that group of patients in whom the kidneys are normal on light microscopy. Such patients have a substantial reduction in proteinuria several months before those who do not have prednisone. Nevertheless during the course of the trial the number of deaths was greater among those patients who were given prednisone, though the difference was not statistically significant.

Very rarely the administration of prednisone to a patient with severe structural changes, in whom renal function is rapidly deteriorating, may induce a dramatic improvement in renal function. Unfortunately it is just as likely to accelerate the rate of deterioration.

CYTOTOXIC DRUGS. For the past few years there has been an increasing use of cytotoxic drugs such as nitrogen mustard, cyclophosphamide, azothioprine, and 6-mercaptopurine in the treatment of immunological diseases of the kidney when they are unresponsive to other forms of therapy.

Control trials are few. One control trial with azothioprine 2·5 to 3 mg/kg/day has shown that it has little effect in any form of nephrotic syndrome. Another control trial with cyclophosphamide, however, has shown that it is of value in patients with minimal glomerular lesions who either relapse frequently after each course of prednisone, or are so dependent on prednisone that oedema re-accumulates as soon as the prednisone is stopped. Cyclophosphamide 3 mg/kg/day is given for eight to 12 weeks together with a small dose of prednisone (e.g. 15 mg) to diminish the incidence of complications from the cyclophosphamide. More recently courses of a little as two weeks have been assessed and they appear to be as efficient as the longer course. There is increasing evidenc however that cyclophosphamide can cause testicular and ovarian changes which may be irreversible. These complications have been described in adults who have been on cyclophosphamide for more than six months. It is not yet known whether the short courses usually advocated for the treatment of minimal change glomerular nephritis in children produce any long-term deleterious effects.

Treatment of the negative protein balance

It is imperative that the negative protein balance should be corrected, and the necessity for a high protein diet cannot be overemphasised.

The only limit to positive nitrogen balance that can be achieved by these patients is their own capacity for protein ingestion. It has been demonstrated that the rate of proteinuria is not affected by high intakes of protein and there is no evidence that renal function suffers in any way, though in patients with an initially depressed glomerular filtration rate it is important to watch the blood urea. A rising blood urea in these circumstances is, of course, no evidence of a further depression in filtration rate but, although a moderate rise to 40–60 mg per 100 ml is permissible, higher concentrations may be associated with anorexia and should be avoided. Adults should, and can, eat 150–200 g of protein a day, which is not difficult if protein concentrates such as Casilan are used, and salt restriction is not too severe (see below). At first anorexia is very frequent, but it can often be abolished by prednisone, even if a short course fails to produce any other immediate benefit. It has been shown that such a diet, continued for several months, and accompanied by a large accumulating nitrogen balance may at first produce no change in plasma protein concentration or oedema, although the plasma volume is gradually increasing. Eventually, when the plasma volume reaches a critical value, the oedema may rapidly recede whether or not plasma protein concentration has altered—additional evidence that the oedema in nephrotic syndrome is more closely related to blood volume changes than to plasma protein osmotic pressure.

Treatment of the low blood volume

This link in the causation of the oedema in the nephrotic syndrome can be treated directly by the intravenous administration of concentrated albumin, dextran or packed red cells. Albumin is reserved for patients in whom the oedema is exceptionally difficult to control. It is expensive to prepare and has little advantage over the other two blood volume expanders. Dextran is used most frequently. It should be salt-free and have either the same or twice the osmotic pressure of normal plasma protein (5 per cent or 10 per cent solutions). The amount given is empirical, but for an adult 1 litre of the 5 per cent solution (or 500 ml of the 10 per cent) is sufficient to produce a diuresis in many patients. Packed red cells are sometimes used; these should increase the blood volume for a longer period than dextran, but it is doubtful whether this is so, for an increase in the red cell mass tends to be associated with a shrinking plasma volume. In addition the nephrotic's liability to pyrexial reactions is a serious disadvantage of red cell infusions, unless the cells are washed with 5 per cent glucose.

Blood volume expanders frequently produce a good diuresis, but shortly after there is usually a period of relative oliguria and a rapid reaccumulation of oedema.

Treatment of the renal tubule's increased salt reabsorption

Salt and water retention can be minimised by decreasing the salt intake, or increasing the excretion of faecal sodium by giving cation exchange resins; or it may be directly countered by increasing the urinary excretion of sodium with diuretics.

DIETARY SALT CONTENT. The amount of salt in the diet should be related to the severity of the oedema and the ease with which it can be controlled with diuretics. In many long-standing cases of the nephrotic syndrome, in whom proteinuria and oedema fluctuate slowly over a period of months, the dietary salt can be adjusted according to the weight chart. When oedema is increasing rapidly it may be imperative to give a "salt-free" diet. Otherwise the ideal is to give as much salt as the patient can easily excrete; it is often an unnecessary burden to give less, and it increases the difficulties of maintaining a high protein diet. One of the great advantages of the wide range of potent oral diuretics now available is that the dietary control of sodium intake need not be nearly as rigid as it used to be. If renal failure supervenes and the oedema clears it may be important to remember to tell the patient to increase his intake of salt, otherwise he may develop salt deficiency which will aggravate the renal failure.

RESINS. The difficulties of giving a diet low in salt and yet high in protein can be overcome to a certain extent by the administration of low-sodium protein preparations such as Casilan, and the use of ion exchange resins or diuretics. Diuretics are more useful and more widely used to deplete the body of sodium while resins are more often used to deplete the body of potassium. A cation resin (Katonium, B.D.H.), 75 per cent in the ammonium phase and 25 per cent in the potassium phase, is given orally 15 g four times a day, for an adult. In the small intestine the ammonium and potassium on the resin are exchanged for an equivalent amount of the patient's sodium; but much of this sodium is again exchanged for potassium in the large bowel. The net result is a negative balance of sodium and potassium, and the production of an acidosis from the absorption of ammonium. In the nephrotic syndrome the negative sodium balance is the aim of the treatment; the negative potassium balance and acidosis are complications to avoid. The potassium loss can be countered by the oral administration of Slow-K (Ciba), a wax sponge slow release preparation containing potassium chloride which is totally absorbed over a period of several hours. The kidney should be able to prevent the tendency to develop an acidosis by increasing the excretion of ammonia and free hydrogen ions; if it is not able to do this adequately an increasing acidosis develops. A cation resin in the calcium phase is also available, this avoids the acidosis but potassium replacements are still necessary, and occasionally, prolonged use may cause hypercalcaemia. Resins, in line with other methods of producing a negative balance of sodium, may cause a fall in glomerular filtration rate and a rise in blood urea, if the oedema is removed too rapidly. When oedema is controlled, but heavy proteinuria continues, it is best to continue resin administration. On occasion the loss of oedema is associated with diminution or disappearance of proteinuria, a rise in glomerular filtration rate, and a return of plasma proteins to normal.

Diuretics. The guiding principle to follow is to use that amount of diuretic which will cause a diuresis that is not too precipitous and which preferably does not cause a negative balance of potassium. Failure to produce a diuresis with one diuretic is an indication to add a second. In order to minimise the urinary loss of potassium, treatment is begun with spironolactone and triampterene. Chlorothiazide can be added later and frusemide or ethacrynic acid later still. The dose of frusemide is doubled each day until a diuresis is provoked or until the dose has reached 4,000 mg per day. If a diuresis has not occurred by this time (which is very exceptional) the large amounts of frusemide are continued (some of it intravenously), while at the same time the blood volume is expanded with an intravenous administration of albumin. A simultaneous intravenous infusion of manitol at this monent gives the *coup de grâce* to any so-called "diuretic resistant oedema". At the onset of treatment body weight must be measured each day; it is a far better guide to water balance than an "input–output" chart. Plasma potassium should also be measured every other day.

Once the oedema has disappeared the diuretics should be rapidly cut back in the reverse order in which they were given so that if it is found necessary to continue with diuretics the patient is discharged on spironolactone and/or triampterene. Spironolactone should be avoided, however, in patients with renal failure for it is apt to cause hyperkalaemia. Chlorothiazide and its derivatives and frusemide are dangerous drugs to use in the treatment of patients suffering from a nephrotic syndrome once they are out of hospital. If diuretics are given, potassium supplements must continue to be supplied, but there is no certainty that such supplements will be either ingested or adequate. Plasma potassium concentrations must therefore be measured from time to time. Chlorothiazide or frusemide are best given to outpatients intermittently, e.g. on two days a week or an alternate days. Sometimes, once a diuresis has been forced by diuretics, there is a spontaneous remission with diminution in urinary protein excretion, a rise in plasma proteins and no further need for diuretics.

Treatment of the increased capillary filtration and local oedema

The increase in capillary filtration which takes place at all capillary surfaces as a result of the decreased plasma protein osmotic pressure can be minimised below the knees by wearing elastic stockings. In some subjects, particularly young women who have a relatively well-controlled nephrotic syndrome, such a measure may enable them to go out in the evening without looking too conspicuous.

Oedema fluid can be removed directly by making multiple superficial skin incisions in the legs through an antibiotic cream such as Neomycin. If the patient is then kept in a sitting posture large quantities of fluid may be removed, but it is a remarkable fact that occasionally these procedures are unsuccessful for the first few days; then losses of 1–2 litres a day may occur through the same sites. This initial delay is most often seen when the accumulation of oedema has been so rapid and extensive that the legs are tense, hard and almost impossible to pit upon pressure. The danger of secondary infection of the skin during these manoeuvres is considerable. For some unknown reason, if a large quantity of fluid is successfully removed in this way it may sometimes initiate the onset of a large diuresis. If ascites and pleural effusions are causing discomfort, the fluid may be removed with a needle and syringe, but otherwise this should be avoided for the protein content of such fluid is sometimes relatively high, and its removal diminishes the already depleted protein stores.

DANGERS OF REMOVING OEDEMA FLUID RAPIDLY. Aside from the dangers of an associated loss of potassium, a rapid loss of fluid, however caused, may lead to an acute reduction of blood volume. There may then be a fall in blood pressure, and a rise in blood urea. The latter is due to a fall in glomerular filtration rate and an increased protein breakdown. Potassium depletion may also occur. Nausea, thirst and faintness are useful premonitory symptoms. The blood pressure should therefore be measured twice a day and a supplement of potassium given. It is also wise to measure the haematocrit each day.

Treatment of the infections

Though the use of antibiotics does not counteract a specific link in the aetiology of nephrotic oedema, their introduction in recent years has nevertheless been the main factor responsible for the longer survival of patients suffering from the nephrotic syndrome. Such patients seem particularly liable to develop infections, and in turn the infections seem to be more severe and are nearly always associated with an acute exacerbation of the nephrotic syndrome. In order to avoid infections oral penicillin is sometimes given daily as a prophylactic; alternatively the patient is given a short course of a wide-spectrum antibiotic (e.g. cephalexin, or trimethoprim/sulphamethoxazole (Septrin)) to take home, to be used at the first sign of an infection.

Synopsis of Treatment

Treatment is started with a low salt, high protein diet. Prednisone is given to children in whom the renal biopsy shows the glomeruli to be normal. The administration of prednisone to adults, whatever the renal histology, is hardly justifiable. When prednisone is given, a remission of the proteinuria should occur within two months. If this does not take place within that time prednisone should be discontinued.

Diuretics are given in sufficient amounts to cause a diuresis. If this is unsuccessful, a plasma expander such as 1 l of 10 per cent Dextran or 5 per cent albumin can be given during the administration of the diuretics.

Ion exchange resins can also be given either as an alternative, or in conjunction with diuretics. Antibiotics should be given at the first sign of infection. They can also be given prophylactically.

If the oedema is painful or incapacitating, even with the patient in bed, and diuretics are slow to take effect, the oedema may be removed with multiple skin incisions.

A high protein diet must be used with some caution when there is renal failure.

In order to be aware of the progress of events it is useful to insist on the following being measured and recorded once a day: (i) body weight; (ii) blood pressure; (iii) fluid intake and output, excluding food and faeces. When there are rapid changes in weight, the haematocrit should be measured every day, and at this time plasma potassium and sodium should be measured on alternate days, with plasma urea and creatinine at least once a week. When the patient is stabilised these estimations can be made less and less frequently. Urinary protein excretion should be measured once a week until the patient is stabilised. Plasma protein concentration should be measured at least once in two weeks; it is probably the best guide to progress.

Long Term Results of Treatment

There seems little doubt that the duration of survival is now longer than it was and that in adults this change is due to the use of antibiotics and a high protein diet. In children, it is still uncertain whether the beneficial effects of prednisone have contributed to the improved survival. There has not yet been a controlled trial of the use of steroids in children.

BIBLIOGRAPHY

ABRAMOWICZ, M., *et al.* (1970). "Controlled trial of azathioprine in children with nephrotic syndrome." *Lancet*, **1**, 959.

AHLINDER, S., BIRKE, G., LILJEDAHL, S. T. O., and PLANTIN, L. O. (1964). "Protein losses studied with double isotope technique. Physiology and pathophysiology of plasma protein metabolism." *Proceedings of the 3rd Symposium held at Grindelwald, Switzerland, Sept.* 1964. Hans Huber Publishers, Bern.

ANDERSEN, S. B., and ROSSING, N. (1967). "Metabolism of albumin and Yg globulin during albumin infusion and during plasmaphoresis." *Scand. J. Clin. Invest.*, **20**, 181.

ARNEIL, G. C. (1968). "Management of the nephrotic syndrome." *Arch. Dis. Child.*, **43**, 257.

BARRETT, T. M., and SOOTHILL, J. L. (1970). "Controlled trial of cyclophosphamide in steroid-sensitive relapsing nephrotic syndrome in childhood." *Lancet*, **2**, 479.

BARRETT, T. M., MCLAINE, P. N., and SOOTHILL, J. F. (1970). "Albumin excretion as a measure of glomerular dysfunction in children." *Arch. Dis. Child.*, **45**, 496.

BLACK, D. A. K., ROSE, G., and BREWER, D. B. (1970). "Controlled trial of prednisone in adult patients with the nephrotic syndrome." *Brit. Med. J.*, **2**, 421.

BLAINEY, J. D. (1954). "High protein diets in the treatment of the nephrotic syndrome." *Clin. Sci.*, **13**, 567.

CAMERON, J. S., and WHITE, H. R. H. (1965). "Selectivity of proteinuria in children with the nephrotic syndrome." *Lancet*, **1**, 463.

CHAMBERLAIN, M. J., PRINGLE, A., and WRONG, O. M. (1966). "Oliguric renal failure in the nephrotic syndrome." *Quart. J. Med.*, **35**, 215.

CHOPRA, J. S., MALLICK, N. P., and STONE, M. C. (1971). "Hyperlipoproteinaemias in the nephrotic syndrome." *Lancet*, **1**, 317.

DIRKS, J. H., CAPP, J. R., and BERLINER, R. W. (1964). "The protein concentration in the proximal tubule of the dog." *J. clin. Invest.*, **43**, 916.

EISENBERG, S. (1963). "Postural changes in plasma volume in hypoalbuminaemia." *Arch. Int. Med.*, **112**, 544.

FAWCETT, I. W., HILTON, P. J., JONES, N. F., and WING, A. J. (1971). "Nephrotic syndrome in the elderly." *Brit. Med. J.*, **2**, 387.

GARNETT, E. S., and WEBBER, C. E. (1967). "Changes in blood volume produced by treatment in the nephrotic syndrome." *Lancet*, **2**, 798.

GITLIN, D. (1957). "Some concepts of plasma protein metabolism, A.D. 1956." *Pediatrics*, **19**, 657.

HILTON, P. J., JONES, N. F., and TIGHE, J. R. (1968). "Nephrotic syndrome in heart disease. An appraisal." *Brit. Med. J.*, **2**, 584.

HULME, B., and HARDWICKE, J. (1968). "Human glomerular permeability to macro-molecules in health and disease." *Clin. Sci.*, **34**, 515.

JENSEN, H. (1969). "Plasma Protein Metabolism in the Nephrotic Syndrome", 1 Vol. Munksgaad, Copenhagen.

KAITZ, A. L. (1959). "Albumin metabolism in nephrotic adults." *J. Lab. clin. Med.*, **53**, 186.

LOUGHRIDGE, L., and LEWIS, M. G. (1971). "Nephrotic syndrome in malignant disease of non-renal origin." *Lancet*, **1**, 256.

LUETSCHER, J. A., HALL, A. D., and KREMER, V. L. (1950). "Treatment of nephrosis with concentrated human serum albumin. II. Effects on renal function and on excretion of water and some electrolytes." *J. clin. Invest.*, **29**, 896.

MORRIS, J. P., GINN, E., and THOMPSON, D. D. (1963). "Unilateral renal vein thrombosis associated with the nephrotic syndrome." *Amer. J. Med.*, **34**, 867.

ROSENHEIM, M. L., and SPENCER, A. G. (1956). "Treatment of nephrotic syndrome with cation-exchange resins and high-protein low-sodium diet." *Lancet*, **2**, 313.

SNASHALL, P. D. (1971). "Gross oedema in the nephrotic syndrome treated with frusemide in high dosage." *Brit. Med. J.*, **1**, 319.

SQUIRE, J. R., BLAINEY, J. D., and HARDWICKE, J. (1957). "Nephrotic syndrome." *Brit. med. Bull.*, **13**, 43.

STANBURY, S. W., and MACAULAY, D. (1957). "Defects of renal tubular function in the nephrotic syndrome." *Quart. J. Med.*, N.S. **26**, 7.

VERE, D. W., and KING, C. E. (1960). "The reaction to subcutaneous drainage in anasarca." *Lancet*, **1**, 779.

14

Acute Renal Failure

ACUTE renal failure can be arbitrarily defined as any condition in which the daily volume of urine passed into the bladder is suddenly reduced below 400 ml.* This definition inevitably includes severe but physiologically normal oliguria, which is sometimes called "acute renal insufficiency".

Aetiology

(1) Severe functional changes without structural damage.
(2) Severe functional changes with acute structural damage.
(3) Functional changes of perhaps moderate severity but occurring in a patient with chronic structural damage.
(4) Acute urinary tract obstruction.

Severe functional changes without structural damage

The most important of these changes is severe but initially reversible renal vasoconstriction, the causes of which have been discussed in Section 9; they are predominantly those which cause acute circulatory insufficiency. Typical examples are the sudden reductions in blood volume which may accompany acute diarrhoea and vomiting, burns and haemorrhage. The reduced renal blood flow which results is associated with a reduced glomerular filtration rate and thus a decreased excretion of solutes. Usually there is a simultaneous stimulation of the supra-optico-hypophyseal system and an increase in the level of circulating antidiuretic hormone. The oliguria which results is thus associated with a urine which at first is highly concentrated. Some of the most severe but rapidly reversible oliguric episodes may occur in the first two days after operation when the 24-hour urine volume may be 150 ml.

Severe functional changes with acute structural damage

A wide variety of conditions may give rise to acute structural changes severe enough to cause acute renal failure; they are illustrated in Fig. 14.1. They include severe forms of certain renal diseases which usually present in a less acute form, i.e. acute nephritis, acute pyelonephritis with acute necrotising

* This excludes a transient form of acute renal failure in which the glomerular filtration rate falls and the blood urea rises, but the urine flow remains normal. The condition has been described in association with burns and has a good prognosis.

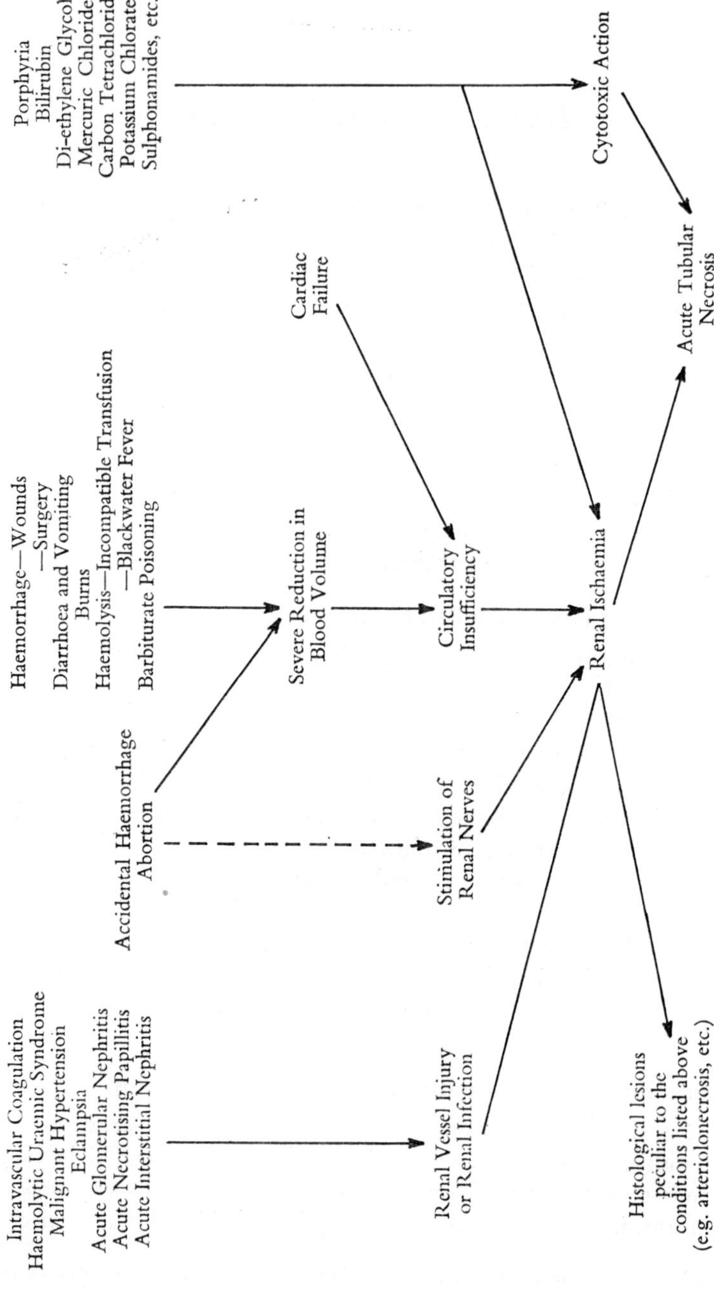

FIG. 14.1. Aetiology of acute renal failure with acute structural changes.

papillitis, malignant hypertension, polyarteritis nodosa and eclampsia. Acute renal failure may also be caused by an acute interstitial nephritis due to a drug sensitivity (e.g. phenindione). Numerically these are not important causes of acute renal failure. The most common form of structural damage is acute tubular necrosis. In the past this condition has been called "lower nephron nephrosis", "shock kidney" and "crush syndrome".

Tubular necrosis may follow directly from the action of poisons or severe prolonged renal vasoconstriction. Poisons act directly by causing the death of those tubular cells which transport the substance from the blood into the lumen of the tubule; they also cause intense renal vasoconstriction and irregularly distributed focal patches of renal ischaemia, which in turn becomes the sites of ischaemic tubular necrosis. Mercury, arsenic, lead, bismuth, carbon tetrachloride, potassium chlorate, propylene glycol, sulphonamides and cephaloridine are some of the substances which have been known to cause acute tubular necrosis; for this reason they are called nephrotoxins. Some endogenous substances such as porphyrins and bilirubin are also liable to produce acute tubular necrosis if present in excess quantities in the plasma.

The causes of renal vasoconstriction which may produce tubular necrosis are the same as those which have been discussed above and in Section 8. Necrosis is due to the intensity and duration of renal ischaemia, i.e. it must be present for a matter of hours, a point of immense importance in trying to prevent the condition. Abortion, multiple wounds and extensive surgery with inadequate blood replacement are the most frequent causes of tubular necrosis. Though it is possible that renal vasoconstriction without a concomitant fall in blood pressure may occasionally be sufficiently intense to cause necrosis, it is clear that necrosis is more likely if there is a combination of vasoconstriction and hypotension. It is not always appreciated that the more intense the vasoconstriction the higher the minimal arterial pressure necessary to keep the vessels open. This is important clinically, for when there is severe renal vasoconstriction minor falls in blood pressure may be sufficient to cause a complete ischaemia.

Whether a shunting of blood through the juxtamedullary glomeruli and away from the cortex ever occurs in any of these situations is not open to demonstration. The meagre evidence that has been obtained in man does not support the idea, and observations made on animals suggest that if there is such a diversion, it is of little consequence compared with the severity of the total renal ischaemia with which it is associated.

Acute functional changes superimposed upon chronic structural damage

Patients suffering from chronic renal failure due to a gradual obliteration of their nephrons may be precipitated into acute renal failure by some disturbance which, in a normal person, would cause only an insignificant change in renal function. This combination of acute functional changes and long-standing structural damage is sometimes very difficult to differentiate from acute structural damage in previously normal kidneys, particularly if the pre-existence of chronic renal disease is unknown. The differential diagnosis is based on obtaining clinical evidence of long-standing renal failure such as a history of polydipsia, polyuria, lassitude, and the presence of pigmentation and anaemia.

Acute urinary tract obstruction

Bilateral pelvic or ureteric obstruction, or unilateral obstruction to a single functioning kidney can obviously cause acute renal failure. This indisputable truth is often forgotten when considering the differential diagnosis of acute renal failure. Pus, clots of blood, crystalluria, tubular debris, and retroperitoneal fibrosis (see below) can cause acute bilateral obstruction. There is also a rare condition known as calculus anuria when acute bilateral anuria results from the presence of a calculus in only one ureter.

The outstanding feature of the acute renal failure due to acute urinary tract obstruction is that the flow of urine is completely suppressed, as opposed to the low flows which are usually found with acute structural damage to the renal parenchyma. The only exception to this rule is in the acute renal failure of acute glomerular nephritis. The therapeutic implication of this fact is that if acute renal failure is associated with complete or almost complete suppression of urine, a cystoscopy should be performed and the ureters catheterised. Obstruction is sometimes relieved by this procedure. But it may be necessary to release the urine above the obstruction by a nephrostomy.

Retroperitoneal fibrosis is the term applied to the presence of a thick mass of fibrous tissue in the retroperitoneal space which spreads outwards from the mid-line. Usually the cause is unknown. It can follow prolonged treatment with methysergide for migraine; and occasionally it is a response to invasion by carcinoma cells. It may be associated with mediastinal fibrosis, oesophageal constriction, and other forms of fibrosis in the chest and abdomen. When the fibrous mass involves both ureters it may give rise to a characteristic form of acute renal failure. The patient is usually a middle-aged man who complains of increasingly severe bouts of unremitting pain in both loins, the attacks come on suddenly and last a few hours or a day or two. A hydrocoele or oedema of the legs may be present, perhaps due to compression of veins and lymphatics. Finally, during a prolonged attack of pain there is oliguria or anuria. This may last a few days. Then there is a profuse polyuria, perhaps only for a few hours, followed by a return of complete anuria. The concentration of blood urea fluctuates wildly with the changes in urine flow, and the urine is free of protein, a most revealing point which excludes a disturbance of the renal parenchyma as the cause of the anuria. Surprisingly ureteric catheters may pass up the ureters without difficulty and urine flows down the lumen of the catheters, but when they are removed, the anuria persists. Radiographic studies may show that the ureters have been pulled inwards towards the mid-line or that they are deformed in a zig-zag pattern along part of their course. The ureteric abnormalities are best seen by filling the ureters with hypaque from below using a bulb Chevasseau type of ureteric catheter. Treatment consists in freeing the ureters and placing them laterally beyond the fibrous mass. The idiopathic form of the disease is thought to be self-limiting.

TUBULAR NECROSIS

The following sections describe the pathological findings, clinical features, treatment and prognosis in acute tubular necrosis. The clinical features and treatment of acute renal failure due to other causes are almost identical.

Pathology of Acute Tubular Necrosis

Macroscopically the kidneys do not look greatly disturbed and may often be passed as normal. When the kidney is incised there is a tendency for the cortex to bulge and to look slightly pale. The only unmistakable macroscopical appearances are those associated with extensive necrosis such as are found with eclampsia and accidental haemorrhage when the condition is called acute cortical necrosis.

Microscopically the lesions are most clearly displayed in nephrons which have been microdissected. By this technique it has been possible to show that there are two distinct lesions; one is due to ischaemia and occurs in a random distribution throughout all nephrons and in any part of the nephron down to the collecting tubule; the other, which is due to nephrotoxins, affects all nephrons equally, and is confined to the same part of each *proximal* tubule. Each ischaemic lesion involves only a relatively short length of the nephron and consists of complete necrosis of the tubule cells and the basement membrane, thus exposing the lumen of the tubule to the renal interstitial space (Fig. 14.2). The nephrotoxic lesion involves a considerable segment of each proximal tubule and consists of necrosis of tubule cells only, without involvement of basement membrane (Fig. 14.3). Nephrotoxins, however, not only cause the death of those tubule cells which transport them, but in addition their presence in high concentrations causes intense renal vasoconstriction. In acute tubular necrosis from nephrotoxins, therefore, both ischaemic and cytotoxic lesions are found.

Ordinary histological sections of the kidney at autopsy show that the glomeruli escape injury while the even distribution of the nephrotoxic tubular lesions are easily recognised; the ischaemic lesions, however, are much more widely spaced and may not be present in a renal biopsy. There are a few foci of round cell infiltration and occasionally some of the tubules are surrounded by a clear "halo"-like area which is thought to be evidence of interstitial oedema. Numerous haemcasts are seen in those cases which follow an incompatible blood transfusion or widespread muscle injury.

Renal biopsy observations have shown that there is little correlation between the light microscopy changes and the functional abnormalities. Indeed most biopsies show little or no light microscopy changes. With the electron microscope, however, it has been possible to demonstrate that even in those specimens

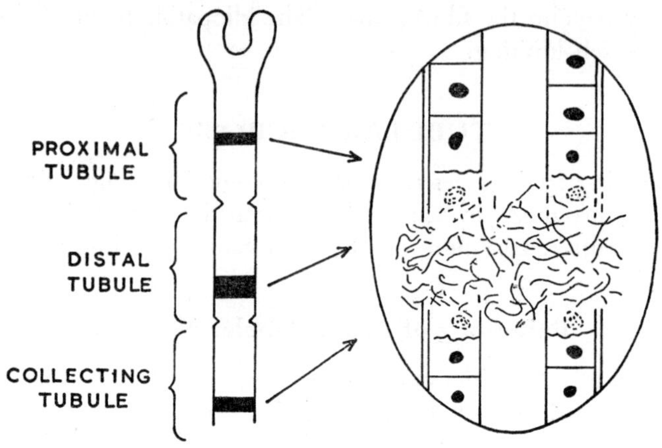

ISCHAEMIC LESION OF

TUBULAR NECROSIS

FIG. 14.2.

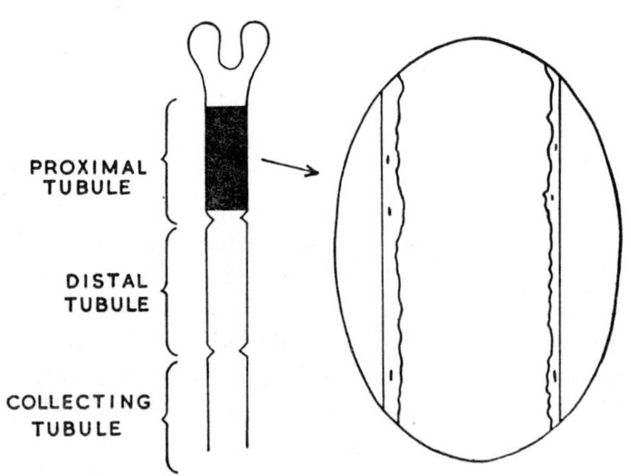

NEPHROTOXIC LESION OF

TUBULAR NECROSIS

FIG. 14.3.

with no light microscopy changes there are pronounced cellular lesions in the tubules with patchy disruption, in the basement membrane and marked intraglomerular deposition of fibrin and platelets consistent with intraglomerular capillary thrombosis.

Clinical and Biochemical Features of Acute Tubular Necrosis

Following the particular episode which has precipitated tubular necrosis and which may be defined at the onset, the natural history of the disorder can be divided into three phases:

(*a*) The oliguric.
(*b*) The diuretic.
(*c*) The postdiuretic.

Oliguric phase

The early part of the oliguric phase is frequently unrecognised, for it often begins during a surgical or medical emergency. In this setting, the fact that the kidneys have almost ceased to function may not immediately alarm, so great is the relief that the patient is still alive. The daily volume of urine excreted varies, but complete cessation of urine flow does not occur with tubular necrosis. At least 50–100 ml is excreted daily; it is often dark and discoloured by breakdown products of blood, and at first may be thickened by the debris of necrosed tubular cells, yet the specific gravity of this small volume of "concentrated"- looking urine is nearly always around 1·010, a paradox which confirms the diagnosis. Proteinuria is always present.

During the oliguric phase renal blood flow is only reduced to about a third of normal whereas glomerular filtration rate is usually less than 1 per cent of normal. The cause of the continuing renal ischaemia is not known. It persists for many days after the situation which precipitated the initial renal ischaemia of the onset has been corrected. It has been suggested that renal ischaemia is caused by a rise in intrarenal pressure, for straight X-rays of the abdomen show the kidneys to be much larger than normal. This hypothesis, however, is no longer tenable, for the intrarenal pressure has been measured and found to be normal. Nor does the persistence of the renal ischaemia appear to be due to a maintained nervous vasoconstriction. It has been proposed that the intra- glomerular coagulation which is present is likely to be an important factor in the prolonged renal ischaemia of tubular necrosis. It is probable that this in turn may be due to the initial ischaemia having caused anoxic damage to the endothelial cells. These therefore swell and obstruct the lumen of the arterioles and capillaries so then the lumen become so small that red cells become wedged and produce complete obstruction and thrombosis. There is good experimental evidence for this sequence. There is also some evidence that the prolonged ischaemia may be due to the high circulating concentration of renin and angiotensin which accompany acute tubular necrosis.

The gross discrepancy between the moderate reduction in renal blood flow and the almost complete absence of apparent glomerular filtration rate is not understood. The electron microscopy changes suggest that perhaps the true filtration rate is not greatly disturbed but that as the filtrate passes down the injured tubule most of it "leaks" back into the peritubular venous capillaries. This is in line with experiments in which a dye which is not reabsorbed by the tubules (lissamine green) has been injected into the renal artery of rats with tubular necrosis. The dye can be seen entering and leaving the glomeruli then passing along some of the proximal tubules but it does not appear in the distal tubules.

The severe reduction in apparent glomerular filtration rate together with the tubular damage cause severe disturbances in function. Urea, creatinine, potassium, phosphate, sulphate and a considerable quantity of unidentifiable anions (which have been aptly called, for want of a better name, "anuric anions") accumulate in the blood and extracellular fluid. There is also an accumulation of hydrogen ions with a fall in plasma pH and bicarbonate. The increase in the concentrations of potassium, phosphate and urea are due to their release from the breakdown of muscle protein; the rate of this release which is greatest during the first few days of the oliguric phase largely determines the course of the illness. The rise in plasma potassium is aggravated by the retention of the hydrogen ions, for these tend to be sequestered intracellularly in exchange for potassium ions which are then released into the extracellular fluid. In addition, a fall in arterial oxygen tension (e.g. with a chest infection) may also cause a rapid shift of intracellular potassium into the extracellular fluid and plasma. The danger to life is that the rising concentration of plasma potassium may cause cardiac arrest. This threat is accentuated by the rise in phosphate which lowers the plasma calcium, and, as potassium and calcium ions have opposing actions on heart muscle, the lowered calcium and the raised plasma potassium summate in their ill effects on cardiac function. There is also a rise in plasma magnesium which potentiates the harmful effects of the rise in plasma potassium. The rate of protein catabolism is greatest following injury to muscle, haemorrhage and trauma in the young and healthy; elderly or debilitated patients break down protein at a slower rate. Infection causes a brisk increase in rate. In most patients protein catabolism is greatest in the first two or three days. On a diet containing about 100 g of carbohydrate per day the average total (endogenous + exogenous) calorie consumption is approximately 2,500 per day, endogenous fat constituting the main source of energy.

The other major electrolyte disturbance which occurs in the oliguric phase is a decrease in the serum concentration of sodium and chloride. In the past this hypotonicity or overhydration was usually due to an attempt to relieve the oliguria by the administration of large quantities of water; an intuitive therapy based on the naive principle that "what goes in must come out". This is a particularly easy trap to fall into for these patients are often excessively thirsty. It has been shown, however, that plasma osmolality gradually falls even if the water intake is limited to an amount which is normally lost by insensible means. At first there was thought to be a shift of sodium into the cells, but it now appears that the most important factor is an increase in the extracellular water. This is derived both from the intake, for the insensible loss of water is below average in these patients, and from "metabolic water" formed by the endogenous breakdown of protein and fat; a quantity which may amount to 300 ml a day. It is important to recognise the origin of this hypotonicity, for its prevention and correction depends on restricting the intake of water, and trying to diminish the endogenous breakdown of protein and fat, *not* in administering large quantities of normal or concentrated saline intravenously; this only expands the extracellular fluid space and may lead to cardiac failure.

Other changes evident in the blood are the development of anaemia and a leucocytosis. The anaemia develops rapidly, fails to progress beyond a certain severity though the oliguria may continue, and often becomes more pronounced when the blood urea concentration is beginning to fall. The cause of the anaemia appears to be a combination of bone marrow depression and haemolysis.

These many changes in the internal environment can only be diagnosed with certainty by laboratory estimations: they are associated with the following rather vague clinical signs. The fall in plasma pH results in deep regular sighing respirations which are easily recognised, but the other electrolyte changes produce signs which are singularly non-specific, even when they are of sufficient severity to threaten the patient's life. Overhydration causes mental dullness and headache, nausea, vomiting and convulsions. It has also been said to cause psychosis and fever. Expansion of the extracellular fluid space is recognised by a rise in jugular venous pressure, oedema, tachypnoea and pulmonary crepitations. The rise in plasma potassium and the fall in plasma calcium concentrations are stated to be responsible for anxiety, restlessness, paraesthesiae and hypotension; these are particularly unreliable signs. Serial electrocardiograms are more valuable in revealing a rise in plasma potassium; initially there is "tenting" of T waves with ST segment depression, flattening of the P wave, and a lengthening of the QRS complex so that it resembles bundle branch block, at higher concentrations of potassium the E.C.G. takes on the appearance of an untidy sine wave and there may be periods of standstill and irregular rhythm. Death occurs from cardiac standstill and ventricular fibrillation. In traumatic cases, particularly those with extensive injury to muscle, the rate of rise of plasma potassium to a lethal concentration may be extremely rapid: a concentration of 6–7 mEq/l rising to 10 Eq/ml overnight. The rise in plasma magnesium probably produces some drowsiness and weakness.

Gastro-intestinal disturbances including hiccoughs are frequent during the oliguric phase; their cause is unknown, but they become more severe as the blood urea rises; both vomiting and diarrhoea may occur and they are usually made worse by oral feeding. Occasionally there is haematemesis and melaena.

As the oliguric phase lengthens there is a gradual clouding of consciousness, nausea and lassitude, fading into a twitching coma. These features seem to be directly due to the retention of some unidentifiable waste products, for they can be relieved by dialysis even if the concentration of blood urea and identifiable electrolytes are left uncorrected.

A rise in blood pressure is infrequent.

Delayed wound healing and haemorrhage often occur in surgical cases. Finally, it is important to be aware that these patients are very liable to develop infections; these are now the commonest cause of death in cases uncomplicated by severe trauma.

Diuretic phase

This phase begins when the 24-hour urine volume reaches 1,000 ml. Together with the onset of diuresis, the renal blood flow and glomerular filtration rate gradually increase. Sometimes, however, the diuresis begins without any marked change occurring in either. At first the urine appears to be pure plasma filtrate, for the total concentration of the urine, and of each of its constituents, is identical with that of plasma. As the urine volume increases, the tubules recover some ability to reabsorb salt and concentrate urea so that the urine now contains less salt and more urea than plasma, but the total osmolar concentration still remains about the same as that of plasma, i.e. isotonic. The delay in the return of the ability to concentrate is paralleled by a similar delay in the ability to acidify the urine.

During the first few days of the diuretic phase the patient's general condition changes markedly; there is an increased awareness, nausea and vomiting cease, and appetite returns. The overall improvement is such that when blood urea estimations are found to be either unchanged or even a little higher than before the onset of diuresis, there is often an atmosphere of disbelief in the accuracy of the estimations. Nevertheless, this is the recurrent pattern of recovery and is another indication that the symptoms of renal failure are not due to the high concentrations of blood urea. The diuretic phase may be a week old before the blood urea begins to fall.

At the height of the diuresis the daily urine volume may be very great (e.g. 6 litre), so that whereas a few days before the patient's life was threatened by an excess of water, salt and potassium, it is now exposed to the perils of dehydration, salt loss and potassium lack. The cause of this extensive diuresis appears to be a combination of three mechanisms: (1) An osmotic diuresis due to the high blood urea; (2) tubular functional inadequacy; and (3) the release of an accumulated surplus of fluid and electrolytes. Obviously if (1) and (2) are responsible for the large diuresis, dangerous electrolyte and water deficiencies may occur, whereas if it is due to (3) it is to the patient's advantage. The urine volume rises to a peak and then falls to normal values; the duration of the diuretic phase is roughly the same as that of the oliguric phase.

Postdiuretic phase

This stage develops imperceptibly from the diuretic phase and is characterised by a normal output of urine although there continues to be some impairment of renal function. Gradually renal blood flow and glomerular filtration rate increase, and the ability to concentrate the urine, and other tubular functions, return towards normal over a period of about one year. Nevertheless, follow-up studies have shown that although renal function is perfectly adequate, full recovery is unusual.

TREATMENT

The first thing to do is to confirm that acute renal failure has indeed taken place, and it is essential to catheterise the bladder to exclude urinary retention. The next step is to decide whether the oliguria or anuria is due to urinary tract obstruction; if this is considered probable, or even remotely possible, cystoscopy and ureteric catheterisation should be performed and any obstruction either dislodged, or relieved by nephrostomy. This is particularly relevant when the acute renal failure follows the taking of sulphonamide or is associated with a high plasma uric acid when tubular debris and crystals can produce complete occlusion of the pelvis and ureters.

Acute tubular necrosis and other forms of acute renal failure should be treated along the following lines.

Treatment of the Onset

During the onset of acute renal failure, when there is severe renal ischaemia, but before tubular necrosis has occurred, it should be possible (except in the case of poisons) to prevent necrosis by prompt transfusion, or electrolyte and water replacement, whichever is appropriate. It is imperative that transfusions should not be withheld on the grounds that, as the patient is already suffering from acute renal failure, he should not be exposed to the risks of a mismatched transfusion. It would be as logical to refrain from throwing a lifebelt to a drowning man for fear it might hit him on the head.

It is wise to try and decide by examining a blood film whether the loss of blood has occurred in an already anaemic person, for if such a patient is transfused so that the haematocrit rises above its usual level, renal failure may be aggravated (p. 107), particularly if there is already some degree of chronic renal structural damage.

If a patient is seen within an hour of a transfusion reaction or the ingestion of a nephrotoxic poison it is possible that renal damage may be less extensive if 500 ml of 10 per cent mannitol is given intravenously in 30 min. If the renal failure is reversible the urine flow should increase by 50 per cent in the next two hours. This is probably useful because (1) it reduces endothelial cell swelling thus opening up obstructed arterioles and capillaries, and (2) it produces an osmotic diuresis with mannitol in the tubule lumen, this may reduce tubule cell swelling and open up obstructed tubules. When acute renal failure follows diarrhoea and vomiting, pyloric stenosis, etc., electrolyte and water losses should be replaced even though the presence of oliguria makes the dangers of overadministration more likely. In order to find out whether the oliguria is reversible, a litre of saline is given intravenously in one hour; if the urine flow rises to 20–30 ml/hr or more it is reasonable to assume that the oliguria is reversible and to continue the saline administration. In any case it is reasonable to continue to give saline, so long as the jugular venous pressure is closely observed, or preferably if the central venous pressure is measured with a catheter in the superior vena cava. The central venous pressure should not rise above 5 cm H_2O. It has also been claimed that if the urine to plasma osmolal ratio is greater than 1·35, or the urine to plasma urea concentration ratio is greater than 6·6, the patient has a potentially rapidly reversible form of acute renal failure; whereas if it is below 1·035 or 2·14 respectively it is not immediately reversible.

Ideally the patient should never be allowed to become oligaemic long enough for severe renal ischaemia to develop. If acute renal failure does supervene it is essential that its time of onset should be determined as accurately as possible, for though rapid intravenous therapy may be life-saving in the first few hours, 24–48 hours later it may only precipitate pulmonary oedema, cardiac failure and death.

Treatment of the Oliguric Phase

The aim of treatment during the oliguric phase is to keep the internal environment normal until the kidneys recover. It is clear that this aim is limited by two factors: (1) the rate at which the internal environment changes, which is mainly dependent on (a) the rate of catabolism, and (b) the efficacy of treatment; and (2) the duration of the oliguria. If the internal environment changes relatively slowly, and the oliguria does not last more than two to three weeks, conservative treatment may be sufficient. But if the internal changes are rapid or the oliguria prolonged then it may be imperative to supplement conservative treatment with artificial dialysis. In practice it is the rate of change which is most liable to vary, and this in turn is largely determined by the extent of the associated trauma and infection. When there is no trauma, e.g. following abortion and poisoning, the rise in blood urea and potassium is often so gradual that conservative treatment is adequate. But with extensive trauma, e.g. gunshot wounds and road accidents, deterioration is so rapid that dialysis is usually necessary. This dissimilarity is not only due to probable differences in the rate of catabolism but also to the fact that traumatic cases, and particularly war casualties, are liable to have large quantities of intracellular products released from non-viable muscles which have been overlooked during debridement.

Whatever means are employed to treat acute renal failure, plasma electrolytes, urea and glucose should be estimated at least once a day; the daily urine volume should be measured and its content of electrolytes and glucose estimated. The patient should be weighed each day if at all possible, and if the patient is being treated by dietary means and not being dialysed he should lose 0·2–0·5 kg per day, for this is approximately the weight of endogenous solids which are metabolised each day.

An indwelling catheter should not be placed in the bladder, for it is likely to cause a urinary infection. If the rate of urine flow is around or above 300 ml per day there will usually be spontaneous bladder voiding once a day, if it is below this it is insufficient to influence decisions about treatment.

Conservative treatment

CONTROL OF WATER INTAKE. As soon as it is considered that the patient is not deficient in water, the intake of water is limited to 500 ml a day, plus a quantity equal to the amount of urine passed in the previous 24 hours. The total amount is increased in very hot weather and if there is much sweating. The amount of water required is best gauged by the weight (see above) and the effective plasma osmolality (i.e. total osmolality less the osmolality due to the urea content); if it is not possible to estimate the plasma osmolality the concentration of sodium is a less exact but useful substitute. The weight should fall gently while the plasma osmolality or sodium concentration should not change. Unfortunately, the patient's persistent thirst is no guide to his needs.

CONTROL OF ELECTROLYTE INTAKE. Following any initial replacement that may be necessary the further ingestion or administration of electrolytes (except for calcium) must be prevented.

The plasma concentration of potassium should be kept below 7 mEq/l. Some authorities have suggested that this can be done by the intravenous administration of calcium gluconate and insulin (50 units per day) throughout the 24 hours. The latter, in association with a high glucose intake (see below), tends to draw the potassium into the cells and so lower plasma potassium. This is certainly true on a short-term basis, but it is impractical over a prolonged period. Resins in the sodium phase or preferably in the calcium phase are used to lower plasma potassium; the dose is 15 g two to four times a day orally, or 60 g as a retention enema. The most satisfactory way to lower plasma potassium temporarily in an emergency is to give 200 ml of molar sodium lactate intravenously in three hours. The rise in extracellular pH induces a compensating shift of hydrogen ions from the intracellular compartment and this in turn causes potassium to pass from the extracellular space *into* the cells.

The fall in plasma sodium and chloride should be treated by limiting the fluid intake for, unless there is a very clear indication of sodium and chloride loss before the onset of renal failure, its administration in order to correct plasma concentrations is potentially dangerous. This also applies to any attempt to correct the acidosis by giving sodium bicarbonate or sodium lactate, for the dangers of expanding the extracellular fluid volume and causing cardiac failure are greater than any benefit gained by a transient change in pH.

CONTROL OF PROTEIN, CARBOHYDRATE AND FAT INTAKE. It is obvious that protein intake should be controlled. Nevertheless a protein-free diet is repugnant. In addition, it has been shown that if the carbohydrate intake can be maintained at a high level (around 200 g per day) 20–40 g of protein per day will not influence the rate of rise of blood urea; and the patient feels much better. The additional potassium intake which this involves can easily be controlled with resins.

Carbohydrates should be free of electrolytes. They are given to slow the rate of endogenous protein breakdown and minimise the rise in plasma potassium concentration (see above). 100 g of carbohydrate per day will reduce endogenous protein breakdown by 50 per cent. Additional amounts up to 400 g per day will further reduce protein breakdown. If the patient can be fed orally the aim is to give as much carbohydrate as can be tolerated. The use of Hycal (Beecham) which contains 400 calories of carbohydrate as disaccharides and dextrose in 180 ml of water is of enormous help, and most patients find this palatable. Caloreen, a soluble glucose polymer, is a useful alternative for patients who find Hycal unpalatable. Anabolic steroids (Nilevar, 16-Ethyl-19-*nor* testosterone or Durabolin, 19-*nor* testosterone-17β phenyl propionate) are sometimes used to delay protein breakdown particularly in obstetric cases.

Fats have a "protein-sparing" effect and can, theoretically, be used instead of, or in combination with carbohydrates. They can be given in relatively large amounts intravenously. Their administration in large amounts by stomach tube is apt to cause diarrhoea.

Administration of water and carbohydrates intravenously

If the patient cannot eat it is necessary to introduce water and carbohydrate requirements intravenously.

PERIPHERAL VEIN. An isotonic solution of glucose is one of 5 per cent; if concentrations of 10–15 per cent are given into a peripheral vein, pain and thromboses are apt to occur after about 6–10 hours, If the patient has many easily accessible veins an attempt can be made to give a 15 per cent solution by changing the site of the intravenous needle at about 8-hourly intervals. In this way thrombosis may be avoided and a continuous administration maintained. If the veins are "poor" then it is unwise to give a concentration greater than 10 per cent, and even with this concentration the veins are more likely to remain patent if the site of the needle is changed at least once a day. Pain and swelling over the vein can sometimes be controlled by placing 10 mg of hydrocortisone in approximately each litre of infusing fluid, and clotting in the needle can be prevented by adding 1,000 units heparin.

It is most unusual to be able to give 100 g glucose per day into a peripheral vein at these high concentrations. When difficulties occur the attempt to give glucose is sacrificed to the need to keep the water intake within the bound described above, and the concentration of the infusions are lowered.

CENTRAL VEIN. Glucose concentrations as high as 50 per cent can be infused intravenously through an indwelling polythene tube placed into the inferior vena cava via a saphenous vein, for the 0·2–0·5 ml per min. of glucose solution is diluted in 2–3 litres of blood. This technique needs the least supervision and causes little overt trouble at the site of the infusion; if heparin (1,000 units per litre) is placed in the solution the tube does not become clotted; the rate of flow is always easily controlled and has no sudden fluctuations; the patient has both arms free and is not subject to recurrent needle punctures and tender veins. Nevertheless, there is one serious complication. A thrombus may form at the saphenous vein incision and spread up through the common iliac vein into the inferior vena cava. There have been some fatalities from pulmonary emboli in patients who have recovered from the renal failure.

CONTROL OF NAUSEA AND VOMITING. These may sometimes be controlled with thiethylperazime preferably by injection.

CONTROL OF ANAEMIA. It is usually inadvisable to try to treat the progressive anaemia by transfusions, for the risk of inducing cardiac failure is very great.

CONTROL OF INFECTION. The likelihood of infection is so great that some centres now treat all patients with acute renal failure in isolation. Antibiotics are not given unless an infection develops. It must be remembered that if the antibiotic that is used is one that is usually eliminated in large amounts in the urine, e.g. streptomycin, it may be dangerous, after the initial loading dose, to give more than small maintenance doses.

Therapeutic measures to avoid

The frustration of seeing a patient gradually dying from acute renal failure, who may have been recently saved from death by an emergency operation, has in the past prompted the use of certain useless and dangerous measures. They are enumerated here, so that their eventual eclipse may be hastened.

(1) The intravenous administration of large volumes of osmotic diuretics or the attempt to force a diuresis by overexpansion of the extracellular fluid space with large quantities of intravenous saline; these will almost certainly cause cardiac failure.
(2) Encouraging the patient to drink large quantities of water while giving 5 per cent glucose intravenously; this causes water intoxication, and pulmonary congestion.
(3) Renal decapsulation and paravertebral block; the trauma of the first procedure hastens the rise in blood urea, while the second may cause hypotension.

None of these measures is beneficial; some are lethal.

Dialysis

Peritoneal dialysis. Now that industry has made available a sterile disposable catheter, and that dialysing solutions for peritoneal dialysis are also available commercially, together with disposable sterile connections, peritoneal dialysis is a relatively simple and safe procedure. The catheter should be placed under aseptic conditions, into the peritoneal cavity in the direction of the pelvis, and a strict aseptic discipline instilled into all those concerned with the dialysis. There are a variety of ways the dialysis can be carried out. There is no doubt that the most convenient is to use a commercially available automatic machine that cycles the dialysis fluid it has warmed into and out of the peritoneal cavity from large prepacked sterile reservoirs. In this way the risks of sepsis are negligible and dialysis can continue for many days and nights without interruption. It is also remarkable that with such a machine the patient can easily be looked after in a general ward without having to have one person continuously at the bedside. There is the added advantage that it is practicable to cycle as little as 1 litre of dialysis fluid, and this can be done about four times an hour. This small quantity in the peritoneal cavity is usually easily acceptable to the patient.

In the absence of an automatic machine the following manual technique has been found useful. Dialysis only takes place from 6 a.m. to 10 p.m.—during the night the peritoneal catheter is left *in situ* but disconnected after clamping. Two litres of a dialysing solution is run in and then as much more as the patient will tolerate, usually not much more than another 2 litres. The fluid is then allowed to run out again immediately until 2 litres has been evacuated. Two more litres are immediately run in and then out again. In this way dialysis takes place continuously for there is always some fluid in the peritoneal cavity. The number of exchanges is usually around one to two per hour. As the fluid is always moving through the connecting tubes the risk of clotting and fibrinous obstruction is greatly diminished. Nevertheless, it is wise to put 500 units of heparin in each of the first two or three exchanges.

The osmolality of commercial dialysis fluid is either near that of plasma or stronger. If it is necessary to remove oedema fluid or there is some difficulty in getting the dialysis fluid to flow out of the peritoneum the stronger solution is used. If possible the patient should be sat up out of bed for a few hours during the day, without interrupting the dialysis, for otherwise the danger of pulmonary collapse at the lung bases with subsequent infection is considerable. All patients lose some protein and amino acids into the dialysis fluid, some lose a great deal. This can be monitored to a certain extent by twice daily haematocrit and frequent estimations of plasma protein concentration, in addition to keeping a watch on the blood pressure and the heart rate. Sometimes it is worth collecting all the dialysis fluid which has been used in a day in one large container and measuring its protein content. Protein loss can be made up by the intravenous administration of suitable quantities of plasma, and by giving a high protein diet, e.g. five eggs per day. The risk of sepsis depends a great deal on how long the

catheter is kept *in situ* and whether the dialysis is being performed automatically
or manually. With the manual technique the rate of infection rises steeply after
36 hours. It is useless to place antibiotics prophylactically into the peritoneal
fluid. If a "mid-stream" sample of the fluid coming from the patient is cultured
once a day, an infection can be treated with the appropriate antibiotic directly

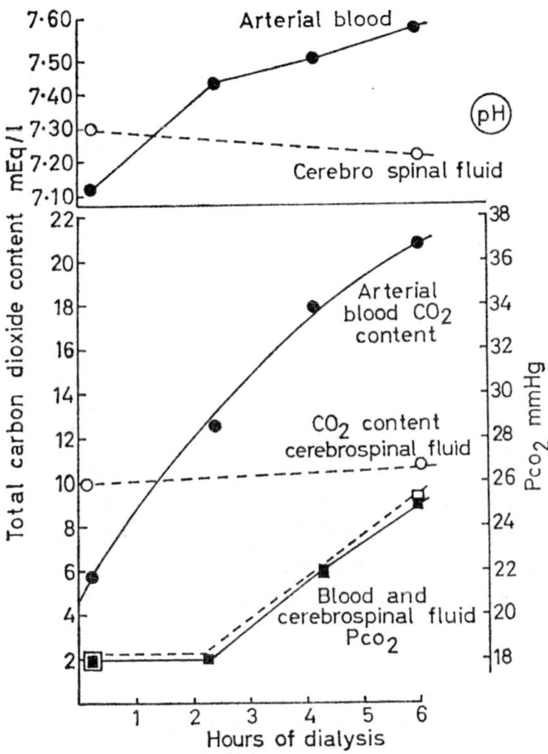

FIG. 14.4. Changes in pH, total CO_2 content of arterial blood and cerebro-spinal fluid
brought about by haemodialysis. (Lambie, Anderton and Robson, 1964, Blackwell
Scientific, Oxford.)

into the peritoneal cavity; and systemically. Some patients, particularly men
who have 2 litre exchanges, suffer much discomfort during peritoneal dialysis.
Considerable quantities of analgesics may have to be given, and in these patients
the risk of pulmonary collapse and infection are particularly great. Dialysates
with a sodium concentration of 130 mEq/l instead of the usual 140 mEq/l
makes control of the hypertension easier.

HAEMODIALYSIS. The main use of haemodialysis is in the treatment of patients
whose kidneys have failed beyond hope of recovery. Its use in acute renal failure
has diminished greatly since the introduction of peritoneal dialysis.

There are many types of artificial kidneys. All of them are suitable for the
treatment of acute renal failure. If such a machine is used sporadically, it is

best to use one that has disposable sterile components, even if they are expensive. The purpose of an artificial kidney is to pass the patient's blood on one side of a semi-permeable cellophane type membrane while a dialysing fluid is passed on the other.

One useful dialysing fluid consists of Na^+130, K^+1, Cl^-90, $acetate^-35$, $Ca^{++}2.5$, $Mg^{++}1$, mEq/l, glucose 200 mg 100/ml. (As acetate is metabolised to bicarbonate, its use greatly simplifies the technical preparation of the dialysing fluid.) The blood gradually equilibrates with the dialysing fluid and the patient should feel better. It is important to note, however, that if this process of equilibration takes place too quickly the patient may have severe headaches, vomiting, fits and become unconscious. This is due to the fact that during the dialysis the changes in the content of urea and bicarbonate in the brain lag behind those in the blood. This causes two cerebral disturbances. The first is due to the content of urea in the brain becoming higher than in the blood. This causes an osmotic gradient. Water diffuses into the brain and there is cerebral oedema. The second is due to the brain bicarbonate rising more slowly than the blood bicarbonate. The rise in blood bicarbonate is associated with a reduction in ventilation and a rise in blood $P{co}_2$ towards normal. As CO_2 is readily diffusible, $P{co}_2$ in the cerebrospinal fluid rises at the same rate as in the blood. In the cerebrospinal fluid, however, there is now a relatively unchanged low bicarbonate but a rising $P{co}_2$, with the result that the already low pH falls to even lower levels (Fig. 14.4). These complications are avoided by not allowing the patient to become too ill before dialysis is begun, by dialysing more slowly, or by dialysing for short periods at frequent intervals. Excess fluid is removed from the patient by having the dialysis fluid in the artificial kidney at a negative pressure, so that water is sucked across the cellophane by ultra-filtration. During dialysis the patient has to be heparinised. If he has recently had a surgical operation, or an accident the heparin will have to be given with great care. The simplest way is to give a small continuous infusion into the blood just as it leaves the patient to enter the artificial kidney. The dose is adjusted so that it keeps the artificial kidney from clotting but is insufficient to cause any important change in the patient's clotting time. Alternatively, heparin is given in the same place but protamine is given into the blood just before it returns to the patient. This is supposed to neutralise the heparin. It is a technique known as regional heparinisation. It is a cumbersome manoeuvre which has little to commend it; it is rarely as satisfactory as the one mentioned above.

Indications for dialysis

It has been established that the higher the blood urea rises, the worse the prognosis, and if the blood urea is allowed to rise above 300 mg/100 ml the patient may have a fatal haemorrhage, either into the pericardium or gastro-intestinal tract. One important indication for dialysis therefore is a blood urea nearing 300 mg/100 ml. As changes usually occur at a uniform rate, it is a fair assumption to extrapolate into the near future from the immediate past, and it is thus possible to anticipate events. Some consider that the blood urea should not be allowed to rise above 200 mg/100 ml. Another indication is a rise in plasma potassium to 7 mEq/l despite other forms of treatment (e.g. resins). A plasma bicarbonate below 10 mEq/l severe acidotic respiration, increasing stupor, confusion or coma are also indications but will rarely be present before the ones already mentioned. There is now an increasing tendency to dialyse early in order to prevent gross changes in the composition of the extracellular fluid from developing.

The artificial kidney is used only in those patients in whom the rate of rise in blood urea or plasma potassium is so great that peritoneal dialysis has either been shown to be inadequate or is likely to be difficult. The first is particularly the case when acute renal failure is associated with multiple injuries in a young man, or when an infection develops; the second when there are abdominal injuries. About 8–12 hours each day, depending on the dialysing capacity of the kidney, should maintain a stable blood urea in most patients.

A tremendous advantage of dialysis, peritoneal or with an artificial kidney (particularly with a Scribner shunt in position), is that if dialyses are performed each day, dietary restrictions are unnecessary and there is no need for fluid restriction. This improves the patient's morale and his physical condition and probably reduces the length of convalescence.

Treatment of the Diuretic Phase

With conservative treatment it is vital that the strict regimen of the oliguric phase should be continued until the blood urea begins to fall. Frequently a partial recovery with a daily urine volume of about 700 ml may progress no further for several days; it is imperative that during this time treatment should not be relaxed.

Once the diuretic phase begins the dangers to look out for and correct are water depletion, salt loss and potassium loss. It has become clear that much of the polyuria which these patients experience is often only the evacuation of excess extracellular fluid, and attempts to replace it only prolong the diuretic phase and may lead to overhydration. An exact replacement should not, therefore, be attempted unless there is evidence of need. It is more important to be guided by the patient's general condition, pulse rate, blood pressure, thirst and plasma electrolyte content than by the urine volume and its content. Intravenous therapy and dialysis are stopped unless there is nausea, vomiting, confusion or coma. The patient is encouraged to eat a high potassium, high salt diet, and given easy access to large amounts of water.

PROGNOSIS

The prognosis of acute renal failure depends on the initiating cause and its associated circumstances (e.g. multiple injuries), the severity of the renal lesion and the efficiency of treatment. It is fair to say, however, that whereas there was a mortality of about 90 per cent before the introduction of conservative treatment and artificial dialysis, it is now nearing 40 per cent. In obstetric and medical cases the mortality is rather less than 15 per cent whereas in surgical cases it is usually greater than 50 per cent. In some of the most advanced centres, however, the mortality in surgical cases has been brought down to between 10 and 30 per cent. Twenty per cent of all deaths are due to infection, and it contributes significantly in another 60 per cent.

BIBLIOGRAPHY

BALSLOV, J. T., and JØRGENSEN, H. E. (1963). "A survey of 499 patients with acute anuric insufficiency. Causes, treatment, and mortality." *Amer. J. Med.*, **34**, 753.

BANK, M., MUTZ, B. P., and AYNEDJIAN, H. S. (1967). "The role of leakage of tubular fluid in anuria due to mercury poisoning." *J. clin. Invest.*, **46**, 695.

BOEN, S. T. (1964). "Peritoneal dialysis in clinical medicine." Charles C. Thomas, Springfield, Ill.

BROWN, J. J., GLEADLE, R. I., LAWSON, D. H., LEVER, A. F., LINTON, A. F., MACADAM, R. F., PRENTICE, E., ROBERTSON, J. I. F., and TREE, M. (1970). "Renin and acute renal failure. A study in man." *Brit. Med. J.*, **1**, 253.

CLARKSON, A. R., MacDONALD, M. K., FUSTER, V., CASH, J. D., and ROBSON, J. S. (1970). "Glomerular coagulation in acute ischaemic renal failure." *Quart. J. Med.*, **39**, 585.

COWIE, J., LAMBIE, A. T., and ROBSON, J. S., (1962). "The influence of extracorporeal dialysis on the acid-base composition of blood and cerebrospinal fluid." *Clin. Sci.*, **23**, 397.

DALGAARD, O. Z., and PEDERSEN, K. J. (1969). "Renal tubular degeneration. Electron microscopy in ischaemic anuria." *Lancet*, **2**, 484.

ELIAHOU, H. E., and BATES, A. (1965). "The diagnosis of acute renal failure." *Nephron*, **2**, 287.

GRANDCHAMP, A., VEYRAT, R., ROSSET, E., SCHERRER, J. R., and TRUNIGER, B. (1971). "Relation between renin and intrarenal haemodynamics in haemorrhagic hypotension." *J. clin. Invest.*, **50**, 970.

JACKSON, R. C. (1970). "Exercise-induced renal failure and muscle damage." *Proceedings of the Royal Society of Medicine*, **63**, 566.

KAPLAN, S. A., and FOMON, S. J. (1953). "Function recovery pattern in acute renal failure following ingestion of mercuric chloride." *Amer. J. Dis. Child.*, **85**, 633.

LIEBERMAN, E., HEUSER, E., DONNELL, G. H., LANDING, B. H., and HAMMOND, G. D. (1966). "Haemolytic-uremic syndrome." *New Eng. J. Med.*, **275**, 228.

LOWE, K. G. (1952). "The late prognosis in acute tubular necrosis." *Lancet*, **1**, 1086.

MUEHRCKE, R. C., and MOSBY, C. V. (1969). "Acute Renal Failure. Diagnosis and Management." Henry Kimpton, St Louis, U.S.A.

MUNCK, O. (1958). "Renal Circulation in Acute Renal Failure." Blackwell Scientific Pubs., Oxford.

OLIVER, J. (1953). "Correlations of structure and function and mechanisms of recovery in acute tubular necrosis." *Amer. J. Med.*, **15**, 535.

OLIVER, J., MacDOWELL, M., and TRACY, A. (1951). "The pathogenesis of acute renal failure associated with traumatic and toxic injury; renal ischaemia, nephrotoxic damage, and the ischaemuric episode." *J. clin. Invest.*, **30**, 1305.

SAVITT, L. H., EVANS, D. J., and WRONG, O. M. (1971). "Acute oliguria renal failure due to accelerated malignant hypertension." *Quart. J. Med.*, **40**, 127.

SAXTON, H. M., KILPATRICK, F. R., KINDER, C. H., LESSOF, M. H., HARDY-YOUNG, S. Mc., and WARDLE, D. F. F. (1969). "Retroperitoneal fibrosis. A radiological and follow up study of 14 cases." *Quart. J. Med.*, **38**, 158.

SHACKMAN, R., and KULATILAKE, A. E. (1971). "Surgical aspects of acute renal failure." *Brit. Med. Bulletin*, **27**, 97.

SHEEHAN, H. L., and MOORE, H. C. (1953). "Renal cortical necrosis and the kidney of concealed accidental haemorrhage." Blackwell Scientific Pubs., Oxford.

SHUBIN, H., and WEIL, M. H. (1965). "The mechanism of shock following suicidal doses of barbiturates, narcotics and tranquillizer drugs, with observations on the effects of treatment." *Amer. J. Med.*, **38**, 853.

SWANN, R. C., and MERRILL, J. P. (1953). "The clinical course of acute renal failure." *Medicine*, **32**, 215.

THIEL, G., McDONALD, M. D., and OKEN, D. E. (1970). "Micropuncture studies of the basis for the protection of renin depleted rats from glycerol induced renal failure." *Nephron*, **1**, 67.

WARDENER, DE, H. E. (1955). "The intrarenal pressure in experimental tubular necrosis." *Lancet*, **1**, 580.

WOLTHUIS, F. H. (1961). "Balance studies on protein metabolism in normal and uraemic men. Effect of diet, bed rest and anabolic steroids." *Acta med. Scand.*, Sppl. 373.

WRONG, O. (1971). "Management of the acute ureamic emergency." *Brit. Med. Bulletin*, **27**, 97.

15

Chronic Renal Failure

Chronic renal failure consists of a persistent impairment of both glomerular and tubular function of gradual onset and of such severity that the kidneys are no longer able to keep the internal environment normal. This definition includes mild asymptomatic functional impairment, which is sometimes called "chronic renal impairment".

Chronic renal failure follows a great number of conditions which devastate the kidney. Its clinical features, however, are remarkably uniform, for usually renal failure is simply due to a deficiency of nephrons, and a fairly fixed combination of disturbances is inevitable. It is in fact the exceptions to this recurring pattern which cause curiosity for example, when the blood pressure has never been raised, and yet at autopsy the kidneys are found to be small and fibrous.

There are certain selective disturbances of tubular function in which initially there is little or no evidence of a decline in the number of nephrons. These syndromes are usually named after the particular disturbance of tubular function involved, i.e. familial nephrogenic diabetes insipidus; they are discussed elsewhere (p. 230).

Causes of Chronic Renal Failure

1. Destructive Diseases due to Some Immunological Disturbance
    Glomerular nephritis.
    Polyarteritis nodosa.
    Disseminated lupus erythematosus.
    Subacute bacterial endocarditis.
    Anaphylactoid purpura.

2. Infection
    Pyelonephritis.
    Tuberculosis.

3. Obstruction to the Urinary Tract
    Prostatic obstruction.
    Bilateral calculi.
    Urethral valves, etc.

4. Congenital Lesions
    Polycystic disease.
    Tubular abnormalities (final stages).

5. HYPERTENSION
>   Malignant.
>   Non-malignant.

6. OTHERS
>   Phenacetin nephropathy.
>   Amyloid.
>   Gout.
>   Diabetic nephropathy.
>   Hypercalcaemia.
>   Chronic intermittent haemoglobinuria: (i) sickle cell; (ii) nocturnal.
>   Renal vein thrombosis.
>   Myelomatosis.
>   Radiation damage.
>   Any other renal diseases which eventually destroy the nephrons, e.g.
>   tubular changes associated with metallic cation loss.

Chronic renal failure is characterised by a wide variety of biochemical disturbances and numerous clinical signs and symptoms. It is one of the outstanding peculiarities of chronic renal failure that some of the biochemical abnormalities do not cause any symptoms, while most of the clinical abnormalities have no known biochemical cause.

The following account of chronic renal failure is divided into two parts. The first describes the biochemical abnormalities which have been identified and the clinical manifestations which they cause; the second describes the many clinical features of unknown cause.

Biochemical Features and their Clinical Manifestations

Water metabolism

Thirst and nocturia occur frequently, polyuria is less common. The symptoms are due to a diminished capacity to concentrate the urine and to a loss of the normal diurnal rhythm of urinary excretion. Often the ability to make the urine hypotonic remains for some time after the ability to concentrate has almost disappeared; later the urine concentration remains fixed at the same osmolality as plasma, a phenomenon known as isosthenuria.

Though inability to make the urine hypertonic may be due in part to a diminished functional capacity of the nephrons which remain, it is mainly due to an increased rate of solute excretion per nephron. This is an explanation which has been advanced earlier (p. 61) but which can be elaborated here. It is evident that in chronic renal failure the total solute output remains almost unchanged, for the patient is usually in normal electrolyte and water balance, and yet nearly always there is a considerable reduction in the number of functioning nephrons. It follows, therefore, that each surviving nephron must be handling much larger quantities of solutes and water than normally. This is a situation similar to that obtaining in each nephron of a dehydrated normal person who has been given a large quantity of a solute, such as sucrose, mannitol or urea which is then promptly excreted in the urine: the rate of solute excreted per nephron increases, and there is a concomitant rise in urine flow and *fall in urine concentration*, i.e. there is an osmotic diuresis (p. 60). There is now increasing evidence that the impaired ability to concentrate the urine in chronic renal failure is mainly due to an osmotic diuresis. It follows that this apparent impairment is not an indication of diseased nephrons but of a deficiency of nephrons.

In chronic renal failure there is frequently an increased turnover of water and the ability to dilute the urine remains normal or better than normal for a considerable time. But there is diminished ability to excrete a water load rapidly. This occurs before, as well as after, the ability to make the urine hypotonic has disappeared. When it is present before, it is presumably due to the diminished number of nephrons, for even if each nephron forms a hypotonic urine at a normal rate there is an insufficient number to increase the total urine flow adequately. This is the reason why polyuria is never gross in chronic renal failure and seldom exceeds 3–4 l/24 hours, in contrast to the 8–10 litres found in diabetes insipidus, or compulsive polydipsia. When the kidneys can no longer form a hypotonic urine the inability to excrete a water load is easier to understand.

These disturbances make patients suffering from chronic renal failure vulnerable to acute changes in water balance. Diarrhoea and vomiting may quickly cause severe dehydration, for the output of water and salt does not drop as sharply as in the normal; conversely, an impetuous intravenous administration of water (5 per cent glucose) may cause overhydration. Sometimes slight nausea with a distaste for eating and drinking is sufficient to cause dehydration, when a vicious circle of increasing renal failure, more pronounced nausea, and further dehydration then occurs.

Sodium metabolism

It has already been pointed out that as the nephron population diminishes each remaining nephron reabsorbs less salt (p. 139) so that the patient remains in sodium balance. The mechanism responsible for this phenomenon is not clear. It is certainly not due simply to a convenient deterioration of function of those nephrons that remain, for often urinary sodium excretion can be altered by changing the dietary salt intake, and by heart failure or haemorrhage. As renal failure advances, however, disturbances of sodium balance may occur. The ability to adjust to sudden changes in salt and water loss becomes progressively less efficient. An attack of diarrhoea or an acute spell of anorexia and vomiting do not cause a compensatory reduction in urinary sodium output. There is instead a continued urinary loss of sodium and water, a contraction of the extracellular fluid volume, an intense renal vasoconstriction and thus a severe deterioration of renal function. This sudden sequence of gross changes is easily recognised. It may cause death.

An insidious change in sodium balance, however, is more common but is usually far more difficult to discern. For instance a gradual retention of sodium without oedema is the main cause of the hypertension which so often complicates chronic renal failure (p. 140). On the other hand there may be a very slowly progressive urinary loss of sodium. This causes a reduction of extracellular fluid volume and a very gradual reduction of renal function. A mild negative

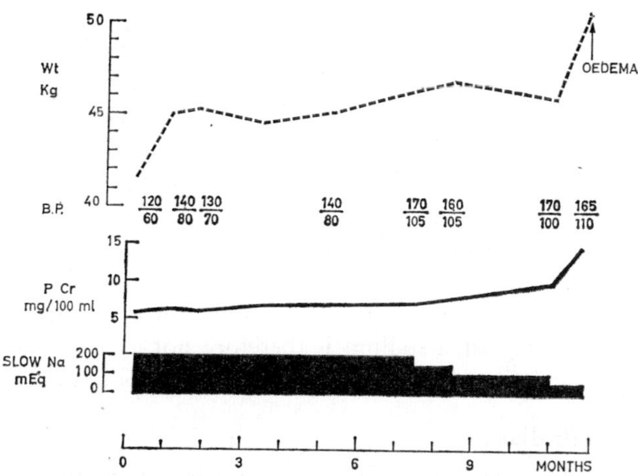

FIG. 15.1. Changes in weight and blood pressure in a patient with chronic renal failure and a sodium leak. Terminally the blood pressure and the weight rose though the sodium supplements were diminished.

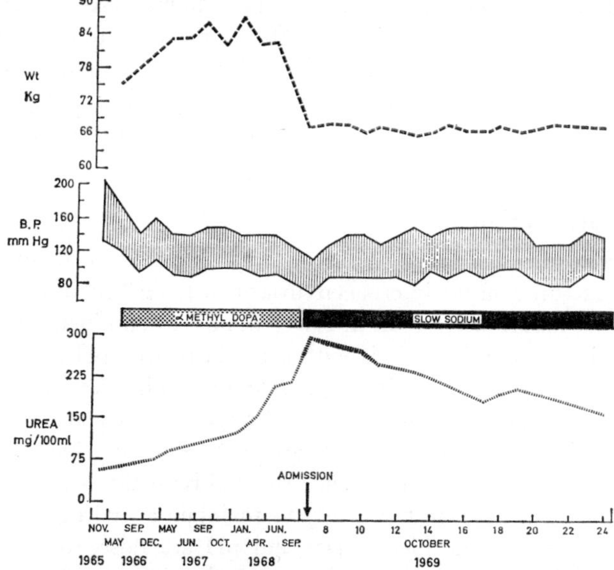

FIG. 15.2. Weight and blood pressure in a patient with chronic renal failure. At first the patient needed methyl dopa to control hypertension. The patient then developed a sodium leak and needed supplemental sodium to control hypotension.

sodium balance in chronic renal failure is associated with an increased secretion of aldosterone, a tendency to a low plasma potassium, and a normal blood pressure. It is, in fact, a useful generalisation that if a patient with advanced renal failure has a normal blood pressure he probably has a urinary sodium leak. More severe urinary sodium leaks which give rise to severe sodium deficiency cause hypotension, rapidly advancing renal failure, thirst and anorexia The syndrome is then called "salt losing nephritis". Patients with urinary sodium leaks often have polyruria. The diseases which tend to cause this syndrome include phenacetin nephropathy, polycystic kidneys, chronic urinary obstruction, and very occasionally chronic childhood pyelonephritis, but only when the urine is infected. Disturbances of sodium metabolism are best detected clinically along the lines outlined above. Some patients may slide from a state of sodium retention to one of urinary sodium leak or vice versa (Figs. 15.1 and 15.2). It is of the utmost importance to be aware of this possibility for the treatment of the two conditions is diametrically opposed. It must be stressed that disturbances of sodium metabolism are poorly reflected by changes in the concentration of plasma sodium which more often reflect changes in hydration. The concentration of plasma sodium is therefore not a safe guide to the size of the extracellular fluid volume, or the exchangeable sodium.

Potassium metabolism

Disturbances of potassium balance occur less frequently than those of sodium. Though a few patients tend to have a urinary potassium leak, hypokalaemia is usually due to an excess of faecal potassium loss due to a high aldosterone secretion secondary to a urinary sodium leak (see above). It is more usual to find that as chronic renal failure becomes terminal there tends to be potassium retention and hyperkalaemia. This may be aggravated iatrogenically by prescribing (1) potassium citrate for a urinary infection, (2) a potassium-diuretic combination for oedema, or (3) the potassium retaining diuretic spironolactone.

Hydrogen ion metabolism

On a normal diet the kidney has to excrete about 40 to 60 mEq a day of hydrogen ions to prevent the internal environment from becoming acid (p. 69). In chronic renal failure there is an impaired ability to eliminate hydrogen ions which results in a systemic acidosis with a fall in plasma pH and bicarbonate. This is due to (1) a reduced ability to excrete ammonia presumably caused by the diminished number of nephrons, and (2) a reduced titratable acid excretion because of a diminished excretion of buffer phosphate, mainly due to a diminished intake and absorption of phosphate. The urine pH is usually below 5·0 and there is therefore no impairment in the ability to maintain a hydrogen ion gradient. Nevertheless, if the plasma bicarbonate and pH are raised to normal by an intravenous infusion of sodium bicarbonate or lactate, and the patient is observed thereafter as he returns to his original acidotic state, it is evident that the urine pH does not fall in a normal manner. In some patients the urine pH does not fall below 5·0 until the plasma bicarbonate is less than 20 mEq/l whereas in a normal individual the urine pH falls below 5·0 when the plasma bicarbonate is less than 24 mEq/l. It is apparent that in chronic renal failure, therefore, the ability to acidify the urine in response to a standard rise in plasma hydrogen ion concentration is in fact below normal. This is due to the nephrons impaired ability to reabsorb bicarbonate which in turn is due to their reduced ability to secrete hydrogen ions and this stems partly from their reduced number but principally from the increased concentration of circulating parathyroid hormone. This phenomenon is sometimes known as bicarbonate wastage or leak.

The most remarkable phenomenon about hydrogen ion metabolism in chronic renal failure is that though the plasma bicarbonate and pH may be depressed, the plasma concentration of these two substances may remain at the same level for many weeks or months. Or in other words, though the patient can only get rid of a fraction of the hydrogen ions he is producing each day, and he is thus in positive hydrogen ion balance, the plasma *does not become increasingly* acidotic. The probable explanation is that the hydrogen ions are being neutralised by calcium carbonate and other calcium buffers in bone.

Kussmaul respiration is the only clinical feature which is undoubtedly due to the acidosis; its severity is determined as much by the rate of fall in pH as by the extent of its reduction. There is also increasing evidence that at least part of the bone changes in chronic renal failure are due to the retention of hydrogen ions. In addition there is a considerable list of signs and symptoms, particularly of the alimentary and central nervous systems, which it is considered may possibly be caused by the acidosis. It is also possible, however, that the pharmacological actions of the unidentified "renal failure anions" are responsible. These clinical disturbances are discussed below.

Calcium metabolism

The disturbances to calcium metabolism in chronic renal failure are multiple. Urinary calcium excretion falls to very low values (10 mg/day or less) and there is little or no calcium absorbed from the gut. Calcium balance therefore is relatively normal. Plasma calcium is either normal or low.

Patients who have suffered from chronic renal failure for several years tend to develop osteomalacia in adults (or rickets in children), hyperparathyroidism, metastatic calcification, and osteosclerosis. Hyperparathyroidism gives rise to the histological and radiological appearances known sometimes as osteitis fibrosis. Soft tissue metastatic calcification may cause tenderness of those muscles in which the calcification has occurred; or it may manifest itself as pseudo-gout. This is an acute arthritis indistinguishable from hyperuricaemic gout but which is due, in this instance, to precipitation of calcium phosphate in the synovial fluid. Histologically, osteomalacia, hyperparathyroidism and osteosclerosis are usually present at the same time though one may be more

G

prominent. The overall effect is one of decalcification. It is not known whether this apparent decalcification is due to negative calcium balance or to redistribution of calcium within the bone; it is probably the latter.

Fig. 15.3 illustrates some of the possible mechanisms responsible for these abnormalities. The retention of phosphate, due to the reduction in glomerular filtration rate, raises the plasma phosphate. This rise tends to lower the plasma calcium, but it raises the product $P_{CA} \times P_P$ (plasma calcium $\times$ plasma phosphate).

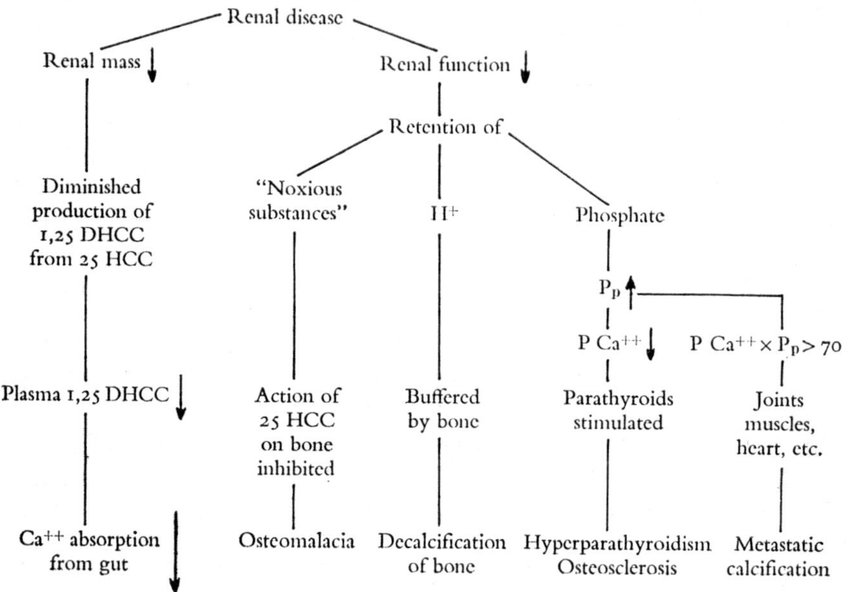

FIG. 15.3. Schema of mechanisms involved in the aetiology of the various disturbances of calcium and phosphate metabolism in chronic renal failure. 1,25 DHCC=1,25 dihydroxycholecalciferol; 25 HCC=25 hydroxycholecalciferol. (de Wardener, 1972, *The Scientific Basis of Medicine Annual Reviews*, Athlone Press.)

If this product rises above 70, metastatic calcification will occur. The retention of phosphate stimulates parathormone secretion (Fig. 15.4), perhaps by transiently lowering the plasma ionised calcium. The raised concentration of parathormone causes osteitis fibrosis and paradoxically also the osteosclerosis. Hyperparathyroidism, however, increases phosphate excretion which tends to return the plasma phosphate towards normal. All four parathyroid glands enlarge, occasionally one becomes adenomatous. In addition, the retained hydrogen ions are buffered in the bone which diminishes the bone's content of carbonate. This may exaggerate the redistribution of osseous calcium.

Renal osteomalacia is due to the retention of some unidentified substance which prevents 25 hydroxycholicalciferol (25 HCC) and other metabolites of vitamin D from acting on the bone. This phenomenon is sometimes known as vitamin D resistance, for the plasma concentration of 25 HCC in chronic renal failure is normal, and the osteomalacia can be cured by the administration of very large doses of vitamin D. There is also some fragmentary evidence that the phenomenon of vitamin D resistance may also affect the function of the

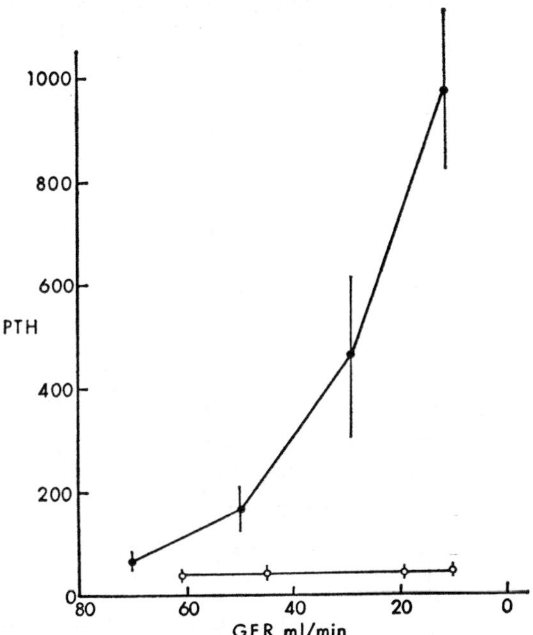

FIG. 15.4. The relationship between parathyroid hormone levels (PTH) and glomerular filtration rate (GFR) in two groups of dogs: those maintained on a diet containing 1200 mg of phosphorus per day (closed circles) and those on a diet containing less then 100 mg of phoshorus per day (open circles). The vertical lines represent $\pm$ S.E.M. PTH is expressed in arbitrary units. (Slatopolsky, Calgar, Pennell, Taggart, Canterbury, Reiss and Bricker, 1971, *J. clin. Invest.*)

parathyroid gland, and be another cause of increased parathyroid hormone secretion.

The diminution of calcium absorption from the gut is due, primarily, to a diminution in plasma 1,25-dihydroxycholecalciferol, a metabolite of vitamin D manufactured only in the kidney. The impaired absorption of calcium is also due, in part, to the tendency of patients with chronic renal failure to ingest only small quantities of dietary calcium (Fig. 15.5). Finally there is some evidence that the hypocalcaemia is due in part to "parathormone resistance" for it occurs in spite of high concentrations of circulating parathormone. Though parathormone levels may sometimes be astronomical the plasma concentration of calcium only rarely rises above normal.

Some patients avoid most of these abnormalities, there being no histological, radiological or clinical evidence of bone disease. In others there is only histological evidence of hyperparathyroidism which in a few, may eventually become radiologically evident. Osteomalacia is the least common abnormality. Clinically symptoms of bone disease are unusual and, except in children, occur very late in the sequence of events. There are vague aches and pains which are frequently disregarded as "rheumatism", or arthritis. Eventually adults may be disabled by the development of the characteristic, bilateral, symmetrical lesions

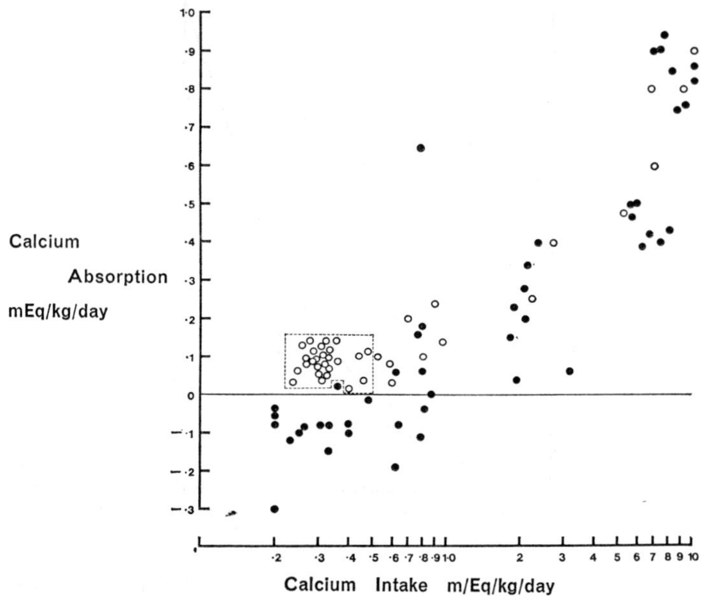

Fig. 15.5. Calcium absorption plotted against a wide range calcium intake in patients with chronic renal failure (●) and normal subjects (○). The normal intake of calcium varies from approximately 0·5 to 1·0 mEq kg day. (Clarkson, Eastwood, Koutsaimanis and de Wardener, 1973, *Kidney International.*

of osteomalacia; in children the classical deformities of rickets develop. Severe hypocalcaemia may cause tetany.

(It must be repeated that, though parathyroid hyperplasia occurs in chronic renal failure, the level of serum calcium is usually *below* normal, that normal levels are unusual, and that levels above 12 mg per 100 ml do not occur unless there is an adenoma of the parathyroid. When a high serum calcium coexists with renal failure the high calcium is not the result of the failure, it is usually its cause.)

Magnesium metabolism

Plasma magnesium and magnesium balance are normal in chronic renal failure whatever the creatinine clearance. There is reduced alimentary absorption and urinary excretion of magnesium due in part at least to the reduced intake of magnesium consequent upon increasing anorexia and medical advice. The ability to excrete a sudden load of magnesium, however, is severely impaired. The use of magnesium sulphate as a purgative may therefore be lethal. Some rise in plasma magnesium has also been claimed in patients taking magnesium trisilicate.

Phosphate metabolism

As glomerular filtration rate falls tubular reabsorption of phosphate also diminishes so that phosphate excretion remains unchanged. This is due in part to an increase in parathyroid hormone secretion which inhibits tubular reabsorption of phosphate. Plasma phosphate therefore does not rise until the creatinine clearance is approximately 10–20 ml/min, even then the rise is usually a modest one. This stability is also due in part to a fall in phosphate intake which accompanies a reduction of protein intake. Occasionally, however, particularly in patients who drink much milk, plasma phosphate may rise to more than 20 mg/100 ml. This may cause tissue calcification including acute arthritis from precipitation of calcium in the synovial fluid (pseudo-gout, see above).

Urea retention

The rise in blood urea is due to the diminished glomerular filtration rate. There is much evidence that urea itself is not responsible for any of the symptoms of renal failure; it has been shown that uraemic patients can be greatly improved by the use of an artificial kidney without necessarily changing the level of blood urea; and it is well known that in acute renal failure, where the blood urea rises to a plateau and then falls, the patient's general condition may be critical as the blood urea is rising, but that at an identical value a week later there may be a vast improvement.

Retention of other substances

It is well established that the longer the blood urea has been raised the greater the discrepancy between the plasma concentration of non-protein nitrogen and urea. This is due to a rise in the concentrations of uric acid, creatinine, phenol derivatives, amines and other nitrogenous metabolites of protein metabolism. Plasma uric acid does not rise until the creatinine clearance is less than 20 ml/min; very occasionally if the concentration rises above 10–15 mg/100 ml it may precipitate an acute attack of gout. The rise in plasma creatinine is not thought to produce any symptoms. The importance of the rise in plasma creatinine is that in advanced renal failure it is a far better guide to the extent of accumulation of toxic protein metabolites than is the level of blood urea. A blood urea of 100 mg/100 ml may be associated with plasma creatinine levels of 3 to 20 mg/ 100 ml depending mainly on the diet the patient is having, the duration of his illness and the glomerular filtration rate. A plasma creatinine of 3 mg/100 ml is of no immediate prognostic importance, whereas with a plasma creatinine of 20 mg/100 ml the patient may die within a few days from a gastro-intestinal haemorrhage, a haemorrhagic pericarditis or some other calamitous complication.

It has been claimed that the increased quantity of circulating phenols is responsible for some of the features of renal failure, such as lassitude, nausea and anaemia but there is no significant correlation between the blood concentrations of phenol and any particular symptom. The rise in amines is probably of more consequence.

There is also a retention of sulphate, some unidentified anions and urochromogen. The retention of sulphate and unidentified anions together with phosphate is responsible for the fact that as the serum bicarbonate falls with the increasing retention of hydrogen ions there is no compensatory rise in plasma chloride; there may even be a fall. This is in contrast to what takes place in the tubular disorder sometimes known as "renal tubular acidosis" (p. 237) where there is hydrogen ion retention with little disturbance in glomerular filtration rate and therefore no retention of phosphates, etc. The fall in plasma bicarbonate which accompanies the accumulation of hydrogen ions is then associated with a compensatory rise in plasma chloride, i.e. hyperchloraemic acidosis.

The diminished excretion of urochromogen is one reason why the urine is pale, even in subjects without polyuria. Urochromogens are lipid soluble pigments which are therefore known as lipochromes. They darken in the sunlight. In chronic renal failure their deposition in the subcutaneous fat causes the characteristic dirty yellow pigmentation of uraemia. And this explains why some patients with chronic renal failure take on such a good tan in the summer and also why it remains relatively unchanged during the subsequent winter. It is not understood why some patients never become pigmented.

Anaemia

The anaemia in chronic renal failure is mainly due to a depression of bone marrow function (p. 115). This is directly related to the plasma creatinine and independent of the blood urea. Blood loss is not important except in advanced cases with a continuous slow leak from ulcers in the gastro-intestinal tract, or following a haematemesis or malaena. In the later stages of renal failure red cell life is shortened. This is directly related to the blood urea and will improve if the blood urea is lowered with a low protein diet.

If the haematocrit in a patient suffering from chronic renal failure and anaemia is suddenly raised by a transfusion there is a transient fall in glomerular filtration rate and rise in blood urea, due to a delay in the normal vasodilating response to a rise in haematocrit (p. 106). This sharp fall in glomerular filtration rate, which often takes place upon transfusing cases of renal failure, may sometimes be fatal if the presence of kidney disease is unsuspected and transfusions are continued until the haemoglobin is normal; the blood urea rises rapidly and the patient dies of acute renal failure. Nevertheless, as acute haemorrhage causes intense renal vasoconstriction, transfusions are occasionally inevitable; and when chronic anaemia is sufficiently severe to cause or contribute to the onset of cardiac failure, there will be an additional depression of renal function which may respond to small transfusions of packed cells.

Proteinuria and urinary cell content

Proteinuria is nearly always present in chronic renal failure, but the concentration of protein in the urine is no guide to the severity of the failure; there are even reports of advanced chronic renal failure without proteinuria. At first protein may appear intermittently and then only after standing in the upright posture. If a nephrotic syndrome has preceded the onset of renal failure the daily protein excretion will sometimes diminish as the glomerular filtration rate falls.

Granular casts and an excess number of red and white cells are also found. The characteristic though uncommon finding of advanced renal failure is the appearance of broad casts; evidence of dilated nephrons.

Clinical Features of Unknown Cause

Gastro-intestinal

The tongue in renal failure is classically described as being brown and dry. Though it is true that such an appearance is frequently seen, it is a change which is by no means confined to those suffering from renal failure. It may occur in any patient who breathes through his mouth, particularly if he has pyorrhoea and bleeding gums, and it is almost inevitable if he is also dehydrated and hyperpnoeic. A foul taste in the mouth is a frequent complaint in chronic renal failure and the patient may notice a taste of ammonia, particularly on waking due to the decomposition of urea.

The breath may smell of urine. This is characteristic of advanced renal failure and is sometimes the first sign to be noticed. It is not present in every case, and often when it has been confidently identified it turns out that the smell has originated from urine in the trousers of a patient with prostatic difficulties, whose blood urea is normal. A person with a normal blood urea but suffering from severe pyorrhoea may also have a uraemic breath.

Hiccough is almost invariably present in advanced chronic renal failure and may cause much fatigue and distress; it appears in episodic attacks of varying length and is usually brought on by eating and drinking.

Anorexia, nausea and vomiting are almost always present. They are often the most prominent and, occasionally, the only symptoms; they are responsible in part, for the extensive loss of weight of chronic renal failure. Nausea and retching may be particularly pronounced in the early morning. All severities of vomiting occur, from two to three times a day to an almost continuous series of painful retches; and both small and large quantities of fluid are brought up. Dehydration follows more or less rapidly and is due to a combination of circumstances which reinforce each other; there is a distaste for fluids by mouth, combined with a loss of fluid from the stomach and an inability to concentrate the urine, so that urine flow tends to remain high. Dehydration in turn causes a further reduction in renal blood flow and glomerular filtration rate, and these aggravate the renal failure so that anorexia, nausea and vomiting become worse.

Sometimes the first complaint is one of fullness after meals with or without vomiting. Such patients are often suspected of having some local stomach condition such as a peptic ulcer. This diagnosis is even more likely to be considered if the patient first appears with a severe gastro-intestinal haemorrhage. Haematemesis and melaena are most frequent towards the terminal phase of renal failure and should not therefore cause any confusion, for by this time the presence of renal failure is usually known. Nevertheless, it is remarkable how often renal failure may progress to an advanced state before the patient decides, or is forced by circumstances, to see a doctor. Gastro-intestinal haemorrhages are due to a combination of increased capillary fragility and local ulceration; the latter is particularly pronounced in the large bowel. The effect of haemorrhage in chronic renal failure is extremely serious, for the accompanying renal vasoconstriction and fall in blood pressure lower the glomerular filtration rate even further and cause a precipitous rise in blood urea. When the haemorrhage is from the gastro-intestinal tract, some of the blood is digested and absorbed so that there is a large ingestion of protein at a time of diminishing renal function.

Constipation is common, but occasionally severe diarrhoea may occur and may quickly cause death from dehydration.

Neurological

CEREBRAL. The commonest complication is an intellectual deterioration. In some patients this is associated with a reluctance to enter into conversation, whereas in others there is a circumlocution which rarely reaches a conclusion. Mental concentration and the making of decisions are difficult. Frequently there are recurrent bouts of depression and apathy, but the tenacity with which most patients will try and overcome their disabilities is remarkable. Headaches, lassitude, languor, muscular fatigue and weakness are all present in the final stages of renal failure. They may occur much earlier. Terminally the patient may become torpid during the day and yet not be able to sleep during the night, when instead he is restless and confused. Finally, there is loss of consciousness, but often even at this late stage there may be short lucid intervals; not infrequently the patient retains a complete understanding of what is happening to him right up to a few hours before death.

Epileptic convulsions in chronic renal failure may be due either to sudden increases in blood pressure in patients with established hypertension, or they may occur without any change in blood pressure. Both types are very rare; the first is called hypertensive encephalopathy; the other has no particular designation. The latter variety is seen mainly in young adults in whom the fits may be the only complaint and yet the blood urea is extraordinarily high, e.g. 400 mg per 100 ml.

In advanced renal failure muscle twitches are often seen; they are caused by anterior horn cell discharges of unknown cause, and are unrelated to any apparent change in calcium metabolism, though they can often be relieved by the intravenous administration of calcium. A few patients have involuntary twitchings and choreiform movements of both legs, a phenomenon appropriately called the "restless leg syndrome". It may herald a fit. A "flapping tremor" which is more frequently described in hepatic failure, often occurs in the terminal stages of chronic renal failure.

PERIPHERAL NERVES. Uraemic polyneuropathy is a rare syndrome which has recently emerged into certain prominence in patients inadequately treated with maintenance haemodialysis (p. 205). It is due to a destruction of the myelin sheath and axons of medullated fibres in the peripheral nerves. The onset may be associated with painful burning feet followed by a progressive numbness and weakness. The feet and legs are affected more than the arms, and the distal segments more than the proximal. Eventually ataxia is prominent with a wide based steppage gait. Sometimes there may be no subjective sensory disturbances. It is not due to a deficiency of vitamin B_1. It is cured by increasing the duration of dialysis, so that it is presumably due to the retention of some injurious substance. There is now some evidence that this is probably guanadino succinic acid which is known to inhibit transketolase activity, a necessary step in the formation of myelin.

MYOPATHY. An unusual condition in which there is a weakness of the proximal muscles, particularly the shoulder girdle, hip flexion and spinal muscles. There is a waddling gait, difficulty climbing stairs and standing upright from the squatting position. Some patients have to go upstairs on their hands and knees. The condition is more often seen in association with renal osteomalacia but it can occur without renal osteodystrophy. The deep tendon reflexes are normal and brisk.

Cardiovascular

HYPERTENSIVE VASCULAR DISEASE. Hypertension and chronic renal failure are closely related (p. 118) and, though hypertension may cause renal failure, the reverse is more common. The blood pressure frequently rises in chronic renal failure, but its rise may produce few symptoms; when they occur they are due to widespread vascular changes or cardiac failure.

The vascular lesions may be acute or chronic. They can nearly always be observed on inspection of the ocular fundus, where they produce certain characteristic disturbances of the retinal arteries and of the retina. The acute changes (i.e. those found in malignant hypertension) produce an appearance called *hypertensive retinopathy*, while the chronic changes are called *arteriosclerotic retinopathy*.

Hypertensive retinopathy is distinguished primarily by the presence of papilloedema which at first may be unilateral. There are also flame-shaped or blotchy haemorrhages fanning out from the optic disc, and multiple areas of white discoloration known as exudates. These have indefinite margins and are of uneven size and colour; a lack of precision and uniformity which has caused them to be called "soft" exudates. They consist of collections of oedema fluid. Sometimes the oedematous retina lies in folds radiating from the macula towards the optic disc, an appearance referred to as a macular star. Soft exudates and haemorrhages may precede the development of papilloedema.

In arteriosclerotic retinopathy the retinal arteries become tortuous and narrow, either irregularly or evenly along their whole length. They characteristically cross the veins at right angles, as opposed to the more usual oblique direction, and at these crossings the veins appear to be compressed by the artery; this appearance is known as arterio-venous nipping. It is due to an accumulation of connective tissue between the artery and the vein, so that in fact the vein, as it approaches the artery, is not compressed but obscured. Exudates are also seen, but they are "hard" as opposed to those seen with the acute vascular changes. They are small and compact, they have definite, sharp margins, and are of a dense yellowish-white colour. Eventually they are found in clusters particularly spreading out radially from the macula; another form of macular star. As chronic vascular changes frequently precede by several years the onset of the acute changes it is not unusual to find arteriosclerotic and hypertensive retinopathy combined.

Hypertensive retinopathy may cause varying degrees of visual impairment, depending on the degree of papilloedema and the site and extent of the haemorrhages and exudates (particularly if the macula has been involved). The striking clinical finding, however, is that often both fundi may be severely affected without the patient being aware of any change in vision; with arteriosclerotic retinopathy visual symptoms are even less frequent.

The changes which hypertensive vascular disease may produce upon renal structure and function have been described on p. 124. When they are superimposed upon chronic renal disease, they will intensify the severity of the renal failure. If cardiac failure occurs there is an additional sharp deterioration in renal function. With malignant hypertension cardiac failure is often one of the presenting clinical features. There are acute attacks of paroxysmal nocturnal and postural dyspnoea, and eventually oedema with a permanently raised venous pressure. Deterioration in renal function is due to (1) the reversible renal vasoconstriction associated with cardiac failure, and (2) the local vascular lesions.

The onset of *acute* vascular changes in the kidney is revealed not only by the sudden change in renal function but also by the onset of haematuria and increased proteinuria. The deterioration in renal function due to the vascular changes associated with malignant hypertension is partially reversible if it has not progressed too far before treatment is started. How far the functional changes produced by chronic vascular changes are reversible is uncertain.

PERICARDITIS. An aseptic, fibrinous pericarditis often develops in the terminal phase of chronic renal failure. Its cause is unknown. It may be painless or excruciatingly painful. Occasionally it is associated with a large bloody effusion, which may cause tamponade.

INCREASED CAPILLARY PERMEABILITY. This manifests itself in many ways. Retinitis in the absence of hypertension; transient attacks of reversible blindness due to cerebral oedema; pulmonary oedema (the uraemic lung) in the absence of a raised pulmonary capillary pressure; skin purpura; and the presence in most patients of a slight excess of peritoneal fluid containing a concentration of protein close to that found in the plasma. One cause for the increased permeability is perhaps an increased concentration of circulating renin which is known to cause increased capillary permeability in experimental animals.

Haematological

Anaemia, leucocytosis and a raised erythrocyte sedimentation rate are all common features of chronic renal failure. The cause of the anaemia has been described above. The mechanisms of the other two are unknown.

Respiratory

The deep sighing respirations of acidosis have already been mentioned. The other respiratory complications of renal failure are (1) "uraemic lung" and (2) infection.

"Uraemic lung" is a radiological diagnosis. It consists of dense bilateral opacities radiating from the hilum into the lung substance, while the upper and lower zones and the outer rim of the middle zones are clear. These appearances are usually due to left heart failure but there is a group of patients in whom they are associated with a normal pulmonary artery pressure when they are presumably due to increased transudation from abnormal capillaries.

Pneumonia is frequently the immediate cause of death, it usually develops only when the patient is already moribund. It is not improbable that the deep respirations of acidosis and the rapid respiration of left heart failure prevent the bronchioles from becoming blocked and the lungs from collapsing, the usual preliminaries to pneumonia in semiconscious patients.

Cutaneous

The characteristic pigmentation of renal failure, together with the anaemia, give patients suffering from chronic renal failure a characteristic colour (p. 190). The eyelids tend to be slightly swollen and an expression of tiredness and depression is common. It is not known why the eyelids should be swollen, this usually occurs in the absence of generalised oedema. Relatively often, patients will develop a moon face like that seen in "Cushing's" disease but it is not associated with an excess secretion of cortisone.

In advanced renal failure there may be purpura, usually preceded and accompanied by bleeding gums; this is associated with gross abnormalities in platelet function, though the number of platelets is normal. This deterioration in platelet function is also related to the retention of guanadino succinic acid.

Pruritus is common and there may also be a variety of unspecific rashes, erythema, vesicles and urticaria. The skin is often very dry because of dehydration. Recurrent boils, carbuncles, and slowly healing scratches and abrasions are not infrequent.

Treatment of Chronic Renal Failure

Treatment of chronic renal failure can be divided into two stages. The first consists of conservative measures which are designed to delay the progressive deterioration of renal function or mitigate its consequences. The second begins when these measures are no longer able to keep the patient at work and leading a normal life. At this point the patient has entered the stage of terminal renal failure when the only effective treatment is either maintenance haemodialysis or transplantation.

Clearly it is of the utmost importance to try and identify the primary cause of the renal failure, for in some instances, e.g. when it is due to the consumption of phenacetin, obstruction of the urinary tract, or malignant hypertension, it may be possible to treat the immediate cause of failure, and so prevent any further deterioration of function; often it may even be possible to obtain a large measure of improvement. Unfortunately, in most instances the cause of chronic renal failure is not treatable, for it is either unknown, or structurally irreversible, as with chronic glomerular nephritis, or congenital polycystic kidneys.

Conservative treatment

This may be very rewarding, for often much of the disturbance in renal function is reversible, having been caused by a vicious circle in which the disturbed renal function causes a change in the internal environment, which in turn leads to a further depression in renal function, e.g. renal failure $\rightarrow$ polyuria and nausea $\rightarrow$ dehydration $\rightarrow$ renal vasoconstriction $\rightarrow$ diminished glomerular filtration rate.

Conservative treatment consists mainly in preventing or correcting disturbances of water and electrolyte balance, controlling the rise in arterial pressure, and delaying the retention of the end products of protein metabolism.

Treatment of biochemical abnormalities

WATER. It has been pointed out on p. 36 that in normal man the amount of urea excreted in the urine is proportional to the urine flow up to urine flows of 2 ml/min (i.e. approximately 3 l/24 hr); in chronic renal failure this relationship is still present and even appears to hold at greater urine flows. There is also evidence that a high turnover of water increases glomerular filtration rate. A large fluid intake and high urine flow will therefore not only prevent dehydration but will also ensure a maximal rate of urea excretion. Unfortunately in many patients thirst is not a sufficient stimulus to prevent their becoming dehydrated. Some patients, particularly women, habitually drink very little, and they must be advised to drink rather more than they are accustomed to, i.e. an extra three to four glasses of water a day. In the average case it is sufficient to point out that the fluid intake should be generous. The dangers of over-hydration are minimal when water is being taken by mouth.

When severe dehydration has occurred through nausea, vomiting or diarrhoea it should be corrected immediately by the intravenous administration of 5 per cent glucose, or half-strength saline.

ELECTROLYTE AND ACID BASE BALANCE. The acidosis of chronic renal failure rarely causes any generalised symptoms. The main reason for trying to correct it is to prevent the bone changes which a persistent and accumulating retention of hydrogen ions may cause (p. 186). In addition, the administration of the sodium ion (if sodium bicarbonate is given) will greatly improve the wellbeing of those patients who may be in negative sodium balance.

Acidosis can be controlled by the oral administration of sodium bicarbonate 3–9 g/day. Calcium carbonate 6–10 g/day can also be given though it is less effective than sodium bicarbonate in raising plasma bicarbonate; it is useful, however, when the intake of sodium must be restricted as in heart failure or severe hypertension. Calcium carbonate also gives rise to a positive calcium balance which may also be of value. When there is a sudden fall in plasma bicarbonate due to a sudden deterioration of renal function and it is thought necessary to treat the acidosis promptly, it may be corrected by the intravenous administration of sodium bicarbonate. The speed of infusion, however, should be carefully controlled for otherwise there may be a sharp fall in the pH of the cerebro-spinal fluid with giddiness, nausea, vomiting and disturbances of consciousness. This is due to the same mechanism as that which causes a similar syndrome during a rapid dialysis for acute renal failure (p. 176).

It should be remembered that sometimes ammonium chloride is given to test renal function, or, in the past, to increase the diuretic effect of mercurial injections, but that in chronic renal failure this may precipitate or aggravate a state of acidosis.

Retention of sodium chloride is associated either with cardiac failure or the nephrotic syndrome; the treatment of the former is discussed on p. 199. Treatment of the nephrotic syndrome when combined with renal failure is awkward and difficult. A high protein diet must not be given, for it will raise the blood urea as will the administration of prednisone. The only procedures which are likely to be useful are the administration of diuretics and a low salt diet.

Gross sodium chloride deficiency arising from excess urinary loss is rare in chronic renal failure; its treatment is dealt with on p. 140. Minor sodium chloride deficiency due to a urinary sodium leak, excess sweating, mild diarrhoea, or glycosuria can be avoided by ensuring that the salt intake is liberal or by giving a slow release sodium chloride tablet (Slow Sodium, Ciba). The latter are extremely useful for they ensure a constant intake of sodium even during periods of anorexia. It is always dangerous to restrict the salt intake of patients suffering from chronic renal failure, particularly if the blood pressure is normal, e.g. the use of a salt-free diet in the treatment of Menier's syndrome. The ability to conserve salt is limited and a contraction of the extracellular fluid space may develop insidiously with all its complications, particularly renal vasoconstriction, *hypotension* and deterioration of renal function.

Potassium retention is unusual in chronic renal failure, and only occurs as a terminal event. It may respond to 15–20 g of cation exchange resin in the sodium or calcium phase, given orally three times a day; potassium deficiency from excess urinary loss is also most unusual; its treatment is discussed on p. 223.

CALCIUM METABOLISM. Metastatic calcification is preventable and should not be permitted to develop. This is achieved by not allowing the product of plasma phosphorous × plasma calcium to rise above 70. As it is the rise in phosphate which usually causes the rise in the product it can be controlled by lowering the dietary intake of phosphate. More acutely it can be lowered by the administration of 50–100 ml of aluminium hydroxide gel per day. This binds the phosphate in the gut and increases the content of phosphate in the faeces. For prolonged treatment it is sometimes useful to give instead 5–10 g of calcium carbonate per day orally. This also lowers plasma phosphate by binding phosphate in the gut, and the small rise in plasma calcium which it causes lowers the concentration of circulating parathormone. This in turn will also lower plasma phosphate, for in advanced renal failure hyperparathyroidism causes the plasma phosphate to rise, in contrast to the fall that occurs when renal function is normal. This is because, in advanced renal failure, the phosphaturic effect of parathormone may not be sufficient to match the effect of the hormone in mobilising phosphate from the bone into the extracellular fluid.

Hyperparathyroidism can be prevented by either reducing the intake of phosphate in the diet, or by increasing the oral intake of calcium. After it has become manifest radiologically, hyperparathyroidism can be controlled to a certain extent by the administration of aluminium hydroxide gel or calcium carbonate. If hypercalcaemia occurs a sub-total parathyroidectomy must be undertaken, for hypercalcaemia causes a deterioration of renal function.

Osteomalacia and rickets can be cured by the administration of large quantities of vitamin D and calcium carbonate. The dose of vitamin D depends on the patient's response, but may have to be of the order of 3 mg of calciferol eight-hourly. The patient's symptoms are relieved within a week or two and radiological improvement is detectable within a few months. It is interesting that eventually the bones are radiologically denser than normal. The administration of calciferol with milk as the calcium supplement as opposed to calcium carbonate, may raise the plasma phosphate and cause metastatic calcification and arthritis. It is important to control the administration of vitamin D by estimating the concentration of serum calcium and alkaline phosphatase at frequent intervals. If the dosage of vitamin D is excessive there will be hypercalcaemia, if it is insufficient the alkaline phosphatase will remain raised.

Treatment of hypertensive vascular disease

MALIGNANT HYPERTENSION. If the patient has malignant hypertension the blood pressure must be lowered immediately; otherwise the prognosis is less than two years. The success of treatment depends not only on the ability of the hypotensive drug to lower the blood pressure but also on the ability of the kidneys to function at the lower pressure (p. 107); the latter probably depends on the extent of irreversible arteriolar narrowing present before treatment is begun. If lowering the blood pressure raises the blood urea the position is hopeless. To avoid this complication it is probably better to lower the blood pressure gently over a matter of days in order to allow the renal circulation time to adapt to the lower pressure. Alpha-methyl dopa, propranolol, hydrallazine and clonidine are all well tolerated antihypertensive drugs. Propanolol is excellent for it causes the least side effects and never causes postural hypotension. Sometimes the blood pressure will not fall unless several of these drugs are given in full dosage simultaneously. In an emergency the blood pressure is most easily reduced with an intravenous or intramuscular injection of 10–20 mg of hydrallazine or an intravenous injection 0·15 mg of clonidine.

The response to treatment, and survival is slightly better in those patients whose malignant hypertension and impaired renal function is superimposed upon chronic renal disease.

NON-MALIGNANT HYPERTENSION. Both in man and animals there is a close association between hypertension and sclerotic vascular lesions. In man the progress of renal damage from "non-malignant" hypertension is so slow that it rarely causes death from renal failure. It is generally agreed, however, that renal function in chronic renal disease deteriorates more rapidly once there is a pronounced rise in blood pressure. Accordingly it is considered reasonable and justifiable to try and lower even a symptomless hypertension if there is any cause to believe that there is underlying renal disease.

The blood pressure can often be brought under control most effectively by combining the administration of hypotensive drugs with a low intake of sodium. In chronic renal failure this causes a substantial sodium depletion more quickly than in a normal person and may lower the blood pressure but it may also induce a rapid deterioration of renal function. Nevertheless, if one is alert and is closely monitoring the patient's progress it is worth attempting. As soon as the blood pressure is under control the intake of sodium must be increased towards normal, the intake then being adjusted according to the patient's weight, blood pressure and renal function.

CARDIAC FAILURE. At first, cardiac failure responds rapidly to bed rest, morphia, digitalis and a low sodium diet; diuretics are also used, but with more restraint than is usual in patients who have heart failure unassociated with renal failure. On the other hand the only diuretic which is likely to cause a diuresis in advanced chronic renal failure is frusemide, and it usually has to be given in single doses of 500 to 1,000 mg orally. It is important however to start with smaller doses for occasionally a patient will respond to much smaller amounts. In advanced renal failure it is best to avoid digitalis for its normal half life of 30–40 hours is prolonged to 4–5 days. To prevent recurrences of cardiac failure it is usually necessary to treat the hypertension (see above) which is the principal cause of the heart's failure.

In advanced renal failure, cardiac failure may be most resistant to treatment. Rest in bed aggravates the dyspnoea so that it is better to sit the patient up in an armchair or a cardiac bed; it is difficult to avoid digitalis overdosage or to induce a saline diuresis; lowering the blood pressure is now almost certain to depress renal function to lethal levels as will any attempt to correct the anaemia.

Treatment of anaemia and blood loss

The anaemia of chronic renal failure is unresponsive to almost all forms of therapy except the transfusion of red cells. Nevertheless, there is little point in giving blood, unless there has been a recent haemorrhage. Transfusions inhibit the bone marrow's production of red cells so that the packed cell volume usually quickly returns to its previous level. It is customary to give iron preparations by mouth, though they are rarely effective.

Haemorrhage must be treated as rapidly as possible with transfusions of whole blood. The dangers to renal function of under- and overtransfusion have already been mentioned. It is essential that patients with chronic renal failure should not become carriers of Australia antigen (the agent responsible for serum hepatitis). The blood for transfusion should therefore have been screened for the presence of Australia antigen.

Treatment of superimposed infection

In patients with chronic renal failure an attack of acute pyelonephritis, however mild, may cause a severe reduction in renal function. Any suspicion of renal infection should therefore be treated promptly with antibiotics (p. 310). The important point to remember about these infections is that clinically they may not be obvious; they should therefore be kept in mind when there is an otherwise unexplained deterioration of renal function.

Infections elsewhere than in the kidney may also cause a deterioration of renal function but, with the exception of subacute bacterial endocarditis, these usually present fewer diagnostic difficulties.

Treatment of hiccough

There are many methods of treating hiccough, including the inhalation of carbon dioxide, and the administration of chlorpromazine or mepyramine (Anthisan). The latter can be given in doses of 100 mg four-hourly by mouth or by injection; it is sometimes useful when all else has failed. Occasionally a drop of oil of peppermint on a piece of sugar is sufficient to stop an attack.

Treatment of nausea, vomiting and dyspnoea

The best treatment is to reduce the intake of protein (see below). Sometimes at the beginning it may be useful to perform one or two peritoneal dialyses to obtain an initial return of appetite. If this is unsuccessful the patient should be placed on maintenance haemodialysis or transplantation. In those patients who cannot eat a low protein diet and for whom maintenance dialysis or transplantation are not available nausea and vomiting can be best controlled by the administration of thiethylperazine or chlorpromazine. In the terminal stages chlorpromazine not only abolishes nausea and vomiting, but it calms the patient's anxiety. It also reduces the quantity of drugs needed to control the other two distressing features of terminal renal failure, dyspnoea, and physical and mental restlessness. Morphia is useful for dyspnoea, and in combination with chlorpromazine will not cause nausea and vomiting. Restlessness and distress can often be controlled with diazepam, if not, chlorpromazine and morphine may be necessary. Barbiturates are also useful in this respect, but they sometimes cause a persistent unhappy, confused drowsiness which aggravates the restlessness. The repeated administration of short and medium acting barbiturates should be avoided because of contamination with barbital which accumulates in patients with renal failure.

Treatment of retention of waste products of protein metabolism

The concentration of urea in the blood is controlled by the rate of protein intake and the glomerular filtration rate. In chronic renal failure glomerular filtration rate falls, the blood urea rises and there is a concomitant deterioration in the patient's general condition. As it is clear that urea is not directly responsible for this change, presumably it is due to the accumulation of other end-products of protein metabolism. For this reason alone the patient will feel better, and may survive longer, if protein intake is limited.

Another, more debatable, reason has been advanced for reducing protein intake. It has been pointed out that in chronic renal failure each remaining nephron has to excrete an increased quantity of solutes (p. 61) and that urea forms a large controllable fraction of this total. It has been suggested that the increased "work" that each nephron must therefore perform may accelerate its eventual destruction. It has been shown that in animals the renal lesions of senescence can be accelerated by a high protein diet; and that following unilateral nephrectomy and the removal of large portions of the other kidney, structural changes in the remaining renal tissue can be hastened by the administration of large quantities of protein. If these results are applicable to man then once renal failure has been diagnosed, protein intake should be reduced, whatever the initial concentration of blood urea. Generally, however, the therapeutic implications of these experiments are not accepted, and protein intake is regulated only to control symptoms.

PROTEIN METABOLISM IN CHRONIC RENAL FAILURE. The stools from both normal men and uraemic patients do not contain urea. This is because the urea in intestinal juice is continually being hydrolysed to ammonia by bacterial ureases. The ammonia nitrogen which is reabsorbed from the gut is then reutilised. It can be found incorporated into serum albumin. In patients with chronic renal failure with a high blood urea, the urea of the intestinal juices is high and therefore the magnitude of this recycling of nitrogen is very great. It has been calculated that with a blood urea of 200 mg/100 ml about 15 g of endogenous ammonia nitrogen is available for protein synthesis.

As chronic renal failure advances there is often a progressive negative nitrogen balance due mainly to a diminished intake of protein. This may be

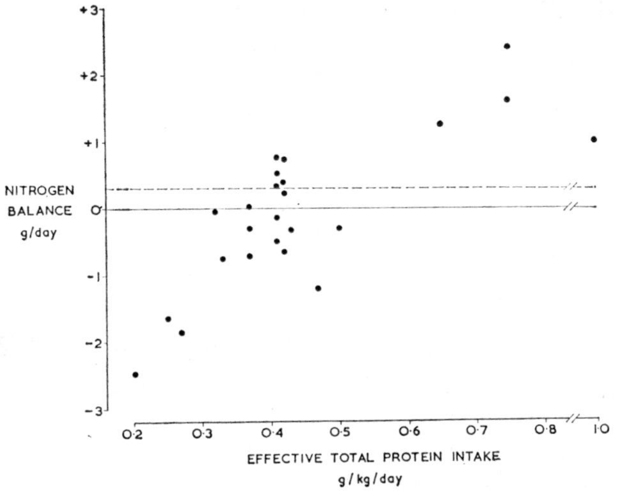

FIG. 15.6. Nitrogen balance in 24 patients with chronic renal failure on varying intakes of protein. The interrupted horizontal line denotes average nitrogen loss per day in sweat in a moderate climate. (Ford, Phillips, Toye, Luck and de Wardener, 1969, *British Medical Journal.*)

due either to anorexia or to the therapeutic use of a low protein diet. In addition it may be aggravated by urinary protein loss or losses into the peritoneal fluid during peritoneal dialysis. As the nitrogen balance becomes negative several adaptive compensatory mechanisms come into play, for instance, the incorporation of ammonia nitrogen into albumin. But these compensatory mechanisms are not so efficient in chronic renal failure as they are in normal man. Whereas normal man can stay in nitrogen balance with a dietary protein intake as low as 0·25 g/kg/day (i.e. about 18 g for a 70 kg man) patients with chronic renal failure need about 0·5 g/kg/day (i.e. 35 g/kg/day) (Fig. 15.6).

Protein catabolism is less the higher the calorie intake. Therefore it is reasonable to suppose that the minimal protein intake needed to maintain nitrogen balance should be lower if the diet includes a high intake of calories. Within the range of calorie intake which is practical, however, these considerations do not seem important. It is also known that the higher the intake of proteins of high biological value (i.e. those which contain a large proportion of essential amino acids) the lower the total protein intake needed to maintain nitrogen balance. Again, however, within the limits imposed in trying to keep the diet palatable this is not an important factor. On the other hand if it is decided that normal food can be renounced the intake of protein can be so arranged that it only contains essential amino acids and then the total protein intake can be drastically reduced. Recently it has been found that ureamic patients can synthesise essential amino acids from their keto-acid analogues (which do not contain nitrogen). In future therefore it may be possible to keep a patient in nitrogen balance with a protein free diet, the nitrogen lost in the urine and faeces being supplied in a non-protein form. Nevertheless the problems of stability, palatability and availability of the appropriate keto-acids are very great.

Low protein diet. The consequences of a persistent negative nitrogen balance are a fall in the albumin pool, hypoalbuminaemia, weight loss, muscle wasting and fatigue. Though a low protein diet may prolong the patient's life it also gives time for the insidious development of many complications including those due directly to protein deficiency. For instance when patients are placed on maintenance haemodialysis they recover their health more quickly if they have not been on a very low protein diet (less than 0·5 g/kg/day) for a long time before dialysis is begun. In contrast full recovery in some protein deficient patients may take up to a year.

The aim therefore of a reduced intake of protein in the management of chronic renal failure is to bring about a reduction in the concentration of nitrogenous waste products without producing a prolonged negative nitrogen balance. On a palatable diet this is achieved by giving about 0·5 g/kg/day of protein (i.e. 35 g per day to a 70 kg man) with as high a calorie intake as is comfortable. It is difficult to be precise when such a diet should be started. Perhaps anorexia and lassitude are the two best guides. In young patients these may not develop until the blood urea is 300 to 400 mg/100 ml whereas in older patients they appear earlier.

If, when a patient is first seen, he is anorexic and vomiting it is usually necessary first to give some saline intravenously. As a result, appetite often returns. It may then be worth while to give a very low protein diet (i.e. 0·2 g/kg/day) for two to three weeks to lower the blood urea. It is important to remember to give at least 100 to 150 mEq of sodium per day at the same time, particularly if the patient is not hypertensive. The blood urea will often fall to below 100 mg/100 ml with creatinine clearances of 5 ml/min. Mental faculties become clear and lassitude diminishes. When the blood urea has stabilised the dietary intake of protein should be increased to 0·5 g/kg/day. This will produce some rise in the blood urea, e.g. from 80 to 120 mg/100 ml but usually the improvement in the patient's appetite and wellbeing will remain. Thereafter treatment depends on whether the patient is eventually going to be treated with maintenance haemodialysis. If he is, the protein intake should not be lowered below 0·5 g/kg/day. If he is not to be treated with maintenance haemodialysis then the protein intake is progressively lowered to control the anorexia and vomiting. The patients who do best are those with normal blood pressures, and they are the ones who tend to have large urine volumes. Patients with severe hypertension do badly. Progress is assessed by measuring plasma creatinine. Whatever the level of blood urea and however satisfactory the patient's clinical condition the outlook is poor if the plasma creatinine continues to rise. Often the plasma creatinine rises while the blood urea remains unchanged. When the plasma creatinine reaches 15 mg/100 ml the patient is liable to die at any moment from a haemorrhage. At this level of plasma creatinine and as it rises further the patient's physical well being begins to be marred by an increasing sense of anxiety, restlessness and insomnia. Nevertheless, protein intakes as low as 0·2 g/kg/day have certainly done much to diminish the protracted periods of severe ill-health which used to accompany the last stages of renal failure.

A transitory fall in blood urea can sometimes be induced by the administration of anabolic steroids. This effect, however, is least noticeable in patients on a low intake of protein, or if there has been much loss of weight.

Maintenance Dialysis and Transplantation

It is important to decide whether a patient is to be treated with maintenance dialysis or transplantation *before* he is moribund. The optimum time to place a patient on maintenance dialysis is when conservative treatment has either failed to enable the patient to stay at work or failed to prevent the plasma creatinine rising to around 13–15 mg/100 ml.

Maintenance dialysis

This can be carried out with either peritoneal dialysis or haemodialysis.

MAINTENANCE PERITONEAL DIALYSIS. This is a useful (if painful) holding manoeuvre for about two to three months. A fresh disposable catheter is inserted into the peritoneal cavity two or three times a week. Dialysis is performed for about 18 hours each time; in some patients the catheter is removed at the end of each dialysis. In others an indwelling silicone rubber catheter is used. Automatic cycling devices have been introduced to simplify the procedure and some patients have been treated at home. Nevertheless, because of the complications mentioned earlier (p. 174) few patients can be maintained on peritoneal dialysis for longer than six months. Dietary restrictions are similar to those for maintenance haemodialysis (see below). Those who do best are middle-aged women with normal blood pressures who are passing large volumes of urine.

MAINTENANCE HAEMODIALYSIS. Either a subcutaneous arterio-venous fistula is made by anastomosing the radial artery to a nearby superficial vein, or an arterio-venous shunt is established into one of the patient's limbs with teflon and silicone rubber tubes. These measures allow repeated, quick, atraumatic access to the patient's arterial and venous circulation at all times. Dialyses are best performed on a modification of the Kiil "kidney" using a cuprophane membrane. The advantage of this "kidney" is that it holds less than 100 ml of blood. It therefore does not need priming with blood before each dialysis and it has a low resistance to blood flow. Patients are dialysed for a total of about 20 to 30 hours a week depending on the dialysance of the particular "kidney". Insufficient dialysis causes the "under dialysis syndrome" which consists of lassitude, anorexia, weight loss, depression and a high incidence of "complications" (see below).

Dietary restrictions depend to a large extent on the daily urine volume residual renal function and the blood pressure. The aim is to keep the weight gain between dialyses down to less than 1·5 kg, and to keep the blood pressure normal. Water and sodium intake are therefore regulated accordingly. Sodium intake has to be regulated more strictly at the beginning of treatment than after a year or two; it is usually limited to 20–50 mEq/day. Potassium intake is limited to around 50 mEq/day, and protein intake to between 40 and 70 g/day depending on the patient's weight. The calory intake is raised to the maximum possible, e.g. 3,000 calories or more. The bone marrow depression of chronic renal failure is relieved to a certain extent by maintenance haemodialysis and most patients will keep packed cell volumes of 20 to 25 per cent without transfusion. Hypertension is brought under control by reducing the patient's weight by 1 or 2 kg at each dialysis, by ultrafiltration. As much as 20 kg may have to be removed before the blood pressure is controlled.

CONTRAINDICATIONS. The patient must be sane and preferably not suffering from some systemic disease. But patients suffering from diabetes and systemic lupus erythematosus have occasionally done well. There should not have been a preceding cerebrovascular accident. Age is not a contraindication to successful dialysis though there are certain socio-financial considerations against treating old people.

COMPLICATIONS. The fistula or shunt may clot or become infected. The other complications include peripheral neuropathy, metastatic calcification, calcium "gout", and hyperparathyroidism. Acute pulmonary oedema and cerebrovascular accident are the commonest cause of death. The former is usually due to carelessness. In addition there is a high incidence of hepatitis both infectious hepatitis (Australia antigen negative) and serum hepatitis (Australia antigen positive). Both are particularly common in patients being dialysed in hospital.

QUALITY OF SURVIVAL. If maintenance haemodialysis is properly carried out, the patient is well, sexually active, fertile, and at work. If maintenance haemodialysis is incompetently performed, particularly if its main purpose is to provide a "pool" of patients for transplantation the patients are impotent, unwell, and unhappy.

Renal transplantation

A kidney is removed from either a living donor or a corpse and transplanted into a patient suffering from terminal renal failure. The functional efficiency of the transplanted kidney mainly depends on the compatibility of the tissue antigens of the corpse and the patient. The greater the incompatibility the quicker the patient's immunological mechanisms cause the kidney to be rejected. If they are completely compatible, as in identical twins, there will be no rejection.

The surgical technique involved in renal transplantation is relatively simple. The prospective patient has usually been kept fit and well by maintenance haemodialysis beforehand. The principal difficulty is to bring the kidney and the patient together rapidly after the donor dies. A variety of techniques have been evolved to prevent the kidney from deteriorating in the interval. Immunological rejection of the transplanted kidney may be particularly violent a few days after the transplant operation. Rejection is suppressed by the administration of cytotoxic drugs such as azathioprine, 6 mercaptopurine, actinomycin and antilymphocyte serum and also by using the immunological suppressive action of prednisone. It is usually necessary to continue two or more of these drugs in small doses indefinitely. In rare instances the transplanted kidney has eventually appeared to be accepted by the recipient and the administration of cytotoxic drugs and prednisone has been discontinued.

CONTRAINDICATIONS. The contraindications to transplantation are (1) the patient is being dialysed at home and refuses to be transplanted; (2) recent exacerbation of tuberculosis; (3) history of angina, myocardial infarction or severe heart failure; (4) over 50 years of age; (5) the presence of circulating antiglomerular basement membrane antibodies; (6) history of treated neoplasms; (7) AB-ve blood group; (8) bronchiectasis; (9) aseptic bone necrosis from a previous transplantation.

COMPLICATIONS. The complications of renal transplantation are those which affect the transplanted kidney or its ureter, and those which are due to the drugs used to suppress rejection. Apart from infection and infarction the kidney may suffer any of five pathological processes. Acute tubular necrosis may occur. It appears immediately after the operation and is due to deterioration of the kidney before it is transplanted. Acute rejection may develop a few days later and is characterised by a heavy infiltration of mononuclear cells, plasma cells and eosinophils together with acute destruction of the renal parenchyma. If these acute hazards are avoided three other more gradual changes may occur, a slowly progressive interstitial nephritis, an occlusive arteritis, or changes which appear to be identical to those of chronic glomerular nephritis. Necrosis of the ureter at its insertion into the bladder is a problem which also appears to be due to a rejection phenomenon.

The complications which stem from the use of cytotoxic drugs are those of immunological and bone marrow suppression including fulminating infections with agranulocytosis, multiple haemorrhages from thrombocytopoenia and the appearance of malignant tumours. The patient may die of infections with various fungi or viruses which are rarely pathogenic in other circumstances. The administration of prednisone often causes the classical florid facies of Cushing's disease, it may also reactivate pulmonary tuberculosis and cause hypertension, cataracts, or a devastating gastro-intestinal haemorrhage from an acute peptic ulcer. It may also cause ischaemic bone necrosis particularly at either end of the femur.

QUALITY OF SURVIVAL. In the absence of complications the patient leads an almost normal life except for the inevitable but gradually diminishing disfigurement of the Cushing's facies. The prednisone administration often contributes a pleasant euphoria.

Duration of Survival

Fig. 15.7 illustrates the survival rates among patients treated in Europe between 1966 and 1971. After five years 75 per cent of the patients treated on maintenance haemodialysis at home were alive, in contrast to 45 per cent of the patients who had received a cadaver kidney. The survival of transplanted patients is much better if the kidney comes from an identical twin or a living related donor. The survival of the grafts is somewhat less than that of the patients. It is clear that the excellence of a transplant centre, as regards its concern for its patients, can be gauged by the ratio of patient survival to graft survival. The further away from unity the better, for this then indicates that the centre is more concerned with the survival of the patients than the graft. There is a temptation, when rejection threatens, to continue to increase the dose of immunosuppressive drugs indefinitely. If this is not resisted the graft may survive but the patient dies from one of the many complications of immu-

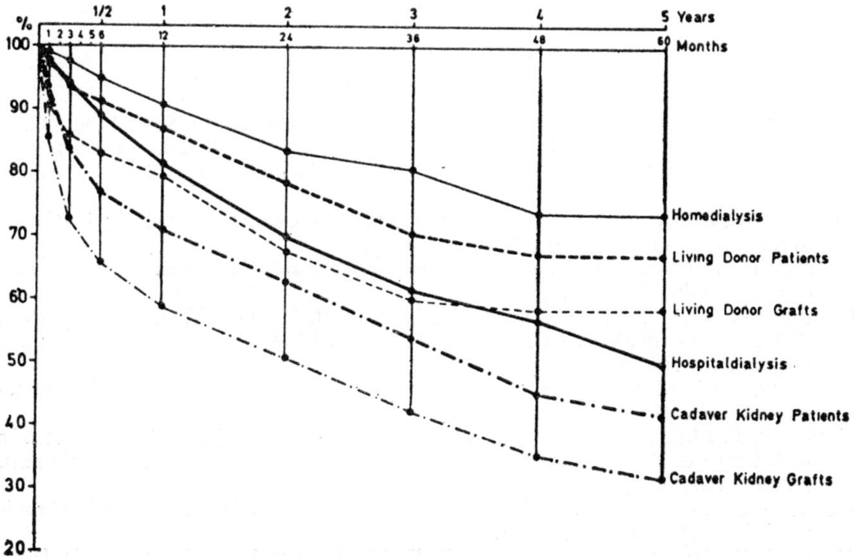

FIG. 15.7. Survival of patients on maintenance haemodialysis and after renal transplantation in Europe. ("Proc. European Dialysis and Transplant Assoc.", 1971, Pitman Medical.)

nosuppression. If rejection is difficult to overcome immunosuppressive treatment would be tailed off and the patient returned to dialysis.

Facilities Needed to Treat Terminal Renal Failure

The number of patients dying of chronic renal failure increases rapidly with age; about 70 per cent are over the age of 50. In England and Wales during 1967 there were approximately 2,000 deaths between the ages of 15 to 59 whereas there were only 1,000 deaths between the ages of 15 to 49. Some of these patients were unsuitable for treatment with maintenance haemodialysis or transplantation, but prospective studies which delineate patients who are suitable have shown total numbers similar to these. The number of patients that are treated falls far short of the number suitable for treatment. Hospital maintenance dialysis centres are the mainstay of the treatment available, for they train, and support the large number of patients who dialyse at home, they also make the patients fit for transplantation and again provide treatment when the graft fails. More patients could be transplanted if the supply of cadaver kidneys became more plentiful. This in turn depends on all doctors becoming aware of the large numbers of deaths that take place from which suitable kidneys can be obtained. Nevertheless the more patients are transplanted the greater the facilities needed to rescue the failures. Any increase in the number of transplantations therefore will increase the requirements for dialysis facilities. Unless, of course, the rate of graft failure is permitted to be the same as that of the mortality rate or the survival of the grafts improves.

BIBLIOGRAPHY

BATCHELOR, J. R., ELLIS, F., FRENCH, M. E., BEWICK, M., CAMERON, J. S., and OGG, C. S. (1970). "Immunological enhancement of human kidney graft." *Lancet*, **2**, 1007.

BERGSTROM, J., and BITTAR, E. E. (1969). "Uraemic Toxicity." Academic Press, London and New York, p. 495.

BLAGG, C. R., KEMBLE, F., and TRAVENER, D. (1968). "Nerve conduction velocity in relation to the severity of renal disease." *Nephron*, **5**, 290.

CHAPLIN, H., and MOLLISON, P. L. (1953). "Red cell life span in nephritis and in hepatic cirrhosis." *Clin. Sci.*, **12**, 351.

CLARKSON, E. M., CURTIS, J. R., JEWKES, R. J., JONES, B. E., LUCK, V. A., DE WARDENER, H. E., and PHILLIPS, M. (1971). "Slow Sodium. An oral slowly released sodium chloride preparation." *Brit. Med. J.*, **2**, 604.

CLARKSON, E. M., MCDONALD, S. J., and DE WARDENER, H. E. (1965). "Magnesium metabolism in chronic renal failure." *Clin. Sci.*, **29**, 107.

CLARKSON, E. M., MCDONALD, S. J., and DE WARDENER, H. E. (1966). "The effect of a high intake of calcium carbonate in normal subjects and patients with chronic renal failure." *Clin. Sci.*, **30**, 425.

COLES, G. A., PETERS, D. R., and JONES, J. H. (1970). "Albumin metabolism in chronic renal failure." *Clin. Sci.*, **39**, 423.

CURTIS, J. R., EASTWOOD, J. B., SMITH, E. K. M., STOREY, J. M., VERROUST, P. J., DE WARDENER, H. E., WING, A. J., and WOLFSON, E. M. (1969). "Maintenance haemodialysis." *Quart. J. Med*, **38**, 49.

CUTHBERT, M. F., and PEART, W. S. (1970). "Studies on the identity of a vascular permeability factor of renal origin." *Clin. Sci.*, **38**, 309.

EASTWOOD, J. B., BORDIER, P., and DE WARDENER, H. E. (1971). "Comparison of the effect of vitamin D and calcium carbonate in renal osteomalacia." *Quart. J. Med.*, **40**, 569.

EKNOYAN, G., WACKSMAN, S. J., GLUECK, H. I., and WILL, J. J. (1969). "Platelet function in renal failure." *New Eng. J. Med.*, **280**, 677.

ELKINGTON, J. R. (1963). "Hydrogen ion turnover in health and in renal disease." *Ann. Int. Med.*, **57**, 660.

FINE, R. N., EDELBROCK, H. H., BRENNAN, L. P., GRUSKIN, C. M., KORSCH, B. M., RIDELL, H., STILES, G., and LIEBERMAN, E. (1971). "Cadaveric renal transplantation in children." *Lancet*, **1**, 1087.

FORD, J., PHILLIPS, M. E., TOYE, F. E., LUCK, V. A., and DE WARDENER, H. E. (1969). "Nitrogen balance in patients with chronic renal failure on diets containing varying quantities of protein." *Brit. Med. J.*, **1**, 735.

GIORDANO, C., DE PASCALE, C., PHILLIPS, M. E., SANTO, M. G., FURST, P., BROWN, C. L., HOUGHTON, B. J., and RICHARDS, P. (1972). "Utilisation of ketoacid analogues of valine and phenylalanine in health and uraemia." *Lancet*, **1**, 178.

GOODMAN, A. D., LEMANN, J., LENNON, E. J., and RELMAN, A. S. (1965). "Production, excretion and nett balance of fixed acid in patients with renal acidosis." *J. clin. Invest.*, **44**, 495.

GOWER, P. E., and STUBBS, R. K. T. (1971). "Some administrative problems in adaption of houses for home dialysis." *Brit. Med. J.*, **1**, 637.

KAYE, M., FRUEH, A. J., SILVERMAN, M., HENDERSON, J., and THIBAUT, T. (1970). "A study of vertebral bone powder from patients with chronic renal failure." *J. Clin. Invest.*, **49**, 442.

MANAGEMENT OF RENAL FAILURE. (1971). Edited by M. D. MILNE. British Medical Bulletin, 27, No. 2. Published by the Medical Dept., The British Council, London.

MASON, E. E. (1952). "Gastrointestinal lesions occurring in uraemia." *Ann. intern. Med.*, **37**, 96.

NUTRITION IN RENAL DISEASE. (1968). Edited by G. M. BERLYNE. D. S. Livingstone Ltd., Edinburgh and London.

PELLEGRINO, E. D., and BILTZ, R. M. (1965). "The composition of human bone in uraemia." *Medicine*, **44**, 397.

PLETKA, P., KENYON, J. R., SNELL, M., COHEN, S. L., HULME, B., OWEN, K., THOMPSON, A. E., MOWBRAY, J. F., PORTER, K. A., LEIGH, D. A., and PEART, W. S. (1969). "Cadaveric renal transplantation. An analysis of 65 cases." *Lancet*, **1**, 1.

RICHARDS, P., HOUGHTON, B. J., and WRONG, O. M. (1969). "Ammonia metabolism in renal failure." *Brit. J. Urol.*, **41**. Supplement to August Number, p. 103.

RICHET, G., NOVALEZ, DE E. L., and VERROUST, P. (1970). "Drug intoxication and neurological episodes in chronic renal failure." *Brit. Med. J.*, **1**, 394.

SCHWARTZ, W. B., HALL, P. W., HAYS, R. M., and RELMAN, A. S. (1959). "On the mechanism of acidosis in chronic renal disease." *J. clin. Invest.*, **38**, 39.

SLATOPOLSKY, E., CALGAR, S., PENNELL, J. P., TAGGART, D. D., CANTERBURY, J. M., REISS, E., and BRICKER, N. S. (1971). "On the pathogenesis of hyperparathyroidism in chronic experimental renal insufficiency in the dog." *J. Clin. Invest.*, **50**, 492.

SLATOPOLSKY, E., GRADOWSKA, L., KASHEMSAUR, C., KELTNER, R., MANLEY, C., and BRICKER, N. S. (1966). "The control of phosphate excretion in uremia." *J. clin. Invest.*, **45**, 672.

STANBURY, S. W. (1972). Bone complications of renal diseases. In "Renal Diseases". Edited by D. A. K. BLACK. Blackwell Scientific Pubs.

STANBURY, S. W., and MAHLER, R. F. (1959). "Salt-wasting renal disease." *Quart. J. Med.*, N.S. **28**, 425.

SYMPOSIUM ON RENAL TRANSPLANTATION (1969). Edited by R. R. ROBINSON. *Arch. Intern. Med.* **123**, No. 5.

SYMPOSIUM ON RENAL OSTEODYSTROPHY (1969). Edited by R. R. ROBINSON. *Arch. Intern. Med.*, **124**, 417.

WATERLOW, J. C. (1968). "Observations on the mechanisms of adaption to low protein intakes." *Lancet*, **2**, 1091.

WARDENER, DE H. E. (1972). Some fresh observations on calcium and phosphate metabolism in chronic renal failure. "Scientific Basis of Medicine." Annual reviews. Athlone Press.

WOLTHUIS, F. H. (1961). "Balance studies on protein metabolism in normal and uraemic man." *Acta med. Scand.*, suppl. 373.

Additional reading on maintenance haemodialysis and renal transplantation:

Transactions of the American Society for Artificial Internal Organs.
Proceedings of the European Dialysis and Transplant Association.

16

The Acute Nephritic Syndrome

THE acute nephritic syndrome consists of a sudden onset of oliguria, oedema, hypertension, raised jugular venous pressure and proteinuria, due to an abrupt generalised disturbance which involves the kidneys. In some patients one or more of these features may be absent, e.g. there may be no proteinuria.

The acute nephritic syndrome may develop in a previously normal person, it may occur as a transient complication in chronic renal failure, or be superimposed upon a nephrotic syndrome. It may also precede chronic renal failure, the nephrotic syndrome or acute renal failure. It is seen in a variety of diseases which affect the kidney, including all stages of glomerular nephritis, polyarteritis nodosa, anaphylactoid purpura, disseminated lupus erythematosus, and following irradiation of the kidneys (Fig. 16.1). It occurs most commonly in acute glomerular nephritis.

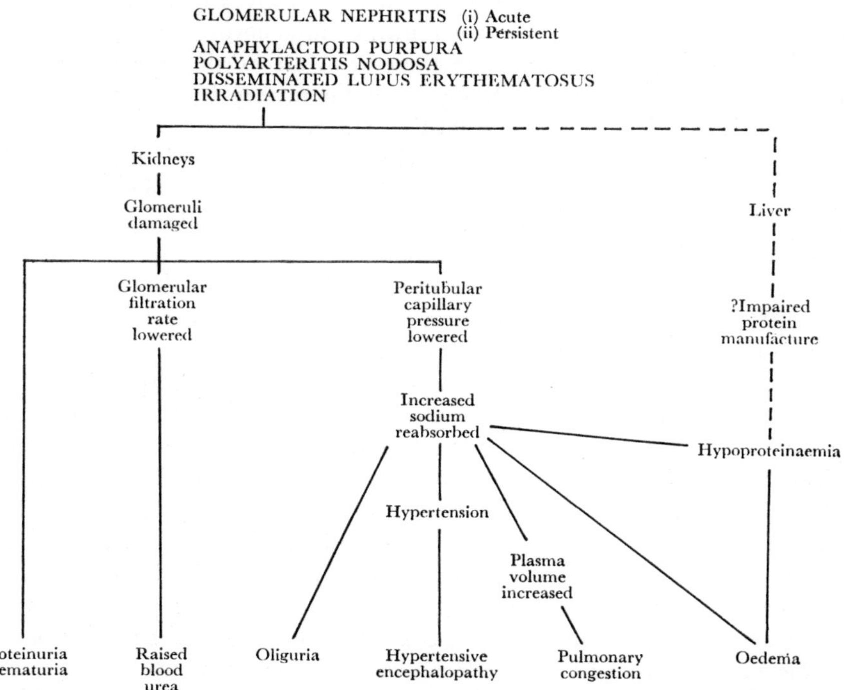

FIG. 16.1. Diseases in which the acute nephritis syndrome may develop and some of the physiological disturbances which take place.

Structural Changes in the Kidneys

The glomeruli usually show diffuse proliferation of mesangial and endothelial cells with narrowing of the capillary lumen, and widening of the capillary walls, with varying degrees of inflammatory cell reaction. In the more severe cases the tubules show focal areas of degeneration associated with clumps of inflammatory cells. On occasion an acute nephritic syndrome may occur without histological lesions.

Functional Changes

Proteinuria is rarely greater than 2–5 g per day, and there is an increased urinary excretion of red and white cells, granular casts and blood casts. The number of white cells sometimes is as great as the number of red cells. As the urine is usually acid the haemoglobin in the red cells changes to acid haematin and, if there is sufficient blood, the urine becomes dark brown. Lesser quantities of blood cause a smoky turbulence when the urine is gently shaken; the presence of blood is confirmed microscopically. These urinary changes are directly related to the histological changes in the glomerular tufts, for when there is no proteinuria the glomeruli are normal.

Glomerular filtration rate is often reduced, but it is remarkable how frequently the blood urea concentration remains within normal limits, if the patient previously had normal kidneys. In those with pre-existing renal disease and long-standing impairment of filtration rate, the further depression in filtration rate associated with the acute nephritic syndrome causes a substantial rise in blood urea. The renal blood flow is usually unaffected except in the most severe cases and in those with pre-existing renal disease; when the blood flow is reduced the decrease is always proportionately less than that of the glomerular filtration rate, i.e. there is a fall in filtration fraction.

The ability to concentrate the urine varies with the degree of tubular damage; if the syndrome complicates established chronic renal failure there is nearly always a complete inability to concentrate.

Salt and water retention is due to an excessive tubular reabsorption of salt and manifests itself as oedema. The increase in tubular sodium reabsorption is possibly due to the endothelial proliferation of the glomerular capillaries obstructing their lumen and thus causing a fall in the peritubular capillary pressure (p. 64). The acute salt and water retention causes an increase in weight, an expanded plasma volume, and consequently a fall in packed cell volume, haemoglobin and plasma proteins. The salt and water retention is also responsible for the concomitant hypertension, rise in jugular venous pressure, cardiac enlargement and pulmonary venous congestion. It has been shown that in spite of these appearances of heart "failure", the arterio-venous oxygen difference is normal both at rest and during severe exercise. There is therefore no evidence that the heart is failing as a pump. In addition, no unequivocal histological lesions in the heart muscle have ever been described. It seems that the retention of sodium and water and the rise in blood volume is associated with redistribution of blood centrally into the heart and lungs. The mechanism responsible for this phenomenon is unknown; it may be due to an increase in peripheral venous tone.

Hypoproteinaemia is usual and occasionally it is severe; it must then also contribute to the formation of oedema. The cause of the hypoproteinaemia is obscure. The retention of water may cause a mild dilution of plasma proteins, and it is possible that on very rare occasions a particularly heavy proteinuria may be partly responsible. Nevertheless, the acute fall in plasma albumin to below 1·0 g per 100 ml which occasionally occurs in patients with acute *anuria* from glomerular nephritis makes it extremely likely that, at least in these cases, there has been a considerable diminution in protein production. It is possible, therefore, that a diminished protein production is a contributory factor in the mild hypo-proteinaemia which is usually found in the acute nephritic syndrome. When there is severe hypoproteinaemia there is also a marked rise in serum cholesterol.

The rise in jugular venous pressure, cardiac enlargement and pulmonary venous congestion occurs in nearly all patients. Paroxysmal attacks of postural and nocturnal dyspnoea are rare, but milder degrees of dyspnoea are relatively common. The heart rate is often either unchanged or slower than normal. In fact this combination of raised jugular venous pressure and bradycardia can be one of the most diagnostic features of the acute nephritic syndrome.

The sudden onset of hypertension probably causes the bradycardia. The extent of the rise in blood pressure varies a great deal and often it is so small that it is only noticed retrospectively, particularly in children. The cause of the rise in blood pressure appears to be related to the salt and water retention, for it does not occur without oedema and a gain in weight; it also seems to be related to the histological changes in the glomeruli, though occasionally the blood pressure may be normal in the presence of extensive glomerular proliferation and exudative inflammation.

Clinical Features

At the onset the patient notices that the face, hands or feet are swelling or that the urine has changed colour to dark brown, or red. Very occasionally dyspnoea may be the presenting symptom; this is more likely in children or when there is pre-existing renal disease. There are few other complaints, though upon direct questioning it may be possible to obtain a history of a recent gain in weight, oliguria, and lassitude. Severe pain in the back often occurs with polyarteritis nodosa, and an ache in the loins seems to be a genuine feature of acute glomerular nephritis. Feverish symptoms and the extent of the rise in temperature vary with the cause of the syndrome. Children often present with loss of appetite, and pallor.

Progress depends a great deal on the disease with which the syndrome is associated, but in the majority of cases the signs and symptoms subside within

7–14 days. There is a brisk diuresis and hypertension and oedema quickly disappear. When the syndrome is superimposed upon pre-existing renal disease, recovery may be much slower and some additional impairment of renal function may be permanent. In patients with previously normal kidneys, recovery is often complete, particularly with acute glomerular nephritis. Death during the acute phase of the syndrome is unusual, but may be caused by pulmonary oedema, acute renal failure or hypertensive encephalopathy.

Treatment

Occasionally it may be possible to influence directly the disease which has precipitated the acute nephritic syndrome; for instance, the use of adrenal steroids in polyarteritis nodosa. Otherwise treatment is symptomatic and is aimed at preventing or minimising the effects of pulmonary oedema, acute renal failure, and hypertensive encephalopathy until there is a spontaneous recovery.

It is convenient to keep a day-to-day chart of the fluid intake, urinary output, blood pressure, weight and 24-hour urinary protein excretion; plasma urea and creatinine should be estimated twice a week.

PULMONARY OEDEMA AND CONGESTION. In most patients there is no necessity to treat this by any other means than the salt and water restriction mentioned above. The dyspnoea of the onset usually settles after a few hours bed rest, but if it increases it may be necessary to use digitalis and morphia, and to sit the patient up in an armchair or cardiac bed throughout the 24 hours. Hypotensive drugs are useful when there is a considerable rise in blood pressure. During a paroxysm of acute pulmonary oedema with deepening cyanosis, 25 mg of either hexamethonium or hydralazine intravenously may be life-saving. On general principles the use of diuretics is not advised and, in any case, they rarely succeed in producing a diuresis in an acute nephritic syndrome.

RENAL FAILURE. As renal failure is usually minimal and of short duration its treatment is not difficult. During the oliguric phase the patient is placed on a salt- and protein-free diet, and the daily fluid intake is limited to a volume equal to the urine passed in the previous 24 hours, plus 500 ml to replace insensible loss. As soon as a diuresis starts, and the glomerular filtration rate returns to normal, these restrictions are relaxed.

In the rare cases when there is acute renal failure with either complete anuria or a daily urine output below 400 ml with a specific gravity around 1·010, treatment is as described for acute renal failure from any other cause, except that measures taken to avoid acute pulmonary congestion have to be more carefully observed than usual.

HYPERTENSIVE ENCEPHALOPATHY. This exceedingly rare complication responds to the intravenous administration of barbiturates (sodium amylobarbitone or thiopentone). After the initial injection it is usually sufficient to continue sedation with large intermittent doses of barbiturates by mouth. The fits are controlled by lowering the blood pressure.

BIBLIOGRAPHY

BLACK, D. A. K., PLATT, R., ROWLANDS, E. N., and VARLEY, H. (1948). "Renal haemo-dynamics in acute nephritis." *Clin. Sci.*, **6**, 295.

EARLE, D. P., FARBER, S. J., and ALEXANDER, J. D. (1950). "Renal function and edema in acute glomerulo-nephritis." *J. clin. Invest.*, **29**, 810.

EARLE, D. P., TAGGART, J. V., and SHANNON, J. A. (1944). "Glomerulonephritis: a survey of functional organisation of the kidney in various stages of diffuse glomerulone-phritis." *J. clin. Invest.*, **23**, 119.

FARBER, S. J. (1957). "Physiologic aspects of glomerulo nephritis." *J. Chronic Dis.*, **5**, 87.

GUZ, A., NOBLE, M. I. M., TRENCHARD, D., GARNETT, E. S., CLARKSON, E. M., McDONALD, S. J., and DE WARDENER, H. E. (1966). "The significance of a raised central venous pressure during sodium and water retention." *Clin. Sci.*, **30**, 295.

HILDEN, T. (1943). "Diodrast clearance in acute nephritis." *Acta med. scand.*, **116**, 1.

PETERS, J. P. (1953). "Edema of Acute Nephritis." *Amer. J. Med.*, **14**, 448.

SCHWARTZ, W. B., and KASSIRER, J. P. (1971). Clinical aspects of acute poststreptococcal glomerulonephritis. In "Diseases of the Kidney". Edited by M. B. Strauss and L. G. Welt. 2nd edition. Little, Brown and Company, Boston, U.S.A.

17

Renal Function and Loss of Metallic Cations

THERE are two important links between loss of metallic cations and renal function: (1) renal failure may be responsible for a negative balance of sodium, potassium, calcium or magnesium, because they are lost in excessive amounts in the urine; (2) a negative balance of sodium, potassium, or an excessive urinary excretion of calcium, may cause renal failure, while a negative balance of magnesium causes changes in renal function.

SODIUM

Sodium deficiency *due to* renal failure

The following renal diseases may sometimes be responsible for an excess urinary loss of sodium:

1. Phenacetin nephropathy.
2. Advanced chronic renal failure.
3. During recovery from acute tubular necrosis.
4. Renal disease of moderate severity combined with dietary salt restriction.
5. Chronic childhood pyelonephritis during relapse of infection.

Sodium deficiency *as a cause of* renal failure

The following conditions may occasionally cause such a loss of sodium that its deficiency contributes materially to the onset of renal failure:

1. Severe diarrhoea and vomiting (e.g. pyloric stenosis).
2. Post-operative gastric suction without replacement.
3. Intestinal and biliary fistulae.
4. Diabetes.
5. Acute pathological processes involving the brain.
6. Hypo-adrenalism (Addison's disease).
7. Diuretics, particularly frusemide and ethacrynic acid.

Clinical Features of Sodium, Chloride and Water Deficiency

Sodium loss is usually accompanied by chloride and water loss, the deficiency of the chloride is usually proportional to that of sodium, but the negative balance of water is usually smaller, for the patient often continues to drink. The extracellular fluid, therefore, tends to become hypotonic, and there is a transfer of water into the cells. The eventual signs and symptoms of sodium deficiency are thus a combination of those due to intracellular overhydration, and decreased extracellular fluid volume. The former gives rise to cerebral and the latter to cardiovascular abnormalities.

The patient is drowsy, restless, apathetic, and sometimes uncooperative. There is thirst (despite the hypotonic plasma), headache, anorexia, nausea and postural giddiness; vomiting may occur and there is a liability to faint on standing; eventually muscle and abdominal cramps develop and the patient may pass into a muttering delirium. There is loss of weight, the face is haggard and the eyes sunken, the skin is clammy and cold and, on pinching it, tends to remain raised; the superficial veins are thin and constricted; the tongue is dry and the eyeballs soft; the pulse is rapid and both the mean arterial and the pulse pressures are decreased. The circulating haemoglobin concentration is raised, but plasma sodium and chloride are lowered. If salt deficiency is not corrected the patient may die rapidly from peripheral circulatory failure.

It must be emphasised, however, that there may be a considerable loss of salt before there is much clinical evidence of deficiency. But even a subclinical deficiency is sufficient to cause renal vasoconstriction with a fall in renal blood flow and glomerular filtration rate, and an increase in blood urea. When salt deficiency is secondary to renal failure the urinary specific gravity is around 1·010 and the urine contains some sodium; whereas if the kidneys were previously healthy, tubular function remains normal, the specific gravity will at first be greater than 1·020 and the urine will contain no sodium. Proteinuria is nearly always present.

Aetiology and Diagnosis

*Sodium, chloride and water deficiency **due to** renal failure.* Phenacetin nephropathy, and chronic childhood pyelonephritis during an acute flare-up of infection are the most common renal diseases to cause florid salt and water deficiency. It has also been reported with chronic glomerular nephritis and polycystic disease. The syndrome is sometimes known as "salt losing nephritis" (p. 183). Very rarely sodium deficiency may also occur during the recovery stage of acute tubular necrosis (p. 168). The chronic renal diseases which cause sodium deficiency may give rise to serious diagnostic difficulties but the salt and water loss following acute tubular necrosis should be anticipated.

*Sodium, chloride and water deficiency **as a cause of** renal failure.* Salt and water deficiency following post-operative gastric suction, intestinal and biliary fistulae should also be anticipated; the onset of renal failure in these conditions is often an indication of mismanagement.

The risk of precipitating renal failure by giving low salt diets to patients suffering from renal disease has been mentioned earlier (p. 198).

Renal failure from loss of water and salt caused by diarrhoea and vomiting

H

or diabetic ketosis does not usually present any diagnostic difficulties. But when it complicates acute cerebral conditions it may easily be overlooked.

The greatest diagnostic difficulty is in differentiating the sodium chloride deficiency and renal failure of Addison's disease from sodium chloride deficiency due to chronic renal disease. In both the deficiency is due to a urinary leak of salt and in both there may be nausea, weakness, loss of weight, pigmentation, hypotension, and a raised plasma potassium. In an emergency the two conditions can be distinguished by the fact that the administration of hydrocortisone and 9α fluorohydrocortisone to patients with renal disease has little effect on the high rate of urinary salt excretion, while recovery occurs rapidly upon giving large amounts of salt and water. When there is more leisure to make the diagnosis it will be found that in sodium chloride deficiency due to renal disease, the concentration of plasma cortisol is normal or raised while the urinary excretion of ketogenic and ketosteroids is normal, and that of aldosterone is raised.

Treatment

If the patient is severely ill treatment consists simply in the rapid intravenous administration of large amounts of isotonic saline, preferably with sodium bicarbonate in a proportion of 2 to 1. Isotonic saline contains 150 mEq/l of sodium and 150 mEq/l of chloride, whereas the extracellular fluid contains 140 mEq/l of sodium but only 100 mEq/l of chloride; the administration of one litre of isotonic sodium bicarbonate (150 mEq of sodium) for every two of saline ensures that sodium and chloride are given in physiological proportions. If acute renal failure has already occurred the rate of infusion must be more moderate, for great care is needed to prevent the onset of pulmonary oedema; it is also essential that sodium bicarbonate be given, for the kidneys are unable to excrete the excess chloride in the sodium chloride solutions. Tablets of Slow release sodium chloride Slow-Sodium (Ciba) 10 mEq can be given orally with water when the need for sodium replacement is less urgent.

Sodium and chloride deficiency with excess water intake

Occasionally patients who are suffering from salt deficiency and oliguria are inadvertently given water (5 per cent glucose) intravenously. They may not excrete this water and they then develop acute overhydration with nausea, vomiting and mental confusion. Treatment consists of the intravenous administration of about 300 ml of hypertonic (3 per cent) saline.

POTASSIUM

Potassium deficiency *due to* renal failure

The following renal diseases may sometimes cause an excess urinary loss of potassium:

1. Chronic glomerular nephritis.
2. Chronic childhood pyelonephritis, during a relapse of infection.
3. Polyarteritis nodosa.
4. During recovery from acute tubular necrosis.
5. Renal tubular acidosis (p. 237).
6. Renal artery stenosis (p. 129).

Potassium deficiency *as a cause of* renal failure

The following conditions may cause such a loss of potassium that its deficiency contributes materially to the onset of renal failure:

1. Prolonged vomiting, e.g. pyloric obstruction.
2. Prolonged diarrhoea, e.g. small bowel insufficiency, excessive use of purgatives or enemas, pancreatic adenomata, and villous tumours of the large bowel.
3. Post-operative gastric suction.
4. Intestinal and biliary fistulae.
5. Uncontrolled diabetes.
6. Injudicious use of ion exchange resins.
7. Aldosteronism.
8. Diuretics.

Clinical Features of Potassium Deficiency

Until potassium deficiency is advanced its signs and symptoms are vague and indefinite. The outstanding and characteristic feature of advanced potassium deficiency is the development of muscular weakness which progresses to paralysis and death from respiratory failure. Otherwise there may be thirst, irritability, nausea, confusion and paralytic ileus. The physical signs are apathy, loss of reflexes, loss of motor power, tetany, gasping respirations and occasionally irregularity of the heart rate. The severity and localisation of the effects of potassium deficiency are influenced to a certain extent by the patient's age. The elderly appear to be more susceptible and tend to have predominantly renal and cardiac complications, whereas the young are less susceptible and tend to have the muscular changes. If the potassium loss is due to renal disease the presence of which is unsuspected, many of these features may at first be thought to be due to hysteria.

A certain diagnosis of low serum potassium can only be made by direct estimation, though some information can be obtained from an electrocardiograph which shows flattened T waves, often with prominent U waves and ST depression. Though the serum concentration of potassium is sometimes of value when the loss of body potassium is severe, it is sometimes misleading, particularly when rapid shifts of potassium are taking place from one fluid compartment to another. The cells may then be severely deficient in potassium though the plasma concentrations are normal or even high. In relatively steady conditions a serum potassium of 3 mEq/l implies a potassium deficit of about 200–300 mEq.

When potassium deficiency is primary and renal failure its consequence, plasma bicarbonate is usually raised; but when potassium deficiency is due to renal disease plasma bicarbonate may be reduced because of the bicarbonate leak and impaired ability to secrete hydrogen ions which accompany chronic renal failure. Alkalosis is initially caused by the diminished amount of potassium in the tubule cells. Sodium reabsorption is then associated with a rather greater secretion of hydrogen than potassium ions from the tubule cells into the tubule lumen. This in turn generates larger quantities of bicarbonate than normal and the plasma bicarbonate rises. A larger load of bicarbonate thus has to be filtered at the glomerulus and a larger reabsorption of bicarbonate results. This active process of bicarbonate reabsorption automatically reduces the passive reabsorption of chloride. Chloride excretion therefore rises. In the final stage there is therefore, a combination of potassium and chloride deficiency and bicarbonate retention. Alkalosis is also due in part to a shift of hydrogen ions into the intracellular fluid, in exchange for intracellular potassium which is released into the extracellular fluid to prevent its concentration from falling to a lethal level. Sodium ions also cross into the intracellular fluid in exchange for potassium so that in pure potassium deficiency there is an overall intracellular sodium retention. Chronic potassium deficiency is often associated with oedema without evidence of heart failure or rise in jugular venous pressure.

Presumably the renal failure which follows potassium deficiency is due to lack of potassium within the tubule cells, for both functional and histological changes are mainly found in the tubules. The ability to concentrate the urine is lost at an early stage though the ability to dilute remains for a considerable time; occasionally the urine may remain at a fixed concentration which is hypotonic to plasma The loss of the ability to concentrate is probably due to the potassium deficiency impairing the sodium pump in the ascending loop of Henle. Polyuria and particularly nocturia are distinctive features of renal failure associated with potassium deficiency. In some patients there is a complete inversion of the normal diurnal rhythm. The polyuria is due to the potassium deficiency stimulating the thirst centre. Following the administration of ammonium chloride, the ability to form a highly acid urine, and to excrete hydrogen ions at a normal rate are impaired though the ability to excrete ammonium remains normal or raised for a considerable time. Changes in glomerular filtration rate follow and are less severe than the tubular changes. The rise in blood urea is also due in part to an increased permeability of the proximal tubule to urea. Nearly always there is a trace of protein in the urine.

The most characteristic histological change found in potassium deficiency in man is extensive vacuolation of the cells of the proximal tubule; this change is rapidly reversible after potassium administration. The more advanced appearances are those of interstitial nephritis and are not reversible. In animals there are extensive changes in the collecting ducts which have not yet been identified in man.

Aetiology and Diagnosis

*Potassium deficiency **due to** renal failure.* This rare phenomenon is characterised by the continued excretion of substantial amounts of potassium in the urine despite depleted body potassium and low plasma potassium. The renal disease responsible for such a deficiency is easy to diagnose when it occurs during recovery from acute tubular necrosis, but it is more difficult to distinguish when it is due to chronic glomerular nephritis, chronic pyelonephritis, polyarteritis nodosa or a selective defect of tubular function. A distinguishing feature of polyarteritis nodosa is pyrexia, which occurs in all cases, even when the only sites overtly involved are the kidneys.

The early stages of potassium deficiency due to a selective error of tubular function (renal tubular acidosis) may sometimes be differentiated from chronic destructive renal disease such as glomerular nephritis by the fact that with the former the impairment in glomerular filtration rate is moderate, and the ability to produce a highly acid urine and to excrete ammonia in response to ammonium chloride is grossly abnormal (p. 237). With chronic destructive lesions, though there is also an impaired ability to excrete ammonia, glomerular filtration rate is severely reduced and the ability to excrete a highly acid urine appears normal until potassium deficiency itself impairs the ability to excrete an acid urine (see above).

*Potassium deficiency **as a cause of** renal failure.* This syndrome is more frequent than its converse and its cause is usually more easily diagnosed. When potassium deficiency causes renal failure the loss of potassium is nearly always from the alimentary tract. Vomiting, gastric suction, diarrhoea, intestinal fistulae and the misuse of ion exchange resins are easily identifiable causes of excessive loss of potassium. Long-continued use of purgatives and small bowel insufficiency may be more obscure, but there is usually some looseness of the bowels. In all these conditions the urine contains only minimal amounts of potassium and except with ion exchange resins, the plasma bicarbonate is raised. This combination of renal failure, low plasma potassium and low urinary excretion of potassium, proves that the renal failure is indeed due to *extrarenal* loss of potassium.

Very occasionally when severe potassium deficiency has been present for some time, the severity of the renal damage which results may impair the reabsorption of potassium. Urinary potassium excretion then rises in spite of the hypokalaemia and it may now be difficult to distinguish whether the renal failure is due to the potassium deficiency or vice versa. Compulsive, depressed, post-menopausal women, who obtain satisfaction and relief by secretly taking large quantities of purgatives, are those most likely to do this to themselves. They are characteristically evasive or downright misleading about their use of purgatives, so that the true cause of the potassium deficiency and renal failure may not be detected for a considerable time, even with the patient in hospital. Others with abnormal personalities who pose the same problems may have anorexia nervosa or they may be surreptitious vomiters or secret users of diuretics (Fig. 17.1).

There are two other situations in which renal failure is caused by excessive *renal* loss of potassium, diabetic ketosis and primary aldosteronism. In diabetic ketosis (p. 341) the potassium deficiency is only an incidental cause of renal failure and no diagnostic confusion is likely.

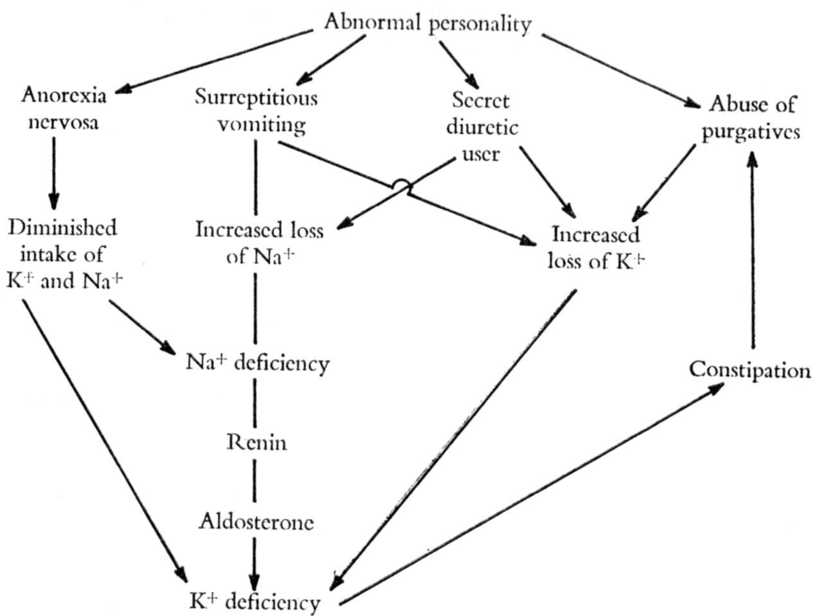

FIG. 17.1. Some causes of potassium deficiency and consequential renal failure in patients with abnormal personalities. (From Wolff, Vecsei, Kruck, Roscher, Brown, Dusterdieck, Lever and Robertson, 1968, *Lancet*, **1**, 257.)

Renal failure due to primary hyperaldosteronism may be extremely difficult to distinguish from renal disease causing secondary hyperaldosteronism, when the associated renal ischaemia causes a release of renin and stimulation of the adrenal glands by angiotensin. In both there may be polyuria and thirst, low plasma potassium, hypertension and a raised blood urea. The blood urea is usually much higher, i.e. about 200 mg/100 ml if renal disease is causing secondary hyperaldosteronism. In primary aldosteronism, malignant hypertension is unusual, whereas it is more often malignant with renal ischaemia. In addition the plasma sodium is higher (137–160 mEq/l) in primary aldosteronism than in secondary aldosteronism (125–141 mEq/l) though there is some overlap. On the other hand, the plasma potassium is lower (1·4 to 3·2 mEq/l) in primary aldosteronism than in secondary aldosteronism (3·1 to 4·2 mEq/l). One method of distinguishing between these two is to measure the plasma renin before and after three days on a low sodium diet; the second blood being taken on the third day, after standing for four hours. In primary aldosteronism the control plasma renin is low and it remains low. In secondary aldosteronism the control renin should be higher but the most characteristic finding is that it rises further after a low sodium diet and standing. A renal biopsy can sometimes help. If the structural changes are characteristic only of potassium deficiency, i.e. there is vacuolation of the tubule cells, particularly of the distal tubules, the hypokalaemia and renal failure may be due to primary aldosteronism. If the lesions are more extensive and include those of interstitial nephritis renal biopsy is of relatively little help, for such changes can follow potassium deficiency or they may be due to a long-standing chronic renal disease which may be the cause of the potassium deficiency.

Treatment

When renal disease is the cause of the potassium deficiency the only effective treatment is potassium replacement followed by the daily oral administration of sufficient potassium to balance the excess urinary loss.

Potassium chloride is clearly what is needed in nearly all instances, particularly at the beginning of treatment when there is a potassium and chloride deficit to be corrected. Solutions of oral potassium chloride however, have an unpleasant taste and enteric coated tablets produce sharply delineated zones of circatricial narrowing of the small bowel which may cause complete or partial obstruction. Slow release tablets of "wax" impregnated with potassium chloride (Slow K, Ciba) are the most suitable preparations to use. Once the initial potassium and chloride deficiency has been corrected, the administration of supplemental potassium chloride may have to be continued to prevent a deficiency of potassium recurring. Other salts of potassium which are also used include a mixture of potassium acetate, citrate and bicarbonate, 1 g of each in 8 ml of water, four times a day which supplies 116 mEq of potassium in a relatively palatable form. Mist. Pot. Cit. (B.P.) contains 3 g of potassium citrate, i.e. 28 mEq of potassium per 15 ml which is about half an ounce; this is also well tolerated.

To prevent the onset of potassium deficiency during the early diuretic phase of acute tubular necrosis, it is usually only necessary to give plenty of orange and tomato juice, figs, apricots, dates and meat extract, all of which contain high quantities of potassium (p. 411).

When potassium deficiency is due to excess alimentary loss all that is required is to replace the potassium and stop any further loss; if the latter is not possible (e.g. intestinal fistulae, gastric suction) potassium should be given intravenously at the same rate as it is being lost.

Potassium is best given intravenously when there is a good urine flow, in order that an excess plasma potassium may more easily spill over in the urine. It is also wise to avoid intravenous administration for 24 hours after any particular stress such as an operation, for at these times the plasma potassium is apt to be raised whatever the concentration in the cells. It should also be borne in mind that in normal circumstances, though the total body potassium is about 2,500 mEq, the amount in the extracellular fluid is only 75 mEq and that death occurs if it rises to 150 mEq. Cardiac arrest from hyperkalaemia occurs at plasma levels of 9–10 mEq/l; it is generally wise not to give potassium intravenously at a greater rate than 25 mEq per hour. It is also best to limit the concentration of the fluid to 40 mEq/l, for higher concentrations are liable to cause painful spasm of the vein.

If a patient suffering from a pure potassium deficiency is given saline instead of potassium there is likely to be increased sodium retention with oedema and an increased urinary excretion of potassium. The administration of sodium bicarbonate should also be avoided for this induces a severe alkalosis.

CALCIUM

A raised urinary excretion of calcium may cause renal failure irrespective of the overall calcium balance. The reason for this is not known, but it is probably related to an intracellular accumulation of calcium ions in the tubules. This is in contrast to the renal failure of potassium deficiency (see above), which is due to an intracellular deficiency of potassium ions, or the renal failure of sodium deficiency which is due to contraction of the extracellular fluid volume and renal vasoconstriction.

The following conditions are associated with a high urinary calcium excretion and renal failure.

Increased urinary excretion of calcium *due to* renal failure

The only renal disease known to cause a great increase in urinary calcium excretion is renal tubular acidosis (p. 237).

Increased urinary excretion of calcium *as a cause of* renal failure

(*a*) Following increased calcium absorption:

    1. Compulsive milk drinking.
    2. Excess vitamin D intake.
    3. Sarcoidosis.
    4. Idiopathic hypercalcaemia of infants.

(*b*) Following an increased rate of bone decalcification:

    1. Hyperparathyroidism.
    2. Diffuse carcinomatosis of bone.
    3. Myelomatosis.
    4. Immobilisation.
    5. Paget's disease.

Effect of Hypercalcaemia on Renal Structure and Function

In the early stages renal biopsy may show no abnormality, but later, precipitated calcium can be seen as clumps between and across the nephrons, and as a fine dusting of the tubule cells and their basement membranes. The early lesions are in the collecting ducts, distal tubules and ascending loops of Henle. Later the whole nephron is involved. Some tubules eventually atrophy, and varying numbers of glomeruli become structureless round eosinstaining masses. In long-standing cases the deposition of calcium in the kidney can be seen radiologically.

Hypercalcaemia from any cause *except hyperparathyroidism* increases urinary hydrogen ion excretion. Ammonia excretion therefore rises and urine pH falls, while plasma bicarbonate and pH rise and there is an alkalosis. (This acceleration of hydrogen ion secretion by the tubule is paralleled by an increase in hydrogen ion secretion by the gastric mucosa so that hypercalcaemia is often associated with epigastric pain, dyspepsia and peptic ulcers.) The cause of this acceleration of hydrogen ion secretion is unknown, it may be due to stimulation of carbonic anhydrase activity. In early hypercalcaemia therefore (with the exception of hyperparathyroidism), there may be the paradoxical finding of a raised plasma bicarbonate with a low urine pH. On the other hand, parathormone inhibits hydrogen ion excretion so that when hypercalcaemia is due to hyperparathyroidism there is a rise in urine pH and a tendency for the plasma bicarbonate to fall.

Hypercalcaemia and hypercalcuria from any cause profoundly impair the kidney's ability to concentrate the urine; frequently the urine concentration remains fixed at a concentration well below that of plasma. The impaired ability to concentrate is related to the hypercalcuria as well as the hypercalcaemia and may therefore occur without hypercalcaemia. It is probably due to the excess intracellular calcium impairing the sodium pump in the ascending loop of Henle. If hypercalcaemia persists there is a fall in glomerular filtration rate, a rise in blood urea and proteinuria. At first the blood urea is only moderately raised to 50–60 mg/100 ml, and there is then a marked discrepancy between the severe impairment in concentrating ability and the modest rise in blood urea. Gradually so many nephrons are destroyed that eventually the findings are the same as those in chronic renal failure from any cause. At this point the increasing impairment of hydrogen ion secretion and ammonia production of renal failure is superimposed upon the effect of hypercalcaemia and if the plasma bicarbonate was raised it now falls to normal or below.

Clinical Features Associated with Hypercalcuria and Hypercalcaemia

As the renal failure is only related to the high urinary excretion of calcium and not to negative calcium balance (unlike potassium and sodium), the general signs and symptoms vary widely from one cause to another. For instance, if the

H§

hypercalcuria is secondary to bone disease there will be a negative calcium balance and signs and symptoms of bone softening or fractures, whereas if hypercalcuria is due to excessive intestinal absorption of calcium there will be calcium equilibrium and no signs or symptoms of bone disease.

There is always thirst, polydipsia and polyuria. These are often of such severity that the patient may at first be thought to be suffering from diabetes insipidus (p. 331). As in potassium deficiency this is mainly due to the hypercalcaemia stimulating the thirst centre.

Hypercalcuria is usually present when the serum calcium is raised; it may also be present without such a rise. Alternatively, if the glomerular filtration rate is sufficiently depressed there may be hypercalcaemia with hypocalcuria. Occasionally, when the urinary excretion of calcium is extremely high, i.e. around 1,000 mg a day (on a normal diet the usual range is 80–400 mg), the urine upon standing will develop a thin white chalky precipitate which is characteristic.

Aetiology and Diagnosis

Increased urinary excretion of calcium **as a cause of** *renal failure*

(a) *Following increased calcium absorption*. In compulsive milk drinking, vitamin D intoxication, sarcoidosis and idiopathic hypercalcaemia of infants there is an increased alimentary absorption of calcium with the following consequences: hypercalcaemia → hypercalcuria → renal failure.

Compulsive milk drinking is a rare condition which, initially, can easily be overlooked, for the patient may fail to disclose his idiosyncrasy, or he minimises its extent. Frequently the milk drinking begins because of recurrent dyspepsia, but as the amount taken increases and hypercalcaemia develops, the dyspepsia becomes worse. The fact that these patients are also apt to take large quantities of alkalis, which often contain calcium carbonate, may increase the liability of calcium to be deposited in the kidney. Compulsive milk drinkers are frequently admitted with advanced renal failure and alkalosis. Diagnosis may be difficult for by this time glomerular filtration rate is so depressed that there is no hypercalcuria, and in addition the patient is now so ill and nauseated that his compulsion for milk is less pressing. Hypercalcaemia is usually present and often there are widespread deposits of calcium in the skin, joints, corneae and lungs.

Excess vitamin D intake is not uncommon. In adults it occurs as a form of food fad, or more usually from taking vitamin D supplements to avoid colds. In infants and children excess vitamin D intake derives from over-solicitous motherly attention. At one time infants and children normally ingested larger quantities of vitamin D than necessary. Not only was it given as concentrated cod and halibut liver oil, but much of the food they ate, such as milk preparations and cereals, often had vitamin D added in substantial quantities. This excess may have been the precipitating cause of the increased calcium absorption of idiopathic hypercalcaemia of infants. In recent years however, the vitamin D content of commercial milk preparations and cereals has been reduced.

The increased calcium absorption of sarcoidosis also appears to be due to vitamin D; not excess ingestion, but rather to a hypersensitivity to normal amounts either in the food or following exposure to sunlight. The increased absorption and hypercalcuria can be controlled by adrenal steroids, 150 mg of cortisone per day for 10 days causes a fall in plasma calcium and in urinary calcium excretion.

(b) *Following increased rate of bone decalcification.* There are three principal conditions to be considered: hyperparathyroidism, diffuse carcinomatosis of bone and myelomatosis.

The diagnosis of hyperparathyroidism depends on the finding of a raised plasma calcium, a low plasma phosphate, and hypercalcuria; the characteristic periosteal erosions in the bones of the hands, bone cysts, a raised alkaline phosphatase and recurrent renal calculi may also occur. It is the condition which gives rise to the highest serum calcium concentrations; sometimes over 20 mg per 100 ml. Acute hyperparathyroidism with severe prostration, muscular weakness, pains and tenderness, vomiting, cardiac failure, dyspepsia, polyuria and polydipsia may not be recognised, unless the diagnosis is suspected on every occasion that there is unexplained thirst and polyuria. Radiological bone lesions may be absent both in acute and chronic hyperparathyroidism, which makes the differentiation from sarcoidosis difficult. The confusion is greatest if renal failure is moderately advanced, for this occasionally causes the plasma phosphate to rise and thus obscure one of the most characteristic signs of hyperparathyroidism.

Diffuse carcinomatosis of bone is identified by X-rays of the skeleton and by bone marrow biopsy; and there may also be a leuco-erythroblastic anaemia.

Renal failure associated with myelomatosis is sometimes due to increased urinary calcium excretion. Hypercalcaemia may precipitate a rapid deterioration of renal function.

Treatment

The treatment of renal tubular acidosis is discussed in Section 18.

The increased calcium absorption in sarcoidosis is treated with cortisone; as this functional peculiarity is often phasic, treatment should be interrupted now and again to see if it is still necessary.

Idiopathic hypercalcaemia of infants will usually respond in a few weeks when treated with either a low calcium diet or cortisone; the latter allows a much greater flexibility in the diet, and calcium ingestion need only be controlled to a limited extent.

Hyperparathyroidism is treated by removal of adenomata or hyperplastic glands. Acute renal failure following operation may occur and is particularly dangerous, for the falling serum calcium and rising potassium summate in their ill effects. Patients suffering from compulsive milk drinking or vitamin D intoxication are usually only in need of advice.

MAGNESIUM

*Increased urinary excretion of magnesium **due to** renal failure*. Very occasionally a severe exacerbation of acute upon chronic pyelonephritis in a patient with established chronic renal failure may cause a reversible urinary leak of magnesium. This is nearly always associated with a simultaneous equally reversible leak of sodium and potassium and a profound hypocalcaemia. The diagnosis is most easily made by measuring the plasma magnesium which will be low. Symptoms of magnesium deficiency develop at plasma levels of magnesium well below 1 mEq/l. These consist of gross tremors, confusion with panic attacks, vomiting, fasciculation, hyporeflexia and usually, but no always, a positive Trousseau and Chvostek's sign. It is interesting that in magnesium deficiency with hypocalcaemia the plasma calcium may rise upon giving magnesium chloride.

Chronic renal failure from other causes such as persistent glomerular nephritis has on rare occasions been described as causing a persistent urinary leak of magnesium.

*Renal failure **due to** magnesium deficiency*. This has not been described in man. In animals magnesium deficiency causes an increased potassium excretion with potassium depletion, together with a hypercalcaemia and hypercalcuria. Renal failure develops eventually. In the earlier stages the potassium deficiency is associated with an unimpaired ability to concentrate. The reason for this is not known. There may be a human paralled. It is known that hyperaldosteronism causes an increased urinary excretion of magnesium, and it is also established that some patients with hyperaldosteronism may have a potassium deficit without an impairment in the ability to concentrate. It is possible that this may be due to the associated magnesium deficiency.

BIBLIOGRAPHY

BURNETT, C. H., COMMONS, R. R., ALBRIGHT, F., and HOWARD, J. E. (1949). "Hypercalcaemia without hypercalcuria or hypophosphataemia, calcinosis and renal insufficiency. A syndrome following prolonged intake of milk and alkali." *New Eng. J. Med.*, **240**, 787.

CANNON, P. J., AMES, R. P., and LARAGH, J. H. (1966). "Relation between potassium balance and aldosterone secretion in normal subjects and in patients with hypertensive or renal tubular disease." *J. Clin. Invest.*, **45**, 865.

DARROW, D. C., PRATT, E. L., FLETT, J., GAMBLE, A. H., and WEISE, H. F. (1949). "Disturbances of water and electrolytes in infantile diarrhoea." *Pediatrics*, **3**, 129.

DAVIES, R. H., MORGAN, D. B., and RIVLIN, R. S. (1970). "The excretion of calcium in the urine and its relation to calcium intake, sex and age." *Clin. Sci.*, **39**, 1.

DENT, C. E., and WATSON, L. (1965). "Metabolic studies in a patient with idiopathic hypercalcuria." *Brit. Med. J.*, **1**, 449.

DENT, C. E., and WATSON, L. (1968). "The hydrocortisone test in primary and tertiary hyperparathyroidism." *Lancet*, **1**, 662.

ELKINTON, J. R. (1952). "Potassium: Physiologic Classification, Diagnosis and Treatment of Clinical Disturbances. Advances in Medicine and Surgery", Graduate School of Medicine, University of Pennsylvania. W. B. Saunders, Philadelphia.

EPSTEIN, F. H. (1960). "Calcium and the kidney." *J. chron. Dis.*, **11**, 255.

FOURMAN, P., and ROYER, P. (1968). "Calcium metabolism and the bone." 2nd Edition. Blackwell Scientific Pubs., Oxford.

GRAEFF, J. DE, and SCHURRS, M. A. M. (1960). "Severe potassium depletion caused by the abuse of laxatives." *Acta Med. Scand.*, **166**, 407.

GRAEFF, J. DE, STRUYVENBERG, A., and LAMEYER, L. D. F. (1964). "The role of chloride in hypokalaemic alkalosis." *Amer. J. Med.*, **37**, 778.

GROSS, F., BRUNNER, H., and ZIEGLER, M. (1965). "Renin angiotensin system, aldosterone, and sodium balance." *Recent Prog. Hormone Res.*, **21**, 119.

GUIGNARD, J. P., JONES, N. F., and BARRACLOUGH, M. A. (1970). "Effect of brief hypercalcaemia on free water reabsorption during solute diuresis. Evidence for impairment of Na^+ transport in Henle's loop." *Clin. Sci.*, **39**, 337.

HOWARD, J. E., and THOMAS, W. C. (1963). "Clinical disorders of calcium homeostasis." *Medicine*, **42**, 25.

LEADING ARTICLE (1960). "Idiopathic hypercalcaemia of infants." *Lancet*, **2**, 138.

LLYOID, H. M. (1968). "Primary hyperparathyroidism. An analysis of the role of parathyroid tumour." *Medicine*, **47**, 53.

MACINTYRE, I., HANNA, S., BOOTH, C. C., and READ, A. E. (1960). "Intracellular magnesium deficiency in man." *Clin. Sci.*, **20**, 287.

MANITIUS, A., and EPSTEIN, F. H. (1963). "Some observations on the influence of a magnesium deficient diet on rats with special reference to renal concentrating ability." *J. clin. Invest.*, **42**, 208.

MCQUEEN, E. G. (1952). "Milk poisoning" and "calcium gout." *Lancet*, **2**, 67.

RICHET, G., ARDAILLOU, R., and CL. ARNEIL (1963). "Alcalose métabolique rénale de l'hypercalcémie." Actualités néphrologiques de l'hopital Necker. Éd. Médicales Flammarion Paris, p. 145.

SHILS, M. E. (1964). "Experimental human magnesium depletion." *Amer. J. clin. Nutrit.*, **15**, 133.

SHULMAN, L. E., SCHOENRICH, E. H., and HARVEY, A. M. (1952). "The effects of adrenocorticotrophic hormone (ACTH) and cortisone on sarcoidosis." *Bull. Johns Hopkins Hosp.*, **91**, 371.

THORN, G. W., KOEPF, G. F., and CLINTON, M. (1944). "Renal failure simulating adrenocortical insufficiency." *New Eng. J. Med.*, **231**, 76.

WALKER, W. G., JOST, L. J., KOWARSKI, A., and DUNN, M. J. (1969). "Aldosterone secretion and sodium balance in salt loosing nephropathy." *Johns Hopkins Med. J.*, **122**, 45.

WALLACE, M., RICHARDS, P., CHASSER, E., and WRONG, O. (1968). "Persistent alkalosis and hypokalaemia caused by surreptitious vomiting." *Quart. J. Med.*, **37**, 577.

WELT, L. G., HOLLANDER, W., Jr., and BLYTHE, W. B. (1960). "The consequences of potassium depletion." *J. chron. Dis.*, **11**, 213.

18

Selective Defects of Tubular Function

Selective functional defects of the renal tubules may be either congenital or acquired.

CONGENITAL DEFECTS OF TUBULAR FUNCTION

Single Defects

Impaired ability to reabsorb:

Water	Renal diabetes insipidus.
Sodium	In proximal tubule (Bartter's syndrome).
Phosphate	Vitamin D resistant rickets, familial hypophosphataemia.
Glucose	Renal glycosuria.
Cystine and other amino acids	Simple congenital cystinuria.
Xanthine	Xanthinuria.
Calcium	Idiopathic hypercalcuria.

Excessive reabsorption of:

Phosphate	Pseudohypoparathyroidism.
Sodium	In proximal tubule (Gordon's syndrome).
	In distal tubule (Liddle's syndrome).

Multiple Defects

Impaired ability to reabsorb:

Phosphate, glucose and amino acids	Idiopathic de Toni–Debré–Fanconi syndrome.
Impaired ability to achieve a high hydrogen ion and osmotic gradient	Renal tubular acidosis. Hyperchloraemic acidosis. Hyperchloraemia nephrocalcinosis.

Familial hypophosphataemia and idiopathic hypercalcuria are now thought to be due to a diminished alimentary absorption of calcium and phosphate, and an increased absorption of calcium respectively. Nevertheless they are included here for traditional reasons.

Impaired Ability to Reabsorb Water

This condition is known as renal or nephrogenic diabetes insipidus. It is described on p. 330.

Impaired Ability to Reabsorb Sodium from the Proximal Tubule, or Excessive Reabsorption of Sodium from the Proximal or the Distal Tubule

Disturbances of sodium reabsorption thought to be due to a specific defect of tubular function are very rare. They do occur however and are of great interest in the study of the pathophysiology of sodium metabolism.

BARTTER'S SYNDROME (DIMINISHED SODIUM REABSORPTION BY THE PROXIMAL TUBULE). These patients present with symptoms due to hypokalaemia. They have a normal or low blood pressure and a reduced extracellular fluid volume. Aldosterone secretion rate and plasma renin are both high. Renal biopsy reveals grossly hypertrophied juxta-glomerular apparati. The most likely mechanism for this syndrome is that a diminished ability to reabsorb sodium from the proximal tubule results in excess sodium reaching the distal tubule which tends to cause a urinary leak of sodium. This shrinks the extracellular fluid volume which reduces the blood pressure and causes the plasma renin and the aldosterone secretion rate to rise. This secondary aldosteronism increases sodium reabsorption by the distal tubule which tends to compensate for the excess sodium delivered to the distal tubule, but at the cost of a high urinary excretion of potassium, which is the cause of hypokalaemia. Treatment consists of supplying sufficient potassium replacements.

GORDON'S SYNDROME (EXCESS SODIUM REABSORPTION BY THE PROXIMAL TUBULE). There is hypertension, an expanded extracellular fluid volume and hyperkalaemia. Aldosterone secretion and plasma renin are low and do not rise normally upon sodium deprivation. It is possible that this syndrome is due to excess sodium reabsorption by the proximal tubule, this expands the extracellular fluid which raises the blood pressure and lowers the plasma renin and aldosterone secretion rate. The increase in sodium reabsorption by the proximal tubule also lowers the delivery of sodium into the distal tubule, which together with the reduced plasma aldosterone, reduces the secretion of potassium by the distal tubule. Treatment consists of a low sodium diet and diuretics.

LIDDLE'S SYNDROME (EXCESS SODIUM REABSORPTION BY THE DISTAL TUBULE). This syndrome is a familial disorder affecting individuals of both sexes and of successive generations. There is hypertension, an expanded extracellular fluid volume and hypokalaemia, with a grossly reduced aldosterone secretion rate. It has been suggested that this syndrome is due to excess sodium reabsorption by the distal tubule of unknown cause. This causes the increase in the extracellular fluid volume which causes the hypertension and the reduced rate of aldosterone secretion. Accordingly the low plasma potassium is due to the excessive secretion of potassium from the distal tubule due to the excess sodium reabsorption. These renal abnormalities are associated with a demonstrable abnormality of sodium transport in the erythrocytes. Treatment consists of a low sodium diet and the diuretic triampterene which acts on the distal tubule without increasing potassium excretion.

Impaired Ability to Reabsorb Phosphate

This condition is also known as vitamin D resistant rickets, or familial hypophosphataemia. These names describe the two main clinical features of the disease and avoid any precipitate precision about its aetiology. In addition to the tubular abnormality, there is also an impaired ability of the intestines to absorb calcium, and occasionally phosphate. The cause of the tubule's impaired ability to reabsorb phosphate is not clear. It is possible that it is due to a secondary hyperparathyroidism compensating for a primary impairment in the ability to absorb calcium from the gut. In favour of this explanation is the fact that (1) in a few cases exploration of the neck has demonstrated parathyroid hyperplasia; (2) secondary hyperparathyroidism is known to occur in nutritional osteomalacia; and (3) if parathyroid function is inhibited by a twelve-hour intravenous infusion of calcium, tubular reabsorption of phosphate rises precipitously until very little phosphate appears in the urine (in one patient there was no phosphate in the urine for twelve hours). If this explanation is accepted familial hypophosphataemia is a disease of the small bowel in which the kidneys are normal. Occasionally familial hypophosphataemia is associated with aminoaciduria and tubular acidosis. Up till now this has made it difficult to accept the hypothesis that the increased phosphate excretion was due entirely to a compensatory rise in plasma parathormone. Recently, however, it has been demonstrated that hyperparathyroidism can cause a reversible aminoaciduria and tubular acidosis. Whatever the true explanation of this syndrome the remarkable ability to reabsorb phosphate which follows an intravenous infusion of calcium makes it most unlikely that there is a primary defect in the tubules capacity to reabsorb phosphate.

The disease is nearly always inherited as a sex-linked dominant characteristic, i.e. it appears to be placed on the X chromosome. This conclusion follows from the fact that all the daughters of the male sufferers tend to be affected but none of the sons, whereas half the sons and half the daughters of the female sufferers are affected. There is a rarer form of vitamin D resistant rickets which is inherited as an autosomal recessive disease.

The classical syndrome is that of dwarfism in a young boy with late rickets (around the age of four to eight years), but many affected individuals, particularly women, are healthy and have no skeletal changes. Regardless of bone changes the presence of the disease in the affected person is recognised by the low concentration of serum phosphorus and the diminished ability of the tubules to reabsorb phosphate. The tubular abnormality is detected by one or more of the several methods described earlier (p. 85). For instance, when the condition is particularly severe urinary phosphate excretion continues when the concentration of serum phosphorus is below the normal phosphate threshold of 2·1 mg/100 ml. Urinary calcium excretion is always low. The glomerular filtration rate is unimpaired and the concentration of serum calcium is usually normal though occasionally it is raised in the affected children (i.e. under the age of 15 years) and usually normal thereafter, and a bone biopsy shows the appearance of osteomalacia. Plasma alkaline phosphatase is raised. The impaired intestinal absorption of calcium has been demonstrated in patients with skeletal changes. There are, as yet, no reports of calcium balance studies in affected individuals with normal bones.

TREATMENT. The aim of treatment is to increase calcium and phosphate absorption and thus increase their deposition in the bones. This is attempted by either giving calcium alone or in combination with calciferol; sometimes calciferol is given with phosphate; and occasionally phosphate alone is given. The short-term efficacy of treatment can be gauged by following the plasma alkaline phosphatase and the urinary excretion of calcium. The former should fall and the latter should rise. At longer intervals series X-rays of bone will demonstrate whether the aim of treatment is being achieved.

Calcium lactate 15–20 g/day may be sufficient. Vitamin D is given in large amounts such as calciferol 2–5 mg per day. Sometimes the calciferol is of most benefit if given with a high intake of dietary phosphate and the administration of $Na_2HPO_42H_2O$ 10 g per day. Calciferol may be difficult to control for it appears that the patient's sensitivity may fluctuate so that he may either develop hypercalcaemia which indicates that too much is being given or a rise in the plasma alkaline phosphatase which means that the dose of calciferol is insufficient. Occasionally the administration of large amounts of phosphate alone without vitamin D has caused a radiological improvement in the bone lesions. This only occurs if the urinary calcium excretion is high or "high normal". As treatment progresses there is usually no significant change in plasma phosphorus or calcium though the tubule's ability to reabsorb phosphate often improves. Frequently the condition does not respond or there is only a transient improvement. In the group of patients in whom the disease is due to an autosomal disorder the administration of vitamin D in large amounts cures the disease so that there is no subsequent dwarfing, and the serum phosphate returns to normal.

Impaired Ability to Reabsorb Glucose

This condition is known as renal glycosuria and is described on p. 340.

Impaired Ability to Reabsorb Cystine and Certain Other Amino Acids

There are two principal conditions in which cystine appears in the urine. In one, which is usually known as cystinuria, the metabolism of cystine is normal, but an isolated abnormality of tubular function allows large amounts of cystine, and the dibasic amino acids arginine, lysine and ornithine to be excreted in the urine. The disease is inherited as an autosomal recessive disorder. Patients suffering from cystinuria also have a defect of intestinal absorption for cystine, arginine, lysine and ornithine. The other condition in which cystine may appear in the urine is best called cystine storage disease, or cystinosis. It is also an autosomal recessive disorder, and is one of the many causes of Fanconi's syndrome. The important disturbance is a defect in protein and amino-acid metabolism which causes a widespread deposition of cystine throughout the body. At the same time there is deposited in tubules an unidentified metabolite which causes the abnormalities of tubular function. These include cystinuria and other amino acidurias, phosphaturia, glycosuria and sometimes an impaired ability to acidify and to retain water.

CYSTINURIA. In this condition cystine appears in the urine together with arginine, lysine, and ornithine. The excretion of cystine averages 0·5 to 1 g per day. A solution of cystine at a pH 5 to 7 becomes saturated around 300 to 400 mg/l and tends to come out of solution when it is acid. In patients with cystinuria it is extremely likely, therefore, that at night when the urine is both concentrated and acid it becomes supersaturated, which explains why the clinical complication of the disease is the recurrent formation of renal calculi made of cystine which are radio opaque. The other amino acids which appear in the urine are freely soluble and do not form calculi, nor does their excess loss seem to cause any detectable clinical abnormality. The first cystine stone commonly presents during childhood or infancy; it is rare for it to do so after the age of 30. It is a surprising feature of cystinuria that though renal calculi may recur over a number of years, renal infection is unusual.

Treatment consists in drinking 3 litres of fluid throughout the 24 hours, including two glasses of water upon going to bed and another two after midnight, when the first two have usually forced the patient out of bed to empty his bladder. It is claimed that such treatment will not only prevent the formation of new stones but it will also "dissolve" those present. Nevertheless it is difficult to maintain a high urine flow during the night. If increased water intake is insufficient to prevent precipitation of cystine, the urine is made alkaline by the administration of 15 g per day of sodium bicarbonate.

Cystinuria can also be treated by the oral administration of D-penicillamine at regular intervals throughout the day. The relatively insoluble cystine is then converted to the highly soluble penicillamine-cysteine-disulphide. The dose of D-penicillamine has to be adjusted to the rate of cystine excretion. This treatment is expensive and can cause a number of unwanted effects including rashes, fever, proteinuria and the nephrotic syndrome. It may sometimes be possible to combine a high intake of water during the day and a moderate dose of penicillamine during the night.

CYSTINE STORAGE DISEASE AND FANCONI'S SYNDROME. This syndrome is discussed on p. 236.

Impaired Ability to Reabsorb Xanthine

This condition is usually known as xanthinuria. It is due to two functional defects. First, an absence of xanthine oxidase in the liver so that the conversion of xanthine to uric acid is blocked; and, secondly, a tubular defect of xanthine reabsorption. The clearance of xanthine equals that of the glomerular filtration rate. Large quantities of xanthine therefore appear in the urine but only traces of uric acid, and the blood uric acid is exceedingly low. Occasionally, xanthine renal calculi, translucent to X-rays, may be formed. As xanthine is much more soluble in alkaline urine, treatment consists in the administration of sodium citrate or bicarbonate to those patients who are apt to form stones.

Impaired Ability to Reabsorb Calcium

This condition is known as idiopathic hypercalcuria. It is characterised by a calcium excretion greater than 400 mg per day. The alimentary absorption of calcium, however, is also raised so that the patient is in calcium balance and there are no bone changes. Plasma calcium is usually normal, but in about 10–20 per cent of patients the plasma phosphate is low (i.e. below 2·6 mg/100 ml). In about 10 per cent of patients there is an intermittent hypercalcaemia due to hyperparathyroidism. A minority of patients with idiopathic hypercalcuria develop renal stones.

The disorder is almost certainly due to an increased absorption of calcium from the bowel. Oral administration of a large dose of calcium produces a significantly greater rise of plasma calcium and urinary calcium excretion in "hypercalcuric" patients than in controls. It is not understood why some patients have a low serum phosphorus. As in familial hypophosphataemia therefore idiopathic hypercalcuria appears to be due to an intestinal abnormality and not to a renal disorder.

Treatment. Unless the patient suffers from renal stones treatment is not required. Otherwise the aim of treatment has been to try and lower urinary calcium excretion in an attempt to prevent the formation of new stones or to produce regression of existing stones. The various ways this has been attempted include: (1) a low calcium diet; (2) the use of oral sodium phytate (6–8 g per day with meals) or sodium cellulose phosphate (12–15 g per day with meals) to bind calcium in the lumen of the intestine, and so reduce calcium absorption; (3) the use of bendrofluezide (5–7 mg per day) which reduces calcium excretion by some unknown mechanism; (4) a low phosphate diet; (5) the administration of oral sodium bicarbonate (5–10 g per day) to alkalinise the urine for this also reduces urinary calcium excretion. Some of these manoeuvres are tedious or unpleasant and some occasionally cause uncomfortable side effects. The best combination is a low calcium diet and sodium cellulose phosphate. It is sometimes capable of lowering urinary calcium excretion to very low levels, e.g. below 50 mg per day. With this treatment about 90 per cent of patients will cease to form stones though a few patients in whom urinary calcium excretion has been persistently reduced to below 50 mg per day will still develop new stones, though these are uncalcified.

Some authorities advise the drinking of large volumes of water to prevent the urine becoming concentrated and thus to minimise the chances of calcium precipitating. This is probably good advice but it is important to remember that some water supplies contain large amounts of calcium (e.g. London, 10 mg/100 ml) and that the ingestion of large amounts of such water may substantially increase urinary calcium excretion.

Excessive Reabsorption of Phosphate

This extremely rare condition is also known as pseudohypoparathyroidism. Most cases are transmitted as a sex-linked dominant disorder. The patient presents with attacks of tetany or fits, and the diagnosis is made by finding a high plasma phosphate concentration and a low serum concentration of calcium which are not influenced by injections of parathormone. There are no other abnormalities of renal function. These patients have characteristic round flat faces with small bulbous noses, thin straight mouths, and strabismus; they also have short stumpy hands with stunted metacarpals. They are usually mentally retarded, of short stature and have cataracts.

Impaired Ability to Reabsorb Glucose, Amino Acids and Phosphate

This combination of functional defects is often defined as Fanconi's syndrome. In nearly every instance it is due to the toxic effects upon the tubule of either a metabolite or an exogenous poison (p. 241). There are a few isolated cases in which up till now it has not been possible to find such a cause. Such patients are sometimes referred to as suffering from an Idiopathic de Toni–Debré–Fanconi syndrome; there is little evidence that this syndrome is inherited.

The best known example of Fanconi's syndrome is the one associated with the widespread deposition of cystine (cystinosis). This is an inborn error of metabolism which is inherited as a simple Mendelian recessive. The tubular defects do not appear until the end of the first six months of life. The amino aciduria includes a wide variety of amino acids, but the amount excreted is much less than in cystinuria (p. 234). In addition there are often other tubular defects including an impaired ability to acidify and concentrate the urine and a renal leak of potassium. These defects may follow from the initial tubular damage and they may in their turn cause further tubular lesions. This vicious spiral can sometimes be arrested and many of the tubular defects reversed by therapeutically correcting their consequences, i.e. if the phosphate loss is corrected with vitamin D and the acidosis with alkalis, the amino aciduria may be lessened or abolished and a potassium leak may be arrested; potassium replacement has sometimes cured the impaired ability to acidify and concentrate.

Apart from these characteristic tubular abnormalities there is always proteinuria; characteristically there is high excretion of α_2 globulin. Glomerular filtration rate is always impaired.

It has been shown by means of microdissection of individual nephrons from patients who have died from cystinosis that the condition is associated with a characteristic structural lesion. The proximal tubule is shorter than normal and is connected to the glomerulus by an abnormally long and narrow neck quite unlike anything seen in normal subjects. The relevance of this finding is equivocal for a similar finding has been found in cases of congenital nephrotic syndrome and other diseases which have none of the tubular defects associated with the Fanconi syndrome.

Cystinosis first makes itself manifest either in infancy or occasionally in childhood. The clinical picture is one of thirst, polyuria, failure to thrive, and rickets. The children are characteristically short and squat, the blood urea is always raised, the plasma potassium often below 3 mEq/l and occasionally there is a hyperchloraemic acidosis. Urinary calcium excretion is low and the alimentary absorption of calcium is impaired. Diagnosis depends upon finding opaque deposits of cystine in the cornea or the finding of cystine in a liver or lymph node biopsy. Infants may die of dehydration with electrolyte imbalance. Those who survive into childhood die of progressive chronic renal failure before puberty.

The defect of phosphate reabsorption is treated with vitamin D, calcium and sodium phosphate; the renal tubular acidosis with alkalis. The treatment of the potassium defect has been mentioned earlier. The administration of potassium should be increased gradually for hyperkalaemia is easily induced.

Impaired Ability to Achieve a High Hydrogen Ion and Osmotic Gradient

This condition is known as Renal Tubular Acidosis. To be correct etymologically this then should include any persistent systemic acidosis due to abnormal tubular function, i.e. inability to lower the urine pH, as well as urinary bicarbonate wastage, and diminished ability to secrete ammonia. In practice the term is restricted to when there is an inability to lower the urine pH. There is often an associated impairment of the ability to concentrate the urine.

The inability to lower the urine pH is not due simply to an impaired ability to transfer hydrogen ions from the cell to the tubular fluid for if an artificially high urinary excretion of phosphate is induced by giving large amounts of phosphates, the rate of urinary hydrogen ion excretion can be raised to normal levels. In these circumstances, of course, the titratable acidity rises without an appreciable change in urinary pH, for the hydrogen ions are buffered by the phosphate as they emerge into the tubular fluid. It seems therefore that the functional impairment in renal tubular acidosis is an inability to produce and maintain a hydrogen ion gradient between the tubule lumen and the cell.

With normal quantities of buffer in the urine the impaired ability to lower the urine pH results in a reduced excretion of titratable acid. Ammonia excretion is usually normal in relation to the urine pH, but as the urine pH cannot be reduced the absolute excretion of ammonia is nearly always low (Fig. 18.1). The combination of a reduced titratable acid and ammonia excretion causes a

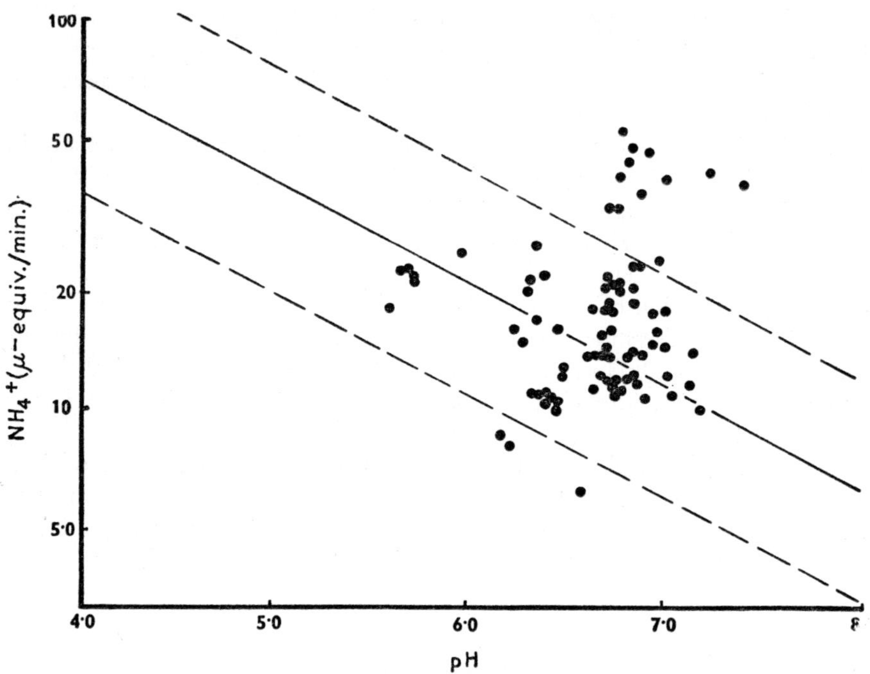

Fig. 18.1. Renal tubular acidosis. Relation between the excretion of ammonium and urine pH. The calculated regression line and 95 per cent range in normal individuals are shown. Each point represents an observation made in a patient suffering from renal tubular acidosis, after the oral ingestion of a single dose of ammonium chloride. (Wrong and Davies, 1959, *Quart. J. Med.*)

serious diminution in total hydrogen ion excretion and a retention of hydrogen ions. In addition to the impaired ability to produce and maintain a high hydrogen ion gradient across the tubule wall the tubules are also unable to produce a high osmotic gradient so that there is an impaired ability to produce a highly concentrated urine.

Renal glycosuria and amino aciduria do not occur and the maximal capacity to excrete PAH and reabsorb phosphate is normal, but other abnormalities of tubular function may be present. There can be an increased urinary calcium excretion, and nephrocalcinosis; often both are present together, but they can occur independently. The hypercalcuria is due to the systemic acidosis for the hydrogen ions tend to be buffered by bone with the release of calcium into the extracellular fluid. The increased calcium excretion is often associated with osteomalacia. The implied abnormality of vitamin D metabolism inherent in this histological diagnosis is not understood. It has been suggested that the nephrocalcinosis is due to the reduced excretion of citrate which accompanies the persistently raised urinary pH.

There may also be an increased excretion of potassium giving rise to potassium deficiency. This is due to many causes including the systemic acidosis itself. Some patients are also inefficient in conserving sodium so that the secondary aldosteronism which develops when they become sodium depleted also increases the renal loss of potassium. And finally some patients have a true potassium-losing renal state which is not due to acidosis or hyperaldosteronism. The distal tubule and collecting duct are responsible for building up ion and osmotic gradients and for secreting potassium into the tubule fluid. It is probable therefore that in renal tubule acidosis there is a biochemical lesion at this site which may lead to an impaired secretion of hydrogen ion against a concentration gradient, a leak of potassium and an impaired ability to concentrate the urine.

The fall in plasma bicarbonate which accompanies the retention of hydrogen ions is accompanied by a compensatory increase in plasma chloride concentration. Often, therefore, the diagnosis is first suspected by a finding of hyperchloraemic acidosis. Usually the creatinine clearance and blood urea are either normal or only moderately impaired so that the fall in plasma bicarbonate is out of proportion to the mild rise in blood urea, e.g. a plasma bicarbonate of 16 mEq/l with a blood urea of 40 mg per 100 ml. The diagnosis is confirmed by finding that though there is a systemic acidosis, the urine pH is around 6·5 and that the urinary excretion of ammonium and hydrogen ions is low. Upon giving a single dose of ammonium chloride by mouth (p. 80) there is usually little change in the urine pH and the excretion of ammonia rarely rises above 50 μEq/min; in children the urine pH is usually greater than 7·4 and there is therefore extremely little excretion of ammonium. The impairment in the ability to concentrate the urine following dehydration or after the administration of vasopressin is equally striking, in contrast to the almost normal glomerular filtration rate, e.g. creatinine clearance 90 ml/min, urine osmolality after vasopressin 420 m.osmole/kg (S.G. 1·013).

Children (usually male infants) are affected mainly by the inability concentrate the urine and the retention of hydrogen ions, so that they usually present with failure to gain weight and dehydration accompanied by vomiting and constipation; nephrocalcinosis, calcium deficiency and potassium deficiency are uncommon. It is interesting that that in Europe the incidence of so-called primary infantile renal tubular acidosis suddenly declined after 1954. This decline and the transient nature of the disturbance in infants, suggests that in many instances it is due to an environmental factor. Nevertheless, none has been discovered except for the occasional case due to mercurial poisoning with dusting or teething powders.

In adults, the most frequent clinical presentation is that of osteomalacia, haematuria and renal infection due to nephrocalcinosis, or renal calculi developing in a woman. In a few adults the disease has only been discovered accidentally because an abdominal X-ray, taken for some unrelated purpose, has shown the appearance of nephrocalcinosis. In some of these patients the tubule's impaired ability to acidify and concentrate the urine has not been accompanied by hydrogen ion retention so that the plasma pH and bicarbonate have been within normal limits. It has been found that this paradoxical situation is due to an increased tubular capacity to excrete ammonia. It is not known whether these findings represent a stage in the chronological progress of the condition or a separate disorder. The incidence of primary renal tubular acidosis in adults, i.e. in the absence of other recognisable associated disease has greatly diminished in recent years. The cause of this phenomenon is unknown.

TREATMENT consists in the administration of alkalis (sodium bicarbonate or citrate) for the acidosis; citrate and citric acid are given to increase the urinary excretion of citrate so as to prevent the further precipitation of calcium in the renal parenchyma, e.g. sodium citrate 98 g, citric acid 140 g, water to 1 litre, 50–100 ml per day. The administration of alkalis also decreases the rate of urinary excretion of calcium. In addition, calcium deficiency is treated with calcium lactate and calciferol, and potassium deficiency with potassium citrate. At first it may be necessary to give as much as 200 mEq of potassium per day; during this time the administration of sodium bicarbonate and citrate is decreased. Later a patient may need 150 mEq of sodium and 50 mEq of potassium as bicarbonate or citrate. Renal infections should be treated with antibiotics, but sulphonamides should be avoided for their inhibiting effect on carbonic anhydrase aggravates the impaired ability to excrete hydrogen ions. Renal tubular acidosis in children can usually be controlled and often there may be a spontaneous recovery. In adults treatment may be more difficult and recovery is unusual.

ACQUIRED FUNCTIONAL DEFECTS OF THE RENAL TUBULE

Single and multiple disorders of tubular function may be caused by a wide variety of conditions. The following list which is not exhaustive shows that most of the disorders are the same as those that are genetically determined.

SINGLE DEFECTS

Impaired ability to reabsorb: Due to:

    Water   .   .   .   . e.g. (*a*) excess intake of water (compulsive water drinking).

                                                      (*b*) sickle cell anaemia.

Sodium . . . e.g. (a) chronic pyelonephritis with infected urine.
(b) cystic disease of the renal medulla.

Potassium . . . e.g. very rarely in cases of persistent glomerular nephritis or pyelonephritis.

Phosphate . . . e.g. (a) potassium deficiency.
(b) acidosis.

Amino acids . . . e.g. galactosaemia.

Impaired ability to secrete ammonia.

MULTIPLE DEFECTS

Impaired ability to reabsorb:
Amnio acids, glucose, phosphate, bicarbonate and water . . . e.g. (a) cystinosis.
(b) heavy metal poisoning
lead
cadmium
mercury
copper (Wilson's disease).
(c) galactosuria.
(d) glycogen storage diseases.
(e) hyperparathyroidism.
(f) hyperglobulinaemia.
(g) amyloidosis.

Impaired ability to achieve a hydrogen ion gradient (sometimes with an impaired ability to achieve an osmolar gradient) . . e.g. (a) potassium deficiency.
(b) chronic pyelonephritis with infected urine.
(c) interstitial nephritis.
(d) mercury.
(e) phenacetin.

Many of these have already been discussed when describing the congenital defects of tubular function. It is not proposed to discuss these conditions further except to stress that it is often difficult to distinguish whether a tubular defect is congenital or acquired; that often acquired lesions are superimposed upon congenital ones; and that treating the metabolic disorder caused by a tubular defect may not only cure the disorder but may also improve or abolish the original tubular abnormality which was its cause.

BIBLIOGRAPHY

ALBRIGHT, F., BURNETT, C. H., SMITH, P. H., and PARSON, W. (1942). "Pseudohypoparathyroidism—example of 'Seabright-bantam syndrome'; report of 3 cases." *Endocrinology*, **30**, 922.

ANDERSON, D. C., PETERS, T. J., and STEWART, W. K. (1969). "Association of hypokalaemia and hypophosphataemia." *Brit. med. J.*, **2**, 402.

BOYCE, W. H., and GARVEY, F. K. (1958). "Abnormalities of calcium metabolism in patients with 'idiopathic' urinary calculi. Effect of oral administration of sodium phytate." *J. Amer. med. Ass.*, **166**, 1577.

BUTLER, E. A., and FLYNN, F. V. (1958). "The proteinuria of renal tubular disorders." *Lancet*, **2**, 978.

CANNON, P. J., LEEMING, J. M., SOMMERS, S. C., WINTERS, R. W., and LARAGH, J. H. (1968). "Juxtaglomerular cell hyperplasia and secondary hyperaldosteronism (Bartter's syndrome). A revaluation of the pathophysiology." *Medicine*, **47**, 107.

COCHRAN, M., PEACOCK, M., SMITH, D. A., and NORDIN, B. E. C. (1968). "Renal tubular acidosis of pyelonephritis with renal stone disease." *Brit. med. J.*, **1**, 721.

DENT, C. E., FRIEDMAN, M., GREEN, H., and WATSON, L. C. A. (1965). "Treatment of cystinuria." *Brit. med. J.*, **1**, 403.

DENT, C. E., and STAMP, T. C. B. (1971). "Hypophosphataemic osteomalacia in adults." *Quart. J. Med.*, **40**, 158.

DENT, C. E., and WATSON, L. (1965). "Metabolic studies in a patient with idiopathic hypercalcuria." *Brit. med. J.*, **2**, 449.

EDWARDS, N. A., and HODGKINSON, A. (1965). "Metabolic studies in patients with idiopathic hypercalcuria." *Clin. Sci.*, **29**, 143.

ENGELMAN, K., WATTS, R. W. E., KLINENBERG, J., SJOERDESMA, A., and SEEGMILLER, J. E. (1964). "Demonstration of the enzyme defect in xanthinuria." *J. clin. Invest.*, **43**, 1303.

FANCONI, G. (1936). "Der frühinfantile nephrotisch-glycosurische Zweigwuchs mit hypophosphatämischen Rachitis." *Jb. Kinderheilk.*, **147**, 299.

GARDNER, J. D., LAPEY, A., SIMOPOULOS, A. P., and BRAVO, L. B. (1971). "Abnormal membrane sodium transport in Liddle's syndrome." *J. clin. Invest.*, **50**, 2253.

GORDON, R. D., GEDDES, R. A., PAWSEY, G. K., and O'HALLORAN, M. W. (1970). "Hypertension and severe hyperkalaemia associated with suppression of renin and aldosterone and completely reversed by sodium restriction." *Aust. Ann. Med.*, **4**, 287.

HIOCO, D., RYCKEWAERT, A., BORDIER, PH., MIRAVET, L., GRUSON, M., LANHAM, C., and MATRAJT, H. (1967). Le métabolisme calcique et phosphoré au cours des ostéomalacies vitamino-résistantes du syndrome de Fanconi et des syndromes apparentés. In "L'Osteomalacie". Edited by D. J. Hioco. Masson et Cie., Paris.

LAFFERTY, F. W., HERNDON, C. H., and PEARSON, O. H. (1963). "Pathogenesis of vit. D resistant rickets and the response to a high calcium intake." *J. clin. Endocrinol.*, **23**, 903.

LATNER, A. L., and BURNARD, E. D. (1950). "Idiopathic hyperchloraemic renal acidosis of infants (nephrocalcinosis infantum). Observations on site and nature of the lesion." *Quart. J. Med.*, N.S. **19**, 285.

LIDDLE, G. W., BLADSOE, T., and COPPAGE, W. S. (1963). "A familial renal disorder simulating primary aldosteronism." *Trans. Assoc. Amer. Phys.*, **76**, 199.

LIGHTWOOD, R., and BUTLER, N. (1963). "Decline in primary infantile renal acidosis; aetiological implications." *Brit. med. J.*, **1**, 855.

LOTZ, K., POTTS, J. T., and BARTTER, F. C. (1965). "Rapid, simple method of determining effectiveness of D-penicillamine therapy in cystinuria." *Brit. med. J.*, **2**, 521.

MASON, A. M. S., and GOLDING, P. L. (1970). "Hyperglobulaemic renal tubular acidosis. A report of nine cases." *Brit. med. J.*, **2**, 143.

McCURDY, D. K., CORNWELL, G. G., and DE PRATTI, V. J. (1967). "Hyperglobulinemic renal tubular acidosis: report of two cases." *Ann. Int. Med.*, **67**, 110.

McGREGOR, M. E., and RAYNER, P. H. W. (1964). "Pink disease and primary renal tubular acidosis." *Lancet*, **2**, 1083.

MILNE, M. D. (1964). "Disorders of amino-acid transport." *Brit. med. J.*, **1**, 327.

MILNE, M. D. (1970). "Genetic aspects of renal diseases." *Progress in Medical Genetics*, **7**, 112.

MUDGE, G. H. (1958). "Clinical patterns of tubular dysfunction." *Amer. J. Med.*, **24**, 785.

MULDOWNEY, F. P., FREANEY, R., and McGEENEY, D. (1968). "Renal tubular acidosis. and amino aciduria in osteomalacia of dietary and intestinal origin." *Quart. J. Med.*, **37**, 517.

PATRICK, A. D. (1965). "Deficiencies of –SH dependent enzymes in cystinosis." *Clin. Sci.*, **28**, 427.

PEACOCK, M., KNOWLES, F., and NORDIN, B. E. C. (1968). "Effect of calcium administration and deprivation on serum and urine calcium in stone-forming and control subjects." *Brit. med. J.*, **1**, 729.

PIERCE, D. S., WALLACE, W. M., and HERNDON, C. H. (1964). "Long-term treatment of vit. D resistant rickets." *J. Bone & Joint Surg.*, **46a**, 978.

PINES, K. L., and MUDGE, G. H. (1951). "Renal tubular acidosis with osteomalacia: report of 3 cases." *Amer. J. med.*, **11**, 302.

RANDALL, R. E. and TAGGART, W. H. (1961). "Familial renal tubular acidosis." *Ann. Int. Med.*, **54**, 1108.

SALASSA, R. M., JOWSEY, J., and ARNAUD, C. D. (1970). "Hypophosphataemic osteomalacia associated with 'non-endocrine' tumours." *New Eng. J. Med.*, **283**, 67.

SELDIN, D. W., and WILSON, J. D. (1965). Renal tubular acidosis. In "The Metabolic Basis of Inherited Disease". Edited by Stanbury. Wyngaardan and Fredrickson. McGraw Hill, U.S.A., 1230.

WINTERS, R. W., GRAHAM, J. B., WILLIAMS, T. F., McFALLS, V. W., and BURNETT, C. H. (1958). "A genetic study of familial hypophosphataemia and vitamin D resistant rickets with a review of the literature." *Medicine*, **37**, 97.

WRONG, O., and DAVIES, H. E. F. (1959). "The excretion of acid in renal disease." *Quart. J. Med.*, N.S. **28**, 259.

19

Renal Function and Metabolic Alkalosis

THE normal kidney's ability to deal successfully with a severe, persistent metabolic alkalosis is now well recognised. For instance, it has been shown that if patients suffering from peptic ulceration are treated with a continuous intragastric drip of 1,000 mEq of sodium bicarbonate (84 g) per day for three weeks there is a persistent rise in plasma bicarbonate, but no apparent change in renal functional efficiency, and in fact the glomerular filtration rate tends to rise and the blood urea to fall.

Excluding increased ingestion of sodium bicarbonate, metabolic alkalosis is caused by either a deficiency of chloride, hydrogen or potassium ions, or very occasionally by a rise in plasma calcium concentration (p. 225). The connection between potassium deficiency and renal failure has been discussed previously (p. 218) while the connection between chloride and hydrogen ion deficiency and renal failure is best discussed in relation to the most common syndrome in which renal failure and alkalosis occur, i.e. pyloric obstruction, in which it will be seen that potassium deficiency may also contribute to the alkalosis, and the renal failure.

Pyloric Obstruction

Gastric juice contains water in which there are approximately 145 mEq/l of chloride, 83 mEq/l hydrogen ions, 50 mEq/l of sodium, and 12 mEq/l of potassium. Following the persistent vomiting of pyloric obstruction there develop deficiencies of water, hydrogen ions, chloride, sodium and potassium and, occasionally, there is the further complication of a gastro-intestinal haemorrhage. Each of these gives rise to its own sequence of disturbance in body fluids, and renal function. It is important to realise that the direction of some of the renal functional disturbances depend on the pattern of the deficiencies, i.e. there may be oliguria or polyuria, an alkaline urine or an acid urine. The relative proportions of these deficiencies determine which functional changes will predominate.

Fig. 19.1 illustrates the changes which may occur.

Factors involved in the renal failure of pyloric obstruction

WATER AND BLOOD LOSS. The continuous loss of water (with sodium and chloride) reduces the volume of all fluid spaces including the blood volume, and this is followed by consequences which have been described previously, i.e. renal vasoconstriction → reduced glomerular filtration rate → rise in blood urea.

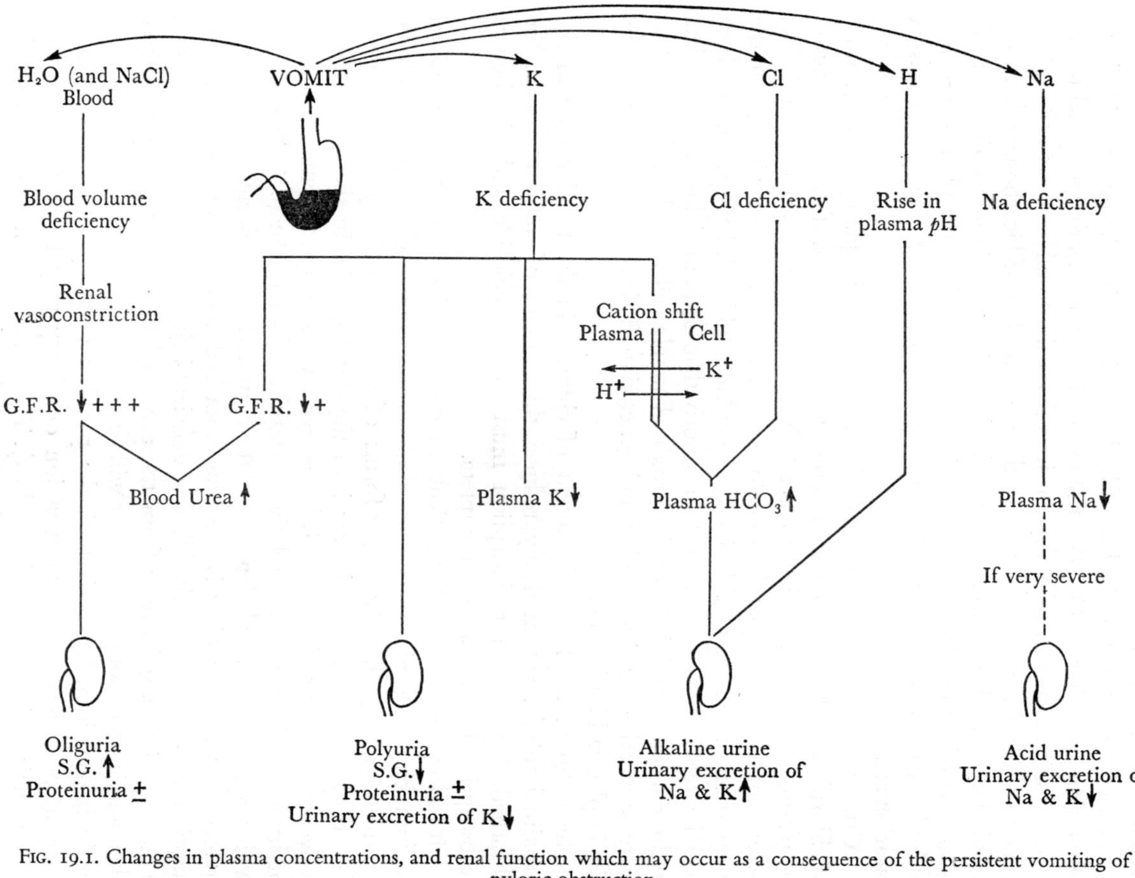

Fig. 19.1. Changes in plasma concentrations, and renal function which may occur as a consequence of the persistent vomiting of pyloric obstruction.

These changes will be more pronounced if there is also gastro-intestinal bleeding; in rare instances acute renal failure develops. Usually the renal ischaemia stops short of tubular necrosis and there is only *oliguria* with a urine concentration which tends to be raised.

HYDROGEN ION LOSS. The loss of hydrogen ions raises the plasma pH, slows respiration and raises pCO_2. The rise in pCO_2 then causes the proximal tubule to increase its secretion of hydrogen ions from the tubule cell into the tubule lumen so that there is an increase in the reabsorption of bicarbonate from the tubule lumen back into the plasma, and also an increase in generation of fresh bicarbonate by the tubule cells which is then secreted into the plasma. The loss of hydrogen ions in the gastric juice is therefore one cause for the rise in plasma bicarbonate.

CHLORIDE LOSS. The loss of chloride ions lowers the plasma concentration of chloride and thus the chloride filtered at the glomerulus. If the concentration of plasma sodium has fallen to a relatively less extent, which is probable, because of the greater quantity of chloride than sodium in gastric juice, then the proportion of sodium to chloride in the tubule fluid will have risen, i.e. there will be relatively less chloride to reabsorb than sodium. This will stimulate hydrogen ion secretion from the proximal tubule cell into the lumen and so increase bicarbonate reabsorption and generation. This is another cause for the rise in plasma bicarbonate.

In addition, the lowered content of chloride in the tubular fluid in the proximal tubule, automatically reduces the amount of sodium that can be absorbed, for sodium reabsorption must stop as chloride and bicarbonate reabsorption become almost complete.

It follows that though the patient is sodium deficient (because of the loss of sodium in the vomit) proximal tubular reabsorption of sodium cannot be complete as it usually is in other forms of sodium deficiency. Sodium therefore continues to be spilled over into the distal tubule. In the distal tubule, however, sodium reabsorption is linked with an exchange for either potassium or hydrogen ions, and the relative quantities of potassium or hydrogen ions which are so exchanged depend on their intracellular concentrations. But in pyloric stenosis the patient is vomiting both hydrogen and potassium ions and his distal tubular cells will therefore be deficient in hydrogen and potassium ions. The sodium that spills over from the proximal tubule into the distal tubule therefore is either not reabsorbed or will be reabsorbed in exchange for potassium or hydrogen ions. There is then the paradox that a patient suffering from sodium, potassium, and hydrogen ion deficiency may be excreting sodium, potassium and an acid urine (see below). The loss of sodium ions contributes to the reduction in extracellular volume and therefore to the precipitation and perpetuation of renal failure. The diminution in extracellular fluid volume increases bicarbonate reabsorption (p. 73) and thus increases the severity of the metabolic alkalosis. The loss of potassium also contributes to the renal failure.

POTASSIUM LOSS. The consequences of potassium loss on renal function have been described on p. 218. There is some reduction in glomerular filtration rate, but the most marked feature is *polyuria* with a urine concentration which remains iso- or hypotonic. Plasma potassium is low, and to compensate for this there is a shift of potassium from the intracellular space to the plasma and extracellular space, and a reverse shift of hydrogen and sodium ions from the extracellular space into the cells. The loss of hydrogen ions from the plasma results in a rise in plasma bicarbonate, one other cause of alkalosis in pyloric obstruction.

SODIUM LOSS. There is an overall sodium deficiency mainly due to the vomiting of sodium in the gastric juice, but compared with the extracellular fluid, vomit contains relatively more water than sodium so that the concentration of plasma sodium sometimes rises. Usually, however, the patient's thirst forces him to drink water, and this selective partial replacement of water to the exclusion of sodium lowers the plasma concentration of sodium below normal.

If sodium and potassium deficiency become sufficiently severe the *urine is acid*, though the plasma is becoming increasingly alkaline. This is due to the lack of available potassium on the cation exchange mechanism in the distal tubule. If sodium reabsorption is nearly complete and there is no available potassium, some of the sodium ions reabsorbed in the distal tubule will be replaced by hydrogen ions and the urine will become acid. This phenomenon must also be related to the raised concentration of hydrogen ions within the tubule cells.

CHRONIC RENAL DISEASE. It is obvious that if there is some antecedent impairment of renal function the onset of pyloric obstruction and vomiting will cause a rapid deterioration of renal function.

ALKALIS AND MILK. The most frequent accompaniment of pyloric obstruction is peptic ulceration, for which patients take both alkalis and milk. Once the glomerular filtration rate begins to fall because of dehydration or potassium deficiency, the continued administration of sodium bicarbonate is not only useless but rapidly aggravates the alkalosis. The high intake of calcium which accompanies the large ingestion of milk and certain alkalis, such as calcium carbonate, may cause hypercalcaemia or at least hypercalcuria which is an additional cause for the renal failure and also for the rise in plasma bicarbonate.

Treatment of metabolic and renal consequences of pyloric obstruction

Upon admission to hospital, most patients with benign pyloric obstruction cease to vomit and quickly begin to correct their electrolyte and water deficiencies almost unaided. During the first few days it is customary to wash out the stomach before meals. Water and food then pass through the pylorus and are absorbed in normal amounts; in such patients it is only necessary to make sure that they are given a mixed diet and that it is relatively low in protein until the glomerular filtration returns to normal levels.

Occasionally, however, it may be necessary to accelerate recovery by giving electrolytes and water intravenously or in additional amounts by mouth.

Isotonic saline is given intravenously in sufficient quantities to correct haemo-concentration, peripheral vein constriction and tachycardia. The administration of isotonic saline not only corrects the depletion of the extracellular fluid volume but also provides at least 40 mEq of chloride per litre to correct the chloride deficiency. (One litre of isotonic saline contains 150 mEq of sodium and 150 mEq of chloride while plasma contains 140 mEq/l of sodium and 100 mEq/l of chloride.) Once the volume of the extracellular fluid is replenished the continued administration of saline rapidly cures any remaining chloride deficiency metabolic alkalosis, for the sodium ion is excreted while the chloride is retained. It is always important to give potassium by mouth even if plasma potassium concentration is normal, for there may be potassium deficiency without much change in plasma potassium. If plasma potassium concentration is unequivocally decreased potassium chloride should be given intravenously in combination with isotonic saline or 5 per cent glucose. When there is severe potassium deficiency, sodium chloride should not be given without giving potassium simultaneously, for the administration of sodium chloride may increase the urinary excretion of potassium.

It is unnecessary and perhaps harmful to use ammonium chloride for the correction of a metabolic alkalosis due to vomiting. Surgery should be avoided until renal function has recovered and there is no longer any evidence of electrolyte deficiency.

BIBLIOGRAPHY

BURNETT, C. H., BURROWS, B. A., COMMONS, R. R. (1950). "Studies of alkalosis: Renal function during and following alkalosis resulting from pyloric obstruction." *J. clin. Invest.*, **29**, 169.

BURNETT, C. H., BURROWS, B. A., COMMONS, R. R., and TOWERY, B. T. (1950). "Studies of alkalosis: Electrolyte abnormalities in alkalosis resulting from pyloric obstruction." *J. clin. Invest.*, **29**, 175.

CLARKSON, E. M., McDONALD, S. J., and DE WARDENER, H. E. (1966). "The effect of a high intake of calcium carbonate in normal subjects and patients with chronic renal failure." *Clin. Sci.*, **30**, 425.

COHEN, J. J. (1968). "Correction of metabolic alkalosis by the kidney after isometric expansion of extracellular fluid." *J. clin. Invest.*, **47**, 1181.

GRAEFF, DE J., STRUYVENBERG, A., and LAMEIJER, L. D. F. (1964). "The role of chloride in hypokalaemic alkalosis." *Amer. J. Med.*, **37**, 778.

KASSIRER, J. P., and SCHWARTZ, W. B. (1966). "The response of normal man to selective depletion of hydrochloric acid." *Amer. J. Med.*, **40**, 10.

KASSIRER, J. P., and SCHWARTZ, W. B. (1966). "Correction of metabolic alkalosis in man without repair of potassium deficiency. A revaluation of the role of potassium." *Amer. J. Med.*, **40**, 19.

SANDERSON, P. H., (1948). "Renal failure following abdominal catastrophe and alkalosis." *Clin. Sci.*, **6**, 207.

SELDIN, D. W., and RECTOR, F. C. (1972). "The generation and maintenance of metabolic alkalosis." *Kidney International*, **1**, 306.

VAN GOIDSENHOVEN, G. M. T., GRAY, O. V., PRICE, A. V., and SANDERSON, P. H. (1954). "The effect of prolonged administration of large doses of sodium bicarbonate in man." *Clin. Sci.*, **13**, 383.

20

Renal Disturbances Following Implantation of the Ureters into the Bowel

WHEN the bladder is severely diseased it may be necessary to transplant the ureters. They can be placed so that they open either on the skin surface, into the large bowel or into an isolated segment of the small bowel.

Ureterosigmoidostomy

This operation is almost inevitably followed by reflux of faecal material up the ureters, and in addition some of the contents of the urine are reabsorbed on their way down the colon. The reflux causes severe renal infections while the reabsorption of urea, hydrogen ions and chloride also cause certain complications. The reabsorption of urea is responsible for a rise in blood urea regardless of any change in renal function. It is distinguished from a rise in blood urea due to a true depression in glomerular filtration by estimating the plasma creatinine, for creatinine is not absorbed from the bowel. The reabsorption of chloride ions is important because in the bowel they are reabsorbed to a greater extent than sodium; this mechanism and the reabsorption of hydrogen ions tend to cause hyperchloraemic acidosis. The acidosis is greatly aggravated by the simultaneous absorption of ammonium salts (p. 80) formed from the urine by urea-splitting bacteria in the urine. The steady infusion of urine into the colon can therefore be looked upon as equivalent to a continuous infusion of ammonium chloride. In addition to the acidosis the other important complications of ureterocolic anastomosis is potassium deficiency from excess loss of potassium in the faeces. It is not clear whether this is due to the inevitable pyelonephritis which accompanies this operation so that increased quantities of urinary potassium are delivered into the lumen of the bowel, or whether it is caused by the loss of large quantities of colonic mucus in the faeces due presumably to irritation of the bowel by urine.

If the patient is not to become acidotic and oedematous (from the sodium reabsorption) the kidneys have to compensate for the intestinal reabsorption by excreting increased quantities of urea, sodium chloride, hydrogen ions and ammonium. After a few months the initial difference between the rates of chloride and sodium reabsorption becomes less marked and the tendency to acidosis ceases. This compensation is accompanied by marked hypertrophy of the kidneys.

Renal infection may be accompanied by partial or complete ureteric obstruction (occasionally both of these may have been present before operation, due to the disease in the bladder). Both infection and ureteric obstruction impair tubular function, including the ability to excrete hydrogen and ammonium, so that they may cause a rapid onset of severe acidosis. Infection may also cause a urinary leak of potassium. The nausea of acidosis diminishes the spontaneous intake of water and potassium and eventually it may cause vomiting, considerable dehydration, and contraction of the extracellular fluid volume. Dehydration, renal infection, ureteric obstruction and acidosis can each depress glomerular filtration rate; together they may rapidly cause death from acute renal failure. Alternatively, the patient may present with hypokalaemic paralysis, the symptoms of potassium deficiency being always more severe if there is an associated acidosis as opposed to the usual accompaniment to potassium deficiency which is an extracellular alkalosis.

These hazards are encountered most frequently immediately, or very soon, after operation. Occasionally a patient may remain well for several months and then suddenly become ill and develop an acidotic coma in a few days. It is probable that these relapses are due to an exacerbation of renal infection.

Treatment

PROPHYLACTIC. Alkalis and antibiotics are given during the post-operative period (e.g. sodium bicarbonate 9 g/day, neomycin and cephaloridine). Plasma electrolyte estimations should be made at frequent intervals and potassium given if necessary. For the first few days a catheter is kept in the rectum to shorten the time during which the urine is in contact with the mucous membrane of the bowel. Later the patient is advised to restrict the quantity of salt in his food and is given about 5 g of sodium bicarbonate to take per day; he is also told to allow the urine to escape from the rectum at frequent intervals. It should be remembered that urinary loss of potassium is greater if a large supply of sodium is available for excretion; in some patients, therefore, a mixture of sodium and potassium citrate may be advisable.

CURATIVE. If the patient subsequently complains of mild nausea, tiredness and headache, the administration of alkalis is increased (e.g. sodium bicarbonate 3 g eight-hourly), a low-salt diet is given, and a course of antibiotics should be given even if there is no overt evidence of renal infection.

When the symptoms are more severe and include vomiting, dehydration and clouding of consciousness, the rapid administration of 1/6 molar sodium bicarbonate intravenously, alternating with 5 per cent glucose, if necessary, will usually cause a quick return of consciousness. If the renal damage is reversible the blood urea will also quickly return to normal, Antibiotics are again administered together with large quantities of sodium bicarbonate by mouth until the plasma bicarbonate is normal.

Ureteroileostomy

If the ureters are placed in an isolated segment of the ileum which opens onto the skin most of the complications listed above can be avoided. The hazards are similar to those in ureterosigmoidostomy and for the same reasons, but they occur less frequently and are less severe. This is because the urine is only in contact with the small segment of the ileum for a shorter time. And the intraluminal pressures in this segment are much lower than in the colon so that reflux is less of a problem.

BIBLIOGRAPHY

ANNIS, D., and ALEXANDER, M. K. (1952). "Differential absorption of electrolytes from the large bowel in relation to uretero-sigmoid anastomosis." *Lancet*, **2**, 603.

CARE, A. D., REED, G. W., and PYRAH, L. N. (1957). "Changes in the reabsorption of sodium and chloride ions after uretero-colic anastomosis." *Clin. Sci.*, **15**, 95.

FOWLER, D. I., COOKE, W. T., BROOKE, B. H., and COX, E. V. (1959). 'Ileostomy and electrolyte excretion." *Amer. J. dig. Dis.*, **4**, 710.

HOPEWELL, J. (1959). "The hazards of uretero-intestinal anastomosis." *Ann. roy. Coll. Surg. Engl.*, **24**, 159.

JUDE, J. R., HARRIS, A. H., and SMITH, R. R. (1959). "The physiologic response to the ideal bladder." *Surg. Gynec. & Obstet*,. **109**, 173.

LEADING ARTICLE (1954). "Uretero-colic anastomosis." *Lancet*, **1**, 866.

LOWE, K. G., STOWERS, J. M., and WALKER, W. F. (1959). "Electrolyte disturbances in patients with uretero-sigmoidostomy." *Scot. med. J.*, **4**, 473.

PARSONS, F. M., POWELL, F. J. N., and PYRAH, L. N. (1952). "Chemical imbalance following ureterocolic anastomosis." *Lancet*, **2**, 599.

PARSONS, F. M., PYRAH, L. N., POWELL, F. J. N., REED, J. W., and SPIERS, F. W. (1952). "Chemical imbalance following ureterocolic anastomosis." *Brit. J. Urol.*, **24**, 317.

PYRAH, L. N. (1954). "Uretero-colic anastomosis." *Ann. roy. Coll. Surg. Engl.*, **14**, 169.

ROSENBERG, M. L. (1953). "Physiology of hyperchloremic acidosis following ureterosigmoidostomy: study of urinary reabsorption with radio-active isotopes." *J. Urol. (Baltimore)*, **70**, 569.

SCHWARTZ, W. B., and KASSIRER, J. P. (1963). "Effects of ureteral transplantation." "Diseases of the Kidney." Ed. Strauss, M. B., and Welt, L. G. J. & A. Churchill, London.

21

Immunological Diseases of the Kidney

THE following conditions are discussed:

(1) Glomerular nephritis.
(2) Renal disturbances in polyarteritis nodosa.
(3) Renal disturbances in diffuse lupus erythematosus.
(4) Renal disturbances in subacute bacterial endocarditis.
(5) Renal disturbances in anaphylactoid purpura.
(6) Shunt nephritis.
(7) Lung purpura with nephritis.
(8) Haemolytic uraemic syndrome.
(9) Renal disturbances in quartan malaria.
(10) Immunological renal disturbances in malignant disease.
(11) Immunological renal disturbances in liver disease.

Some Immunological Mechanisms Responsible for Renal Lesions in Man

In animal experiments two immunological mechanisms have been found to cause renal lesions. There are some grounds for thinking that both cause renal lesions in man. They are:

1. Immune complex disease.
2. Antibodies to glomerular basement membrane.

Immune complex disease

ANIMAL EXPERIMENTS. The pattern of events is one which was originally delineated in serum disease. When a foreign serum (the antigen) is injected into an animal it diffuses throughout the blood and extracellular fluid so that its concentration in the plasma at first falls rapidly. The plasma concentration then falls more gradually as the antigen is slowly metabolised. But at the end of 10 to 15 days there is a sudden disappearance of the antigen from the plasma, the animal develops an acute illness and circulating antibodies to the antigen make their first appearance. The disappearance of the antigen is due to the formation of a specific antibody, such as IgG or IgM to the antigen. The antibody binds on to the circulating antigen to form what are known as immune complexes. These vary in size depending on the relative concentrations of antigen and antibody. When antigen predominates in great excess the complexes are small, they remain in the circulation and do no harm. When antibody is in excess the complexes are very large, they are precipitated and disposed of by phagocytes into the reticulo-endothelial system. When the concentrations of plasma antigen and antibody are near equivalence, however, the intermediate sized complexes that are formed become attached to capillary walls and combine with serum complement. This activates complement so that a series of cascade-like enzyme substrate interactions with each of the various fractions of complement then takes place. Each successive step causes the release of active split products which cause local damage to the capillary wall. Some cause vasodilatation and increase permeability. Others induce polymorphonuclear leucocytes to come towards the immune complexes, and yet others make the polymorphonuclear leucocytes adhere to the capillary wall. Platelets also become adherent and attach themselves to the capillary wall. The adherent leucocytes discharge their lyzosomal enzymes and strip up the endothelial cell cytoplasm from the basement membrane. The clumped platelets release histamine, initiate clotting and cause the deposition of fibrin. The presence of fibrin causes both endothelial and epithelial cell to proliferate, particularly the epithelial cells of Bowman's capsule, where proliferation develops into capsular crescents.

The administration of a single dose of foreign serum causes an acute reversible proliferation of the glomerular tufts. The daily administration of serum for several weeks produces chronic renal disease with a variety of histological changes similar to those seen in man. With fluorescein-conjugated anti-sera to, (1) the antigenic components of the foreign serum (e.g. the albumin), (2) the recipient animals' own immunoglobulins, and (3) to complement it is possible to demonstrate the presence of antigen–antibody-complement complexes bound to the glomerular tufts. The presence of fibrin can be detected in the same way. The antigen, antibody and complement are found to be distributed either in the walls of the capillary or in the mesangial areas. The pattern of distribution along the capillary walls is characteristic. It consists of finely granular or lumpy deposits laid down on the epithelial side of the basement membrane (p. 26).

IMMUNE COMPLEX DISEASE IN MAN. This mechanism is probably responsible for more than 99 per cent of all the immunological lesions which affect the kidney in man. In order to be able to delineate its presence in man antibody, antigen and complement must be detected in the glomerular capillary deposited in the characteristic pattern described above. And it is preferable, if in addition, immune complexes can also be detected in the plasma.

Most of these criteria have been met for the renal lesions of disseminated lupus erythematosus, quartan malaria, and in nephritis associated with thyroiditis and malignant disease. In lupus erythematosus the antibody (IgG) is directed against nuclear debris, mainly DNA. In the glomerular tufts it is possible to demonstrate the presence of IgG, DNA and complement. And in quartan malaria it is malarial parasite antigen, IgG and complement which are deposited. In all these conditions the immunological deposits are laid down in the characteristic granular or lumpy pattern which experimentally induced immune complex disease causes in animals. In disseminated lupus erythematosus and quartan malaria it has also been possible to detect the presence of circulating immune complexes.

There are many other renal diseases in which immunoglobulin and complement are found in the glomerular tufts but in which it has not yet been possible to identify the antigen. Nevertheless these are usually included as probably being due to some immunological disturbance in the confident expectation that sooner or later the appropriate antigen will be detected. The lesions of diabetic nephropathy contain insulin, insulin antibody and complement. Perhaps they are also due to an immune complex disease which affects the small vessels and capillaries of many organs.

Anti-glomerular basement disease

ANIMAL EXPERIMENTS. An animal is immunised with an extract of kidney tissue obtained from an animal of a different species. The antiserum is then harvested and injected into an animal of the same species as that from which the extract of kidney was obtained. The exogenous immunoglobulins contained in the antiserum bind on to the glomerular tuft and cause complement to be fixed and activated at the same site. This is in turn leads to the sequence of events described above which cause tissue damage. A diffuse glomerular nephritis then develops which is usually chronic and self-perpetuating. It was eventually discovered that the critical antigen in the kidney extracts which were used to produce anti-kidney serum is glomerular basement membrane. And that therefore the active component of the antiserum is an anti-glomerular basement membrane antibody. More recently it has been demonstrated that glomerular basement material is normally excreted in the urine. It is possible therefore to inoculate an animal with its own glomerular basement membrane material. This manoeuvre causes the animal to develop anti-glomerular basement membrane antibodies and a diffuse glomerular nephritis which is self-perpetuating. The perpetuation of the disease process is due to the antigenic properties of the anti-glomerular basement membrane antibody itself. This creates a vicious cycle in which the more anti-glomerular basement membrane antibody is present the more anti-glomerular basement antibody is formed.

IgG and complement are laid down along the glomerular capillary walls in a characteristic pattern. With immunofluorescence the immunoglobulin and complement are found distributed in a smooth manner along the capillary wall as if they had been painted on with one continuous stroke of a brush (p. 26). This is in contrast to the granular interrupted pattern seen in immune complex disease. A few minutes after the injection of anti-glomerular basement membrane antibody labelled with ferritin, electron microscopy reveals that the ferritin has been deposited between the endothelial cell cytoplasm and the basement membrane as a fine evenly distributed dust.

ANTI-GLOMERULAR BASEMENT DISEASE seldom causes renal lesions in man. To demonstrate its presence in man it is first necessary to show that immunoglobulin and complement are laid down in the characteristic smooth lines on the glomerular capillary walls. It must also be shown that the immunoglobulin fixed in the kidney is an anti-glomerular basement membrane antibody, and that anti-glomerular basement antibody can be detected in the blood. Both of these criteria have been met in a small group of patients which have been intensively studied. Elution of homogenates from human kidneys in which the characteristic smooth distribution of immunofluorescence was demonstrable has yielded anti-glomerular basement antibody. It was identified by applying the eluted material on to frozen sections of normal kidney and then showing with a fluorescence labelled anti-human globulin serum, that a globulin had become fixed to the capillary wall in a smooth linear pattern. The eluted material was also injected into monkeys in which it caused a persistent glomerular nephritis. And in the kidneys of these monkeys immunofluorescence showed the presence of immunoglobulin and complement laid down in a smooth linear fashion along the capillary wall. In man circulating anti-glomerular basement membrane antibody has been detected on rare occasions. This is most easily done after bilateral nephrectomy, the patient being kept alive on maintenance haemodialysis. Presumably this is because, when the kidneys are *in situ.* they mop up the anti-glomerular basement membrane antibody and keep its circulating concentration below detectable levels. Anti-glomerular basement membrane disease is responsible for the renal lesions in the syndrome of lung purpura with nephritis (sometimes called Goodpasture's syndrome), and in some patients without haemoptysis in whom the combination of multiple capsular crescents and rapid downward clinical course places them in that category of glomerular nephritis called rapidly progressive glomerular nephritis.

GLOMERULAR NEPHRITIS

This disease is sometimes referred to as primary glomerular nephritis. It is a most difficult disorder to define or describe. It encompasses all immunological diseases of the kidney not associated with obvious lesions in other organs. It therefore excludes such diseases as disseminated lupus erythematosus, polyarteritis nodosa, sub-acute bacterial endocarditis, etc. The difficulty in describing the disease derives mainly from the lack of precise information about its aetiology and its variegated clinical and histological patterns. It is very probable that eventually it will be found to consist of several separate conditions. The several light microscopy and immunofluorescent patterns which can already be discerned support this hypothesis. The description of the disease is much influenced by whether the narrator is a clinician, a histologist, or an immunologist. In the following account glomerular nephritis is described primarily according to the many ways it may present clinically. An attempt is then made to describe which light microscopy and immunofluorescent pattern accompanies these

Clinical Features, Light Microscopy Appear

Clinical features	Light microscopy appearances
ACUTE GLOMERULAR NEPHRITIS Acute nephritic syndrome Acute renal failure	Diffuse proliferative — Exudative / Mesangial
PERSISTENT GLOMERULAR NEPHRITIS *Rapidly progressive*	Diffuse proliferative with crescents
Chronic Recurrent macroscopic haematuria Persistent proteinuria with r.b.c. Persistent proteinuria without r.b.c.	Focal proliferative
Nephrotic syndrome Persistent proteinuria without r.b.c. Persistent proteinuria with r.b.c.	Nil change
Persistent proteinuria with and without r.b.c.	Focal proliferative
Nephrotic syndrome	Diffuse proliferative — Exudative / Mesangial
	Diffuse proliferative with crescents
	Membrano-proliferative
	Focal sclerosis
	Extra-membranous
Chronic renal failure	Intramembranous
	Advanced lesions

TABLE 21.1. The clinical features, light microscopy appearances and immunofluorescence in 425 basement membrane.

various clinical presentations. The task is not easy for though the clinical syndromes of acute glomerular nephritis, rapidly progressive glomerular nephritis, and recurrent haematuria are each accompanied by a relatively clear-cut histological and immunofluorescent pattern, these same patterns can be found in association with almost any of the other clinical presentations. Conversely, when the light microscopy appearances are normal the patient may have a nephrotic syndrome or persistent proteinuria, but either of these clinical presentations may be accompanied with several other histological patterns.

Table 21.1 illustrates the various clinical and histological combinations that are found in glomerular nephritis. The gross overlap between the many clinical syndromes and histological appearances is immediately apparent.

It is interesting to note that Richard Bright's own speculations about the aetiology of glomerular nephritis are remarkably topical: "the structure of the

ances, and Immunofluorescence in Glomerular Nephritis

Number of patients*	Type	Immunofluorescence Pattern
22	B_1C++ IgG+	Lumpy deposits scattered along GBM Occasionally smooth linear deposits
12	B_1C++, IgG++ or None	
22	Fibrinogen++ B_1C+ (IgA, IgM, IgG)	Coarse granular deposits of fibrin in crescents. Occasionally smooth linear deposits of immunoglobulins
88	IgA++ (B_1C+, IgG+) Fibrinogen±	Diffuse in all glomeruli, mainly mesangial
96	None	
30	B_1C+ or None (IgM, IgG)	Diffuse, or focal granular scattered
6	(see above)	(see above)
18	(see above)	(see above)
10	(see above)	(see above)
33	B_1C+ IgM and Fibrinogen	B_1C coarse granular focal or diffuse along GBM and mesangium. IgM coarse deposits—focal
30	IgM±B_1C	Focal only in sclerosed areas
42	IgG+++ B_1C+++	Diffuse finely granular along GBM *not* in mesangial areas. Occasionally smooth linear
4	B_1C++, IgM±	B_1C diffusely laid granular
12	B_1C	Coarse granules

patients described by Morel-Maroger, Leathem and Richet (1972). *Amer. J. Med.* GBM= glomerular

kidney becomes permanently changed, either in accordance with, and in furtherance of that morbid action; *or by a deposit which is a consequence of the morbid action*". His description of a patient with glomerular nephritis is given below. It is noticeable, that it is principally a description of acute glomerular nephritis developing into persistent glomerular nephritis; a nephrotic stage is just discernible.

Bright's Description

"A child or an adult is affected with scarlatina, or some other acute disease; or has indulged in the intemperate use of ardent spirits for a series of months or years; he is exposed to some casual cause or habitual source of suppressed perspiration: he finds the secretion of his urine greatly increased [*sic*], or he discovers that it is tinged with blood; or, without having made any such

I§

observation, he awakes in the morning with his face swollen, or his ankles puffy, or his hands oedematous. If he happens, in this condition, to fall under the care of a practitioner who suspects the nature of his disease, it is found that already his urine contains a notable quantity of albumen: his pulse is full and hard, his skin dry, he has often headache, and sometimes a sense of weight or pain across the loins. Under treatment more or less active, or sometimes without any treatment, the more obvious and distressing of these symptoms disappear; the swelling, whether casual or constant, is no longer observed; the urine ceases to evince any admixture of red particles; and, according to the degree of importance which has been attached to these symptoms, they are gradually lost sight of, or are absolutely forgotten. Nevertheless, from time to time the countenance becomes bloated; the skin is dry; headaches occur with unusual frequency; or the calls to micturition disturb the night's repose. After a time, the healthy colour of the countenance fades; a sense of weakness or pain in the loins increases; headaches, often accompanied by vomiting, add greatly to the general want of comfort; and a sense of lassitude, of weariness, and of depression, gradually steal over the bodily and mental frame. Again the assistance of medicine is sought. If the nature of the disease is suspected, the urine is carefully tested; and found, in almost every trial, to contain albumen, while the quantity of urea is gradually diminishing. If in the attempt to give relief to the oppression of the system, blood is drawn, it is often buffed, or the serum is milky and opaque; and nice analysis will frequently detect a great deficiency of albumen, and sometimes manifest indications of the presence of urea. If the disease is not suspected, the liver, the stomach or the brain divide the care of the practitioner, sometimes drawing him away entirely from the more important seat of the disease. The swelling increases and decreases; the mind grows cheerful or sad; the secretions of the kidney or the skin are augmented or diminished, sometimes in alternate ratio, sometimes without apparent relation. Again the patient is restored to tolerable health; again he enters on his active duties; or he is, perhaps, less fortunate; the swelling increases, the urine becomes scanty, the powers of life seem to yield, the lungs become oedematous, and, in a state of asphyxia or coma, he sinks into the grave; or a sudden effusion of serum into the glottis closes the passages of the air, and brings on a more sudden dissolution. Should he, however, have resumed the avocations of life, he is usually subject to constant recurrence of his symptoms; or again, almost dismissing the recollection of his ailment, he is suddenly seized with an acute attack of pericarditis, or with a still more acute attack of peritonitis, which without renewed warning, deprives him in eight and forty hours, of his life. Should he escape this danger likewise, other perils await him; his headaches have been observed to become more frequent; his stomach more deranged; his vision indistinct; his hearing depraved: he is suddenly seized with a convulsive fit, and becomes blind. He struggles through the attack; but again and again it returns; and before a day or a week has elapsed, worn out by convulsions, or overwhelmed by coma, the painful history of his disease is closed."

Acute Glomerular Nephritis

Aetiology

INFECTING ORGANISM. Acute glomerular nephritis usually follows infection with a β haemolytic streptococcus, usually types 4 and 12, though a few other strains are occasionally involved. It is possible that the predilection of these strains to affect the kidneys is due to their having antigens in their cell walls which are the same as those in the basement membrane of the kidneys. This specificity of strain accounts for the irregular manner in which cases of acute glomerular nephritis appear. Until this was recognised, it was difficult to know why the incidence of acute glomerular nephritis varied so widely among epidemics of streptococcal infection: particularly why several members of a family should suddenly develop the disease almost simultaneously.

SITE OF INFECTION. This is usually the throat or the skin. Typically there is such a severe sore throat that the patient has to retire to bed for several days; in children, scarlet fever was at one time a major cause of acute nephritis, but it is now less frequent, probably because of the use of penicillin. The proportion of cases in whom it is possible to obtain a satisfactory history of previous infection is about the same in children as adults.

INTERVAL BETWEEN INFECTION AND ONSET. This interval varies from 2–3 days to more than a month; it averages 14 days. It is usual for the patient to have returned to work or school before the onset of acute glomerular nephritis.

SEX AND AGE. Acute glomerular nephritis is more common in males, and is seen most often below the age of 20 years; however, it is by no means confined to this age group and is frequently seen at all ages, including the elderly.

Pathology

Characteristically, the kidneys are normal in size, shape and colour, although occasionally there may be punctate haemorrhages on the surface. Microscopically the structural changes are principally in the glomeruli, and are those of diffuse proliferative glomerular nephritis (Table 21.1(b)). Often all glomeruli are equally affected, but frequently the changes vary in intensity not only between one glomerulus and another but in different parts of the same glomerulus. There is a great increase in the number of the endothelial and mesangial cells, but what is even more striking, they have a considerably greater quantity of cytoplasm, and their nuclei are enlarged. If this change is diffuse throughout a glomerulus it then loses its normal rather delicate tracery and instead appears stuffed with nuclei and cytoplasm.

This is accentuated by a focal swelling of the capillary walls, and the appearance of numerous fragmented P.A.S. staining "fibrils". One of the most characteristic features is an infiltration of the glomerular tufts with numerous polymorphonuclear leucocytes. When this is seen the appearances are called acute exudative diffuse proliferative glomerular nephritis (Fig. 21.1(c)). Occasionally there are small foci of intracapillary thrombosis. The cells of

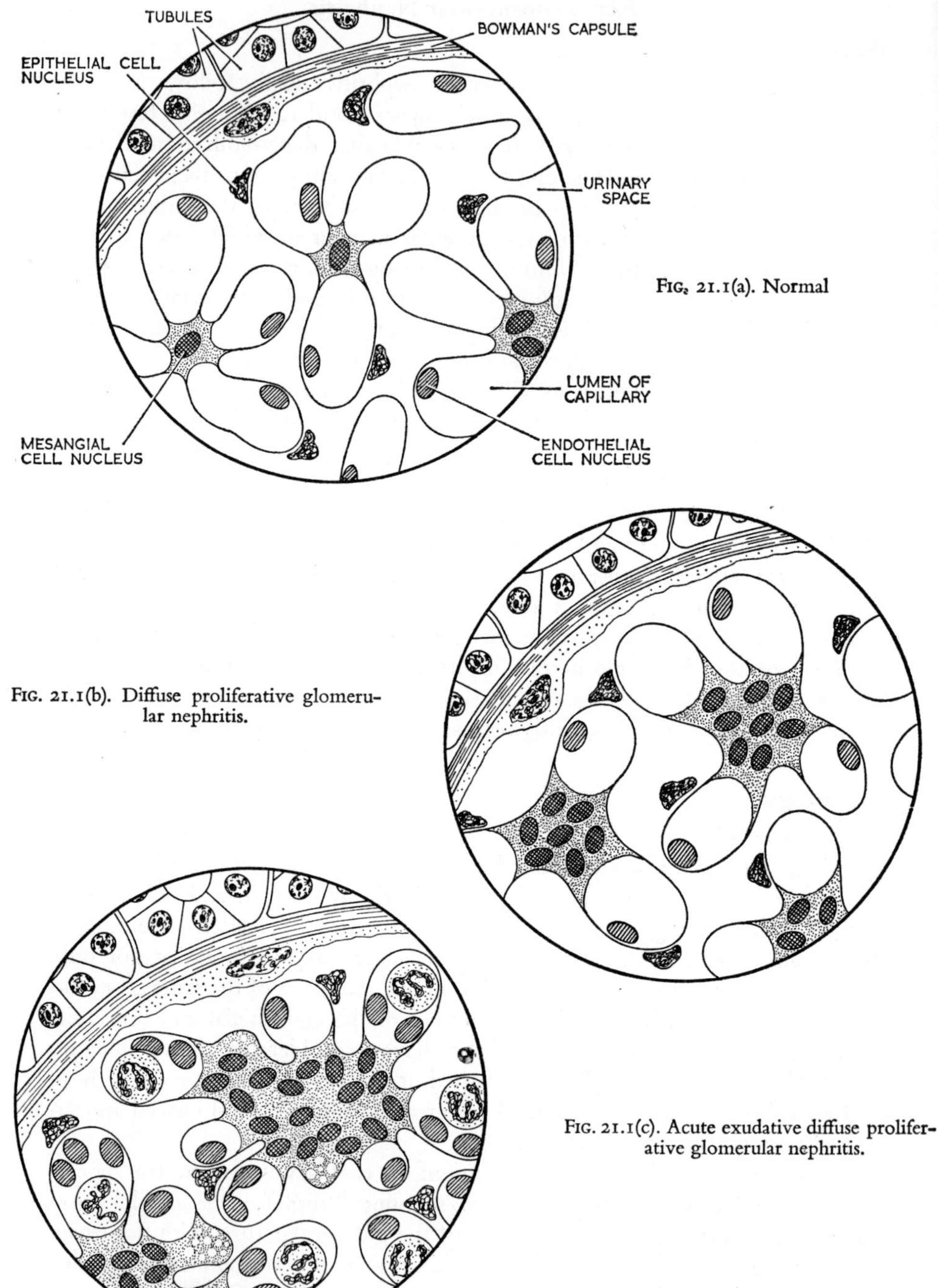

Fig. 21.1(a). Normal

Fig. 21.1(b). Diffuse proliferative glomerular nephritis.

Fig. 21.1(c). Acute exudative diffuse proliferative glomerular nephritis.

the glomerular capsule sometimes enlarge, become cuboidal and histologically resemble the cells of the proximal tubule; the loose shredded cytoplasm of these capsular cells is sometimes thought to represent precipitated protein which has leaked through the damaged glomerulus. Proliferation of the capsular epithelium into crescents is unusual. Unequivocal evidence of inflammatory exudate in the capsular space is rarely seen.

Electron microscopy reveals that the cell proliferation is indeed mainly endothelial and mesangial in origin. The swelling of the capillary walls consists of extensive fragmentation and shredding on the luminal, or endothelial side of the basement membrane. The changes suggest that the endothelial cells are laying down basement membrane-like material at an increased rate and that the vast numbers of redundant new layers that are formed fail to bind together in a normal manner. The appearances are not unlike those of flaky pastry. With light fluorescent microscopy it is possible to show that fibrin has been deposited on the endothelial surface of the glomerular capillaries. Presumably this is secondary to the injurious effect on the basement membrane of the abnormal antigen-antibody reaction. It is this deposition of fibrin which causes the proliferation and swelling of the endothelial cells. Electron microscopy also shows the presence of small "humps" of electron-dense material lying between the basement membrane and the overlying epithelium (Fig. 3.2). Whatever the outcome of the disease these "humps" disappear within six weeks of the onset of acute glomerular nephritis. It is likely that they are due to depositions of antigen, antibody and complement though antigen has not yet been identified. Immunofluorescence demonstrates granular, lumpy deposits of B_1C and smaller amounts of IgG scattered along the capillary walls. Small amounts of fibrinogen are seen occasionally. Very occasionally IgG is found lying as a smooth line along the capillary wall. Frequently there is no fixation of any of the antisera used.

In approximately half the cases, renal biopsies have shown the presence of focal areas of tubular degeneration. These are situated throughout the nephron, but are found most often in the distal tubules. A few patients have focal areas of complete tubular necrosis. Each site of tubular damage is surrounded by inflammatory cells, including lymphocytes, plasma cells, eosinophils and polymorphs. Occasionally, the most severe cases show a generalised separation of the tubules by a thickening of the interstitial tissue. In the interstitial spaces there are scattered small collections of inflammatory cells, and sometimes a glomerulus may be surrounded by a band of inflammatory cells including polymorphs, eosinophils and lymphocytes. Arteriolar necroses have occasionally been seen at *post-mortem.*

In some cases of acute glomerular nephritis without proteinuria or haematuria there are no structural changes except for the occasional presence of cuboidal capsular epithelium.

The first lesion to resolve is the diffuse endothelial proliferation. But focal areas of mesangial proliferation remain for a considerable time thereafter, even in those patients who eventually make a complete recovery. These focal collections lie along the stalks of the glomeruli and are particularly noticeable at the periphery of the stalk. A peripheral lesion of this kind then consists of a collection of mesangial cell nuclei surrounded by a relatively large common "eosinophilic" mass in which no cell boundaries can be discerned. Around the periphery of this lesion there lies a group of capillaries with normal walls. This residual focal mesangial proliferation is stated to be characteristic only of post-streptococcal nephritis.

The mass which surrounds the proliferated mesangial cells is composed mainly of mucopolysaccharide matrix which has been secreted in excess by mesangial cells in response to the inflammatory stimulus. The term "lobular stalk thickening" has been coined to describe the appearances produced when this material is deposited along the long axis of the glomerular stalk.

Clinical features

The clinical features of acute glomerular nephritis are those of an acute nephritic syndrome (p. 211). Clinically the cardinal points are the sudden onset of oedema, gain in weight and oliguria; raised blood pressure and bradycardia; raised jugular venous pressure and dyspnoea; haematuria, proteinuria and discoloured urine. Acute glomerular nephritis is the commonest cause of "heart failure" in children. It is important not to be confused by finding that in most patients there is a high urinary white cell excretion rate, and in about a third of patients an asymptomatic persistent bacilluria. The white cells presumably come from the acute inflammatory lesions in the kidneys which are themselves due to the deposition of antigen, etc. The organisms responsible for the bacilluria are ordinary urinary pathogens such as *E. coli*; their relevance, if any, to the primary renal lesions is unknown.

Relationship between certain clinical and structural features

Renal biopsy studies have shown that in acute glomerular nephritis the presence of proteinuria and haematuria is evidence of widespread and pronounced proliferative and inflammatory changes in the glomerular tufts, though the severity of these structural changes bears no relation to the extent of the proteinuria or haematuria. Surprisingly, there is only an uncertain relationship between the creatinine clearance and the structural changes in the glomeruli; and the concentration of the blood urea is the poorest guide to the presence or extent of such changes. Impairment in the ability to concentrate is certain evidence of widespread focal degenerative lesions of the tubules, though these can be present without gross changes in concentrating ability; a raised erythrocyte sedimentation rate above 50 mm in the first hour (Westergren) is highly suggestive of tubular degeneration. Widespread necrosis of glomeruli is always associated with acute renal failure but otherwise there is little correlation between the presence of acute renal failure and the severity of the structural lesions.

Course

In some series in children there have been no deaths, with complete recovery in almost 100 per cent. In adults complete recovery occurs in approximately 80 per cent of patients; 5 per cent die within one or two weeks of acute pulmonary oedema, renal failure or hypertensive encephalopathy, while the remainder develop persistent glomerular nephritis. The persistent stage may either develop as a rapid deterioration of the acute phase with increasing failure, oedema and hypertension and death within a year (5 per cent), or there may be almost complete recovery, except for the continued presence of proteinuria which persists for up to 25 years before the onset of chronic renal failure (10 per cent). A superimposed nephrotic syndrome occurs particularly in those who develop and die of persistent glomerular nephritis within a year.

Differential diagnosis

The onset of acute streptococcal glomerular nephritis is sometimes indistinguishable from that of other conditions which give rise to an acute nephritic syndrome. The history of recent infection, the identification of the streptococcus, an antistreptolysin titre greater than 1 in 300 and the low level of serum complement are useful distinguishing points. Occasionally a patient may present with acute renal failure following the use of sulphonamide for a streptococcal infection. It may then be extremely difficult to decide whether the patient has acute glomerular nephritis or acute tubular necrosis. In such cases it is essential that the ureters be catheterised to make certain that they are not plugged with crystals of sulphonamide and tubular debris (p. 169).

The two conditions which cause most confusion are some cases of polyarteritis nodosa, and disseminated lupus erythematosus; often the correct diagnosis is only made retrospectively. A pyrexia for longer than the first two to three days, or the continued presence of macroscopic haematuria are highly suggestive of a diagnosis of polyarteritis nodosa.

Prognosis

At the beginning, acute renal failure is the complication most likely to destroy the patient. Acute glomerular nephritis is one of those rare causes of acute renal failure in which there is often complete cessation of urine flow. In adults acute renal failure due to acute glomerular nephritis nearly always causes death even if life is prolonged by appropriate measures. In children, however, haemodialysis is accompanied by recovery in most cases. Acute pulmonary oedema and hypertensive encephalopathy should respond to treatment whatever the age of the patient.

Recurrent exacerbations of haematuria and hypertension, with violent fluctuations in glomerular filtration rate and blood urea, carry an increasing risk that the patient may develop rapidly progressive persistent glomerular nephritis. Nevertheless a guarded prognosis should be given for a considerable time, for recovery may take place even if the disease has persisted in this manner for several weeks. It has been claimed that rapidly progressive glomerular nephritis never follows an attack of acute glomerular nephritis due to an infection with β haemolytic streptococci. If the onset of acute glomerular nephritis is associated with a petechial rash, complete recovery is unusual.

The proteinuria which follows any attack of acute glomerular nephritis constitutes the most difficult prognostic problem. It is generally considered that

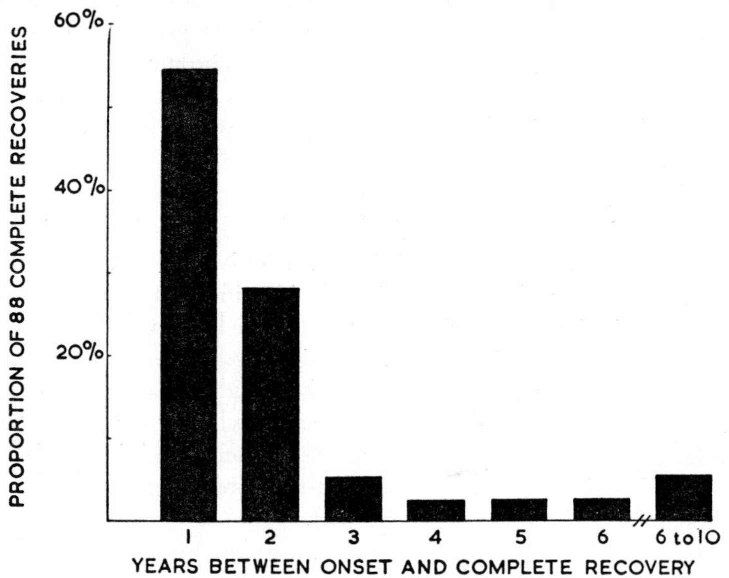

FIG. 21.2. Interval between onset and healing of acute glomerular nephritis in 88 cases who recovered completely. (After Addis, 1949.)

the patient has an active renal lesion until proteinuria ceases, and that the longer this continues the more likely it is that he will develop persistent glomerular nephritis and renal failure. Complete recovery, therefore, has not taken place until proteinuria ceases. But for how long may it continue and yet recovery occur? Fig. 21.2, drawn from Addis's observations, gives the most comprehensive answer. It can be seen that whereas in the majority proteinuria ceases within two years, there are some patients in whom it continues for six to ten years before it disappears.

Treatment

PROPHYLACTIC. It is reasonable to try and eradicate the β haemolytic streptococcus from a small community (i.e. a family), in which a case of acute glomerular nephritis has occurred. The organism is highly sensitive and easily removed by one injection of long-acting penicillin.

CURATIVE. There is no known way of preventing acute glomerular nephritis developing into persistent glomerular nephritis. Accordingly, treatment is directed solely at saving the patient's life and shortening the duration of the acute attack.

An attempt should be made to isolate the β haemolytic streptococci immediately on the day of admission. Penicillin administration is begun on the same day and continued for a considerable time thereafter. Opinions differ, but some authorities consider that penicillin should be continued until proteinuria disappears, however long that may be.

Bed rest is essential, for it is remarkable how often a diuresis and recovery will begin within a few hours of the patient's retiring to bed, irrespective of the duration of the illness up to that time. Rest in bed also diminishes the risk of acute pulmonary oedema and hypertensive crises. For the first 24 hours it is well to allow only 500 ml of sweetened fruit juice by mouth and nothing else. This allows time to observe the direction the illness is taking and its severity. If during that time a diuresis has begun, i.e. if the urine volume is greater than 1,000 ml and there has been a loss of weight, then a normal diet and unrestricted intake of fluids is allowed. If a diuresis has not begun but the urine volume is greater than 400 ml, the intake of fluids for the next 24 hours should be limited to 500 ml plus a volume equal to that which has been passed in the preceding 24 hours; a low-salt, low-protein diet is also started. By these means it is hoped to prevent the onset of acute pulomary oedema and to minimise the rise in blood urea. If the urine volume has been lower than 400 ml the patient is considered to have acute renal failure and treated accordingly (p. 170).

The treatment of acute pulmonary oedema and hypertensive fits has been described on p. 214.

Once a diuresis has begun there is no evidence that the speed of recovery thereafter is influenced by the amount of protein in the diet. For instance, it has been shown that the duration of proteinuria following acute glomerular nephritis is the same whether abnormally high or low protein diets are given for some weeks after the oliguria and the urea retention have ceased.

How long the patient should remain in bed once the oedema, the raised jugular venous pressure, hypertension and raised blood urea have disappeared is determined by the number of red cells or the amount of protein being excreted in the urine. Progress is best guided by the red cell excretion. The aim is to allow the patient to get up once the red cell excretion, *though still raised*, has reached a relative plateau. The excretory rate should have fallen to somewhere near 1,000,000/hr. Usually, however, progress is judged by the extent of the proteinuria, and again it should reach a steady level before the patient is allowed to get up. As a rough approximation, it should fall below 1 g/24 hours, or be no greater than + in a sample of urine with specific gravity above 1·016.

It is clearly a useless and unwarrantable interference with the patient's liberty to keep him in bed until proteinuria disappears, for (1) proteinuria will persist for over a year in about half of the 90 per cent of patients who eventually make a complete recovery (Fig. 21.2), and (2) in those in whom the disease remains active it may persist as the only abnormality for 25 years. There is no evidence that the duration of rest in bed influences the eventual course of the disease.

Persistent Glomerular Nephritis

Clinically, persistent glomerular nephritis either (1) follows an attack of acute glomerular nephritis in a clinically recognisable manner, or (2) more commonly it presents without any previous known history or evidence of renal disease.

Presenting renal syndromes

Persistent glomerular nephritis may present as a rapidly progressive renal failure, recurrent haematuria (usually with persistent proteinuria), persistent proteinuria, a nephrotic syndrome, or chronic renal failure.

Rapidly Progressive Glomerular Nephritis

Pathology

The rapidly progressive form of persistent glomerular nephritis causes death within one or two years. At autopsy it is unusual for there to be more than some cortical narrowing to be seen with the naked eye. The macroscopical appearances of the kidney in patients dying during a nephrotic syndrome may either resemble those found in patients dying of persistent glomerular nephritis with chronic renal failure, or both kidneys are pale, smooth and enlarged. Death from chronic renal failure is associated with bilateral, symmetrical, shrunken, irregular and firm kidneys, the surfaces of which are pitted from contraction of underlying fibrous tissue, and raised by areas of hypertrophied nephrons.

In the glomeruli the outstanding feature is one of diffuse but not particularly marked mesangial and endothelial cell proliferation. The epithelial cells of the glomerular tuft also proliferate and swell. The distinguishing feature is the extensive proliferation of the cells of Bowman's capsule with the formation of numerous large, thick crescents (Fig. 21.3). The prognosis is directly related to the number of crescents. If they are present in less than 60 per cent of the glomeruli the course of the disease is not rapidly progressive whereas if more than 80 per cent of the glomeruli have crescents death occurs within two years. Often the crescents are so wide that they seem to compress and obliterate the tuft. The capillary wall changes are similar to but more pronounced than those found in acute glomerular nephritis. Some glomeruli are replaced by collagen. The tubules are invariably widely separated by a marked increase of interstitial material which is heavily infiltrated with chronic inflammatory cells. As in acute glomerular nephritis there are scattered foci of tubular necrosis.

The outstanding immunofluorescent finding is the presence of fibrinogen in the crescents, in the necrotic areas within the tuft and in intramembranous

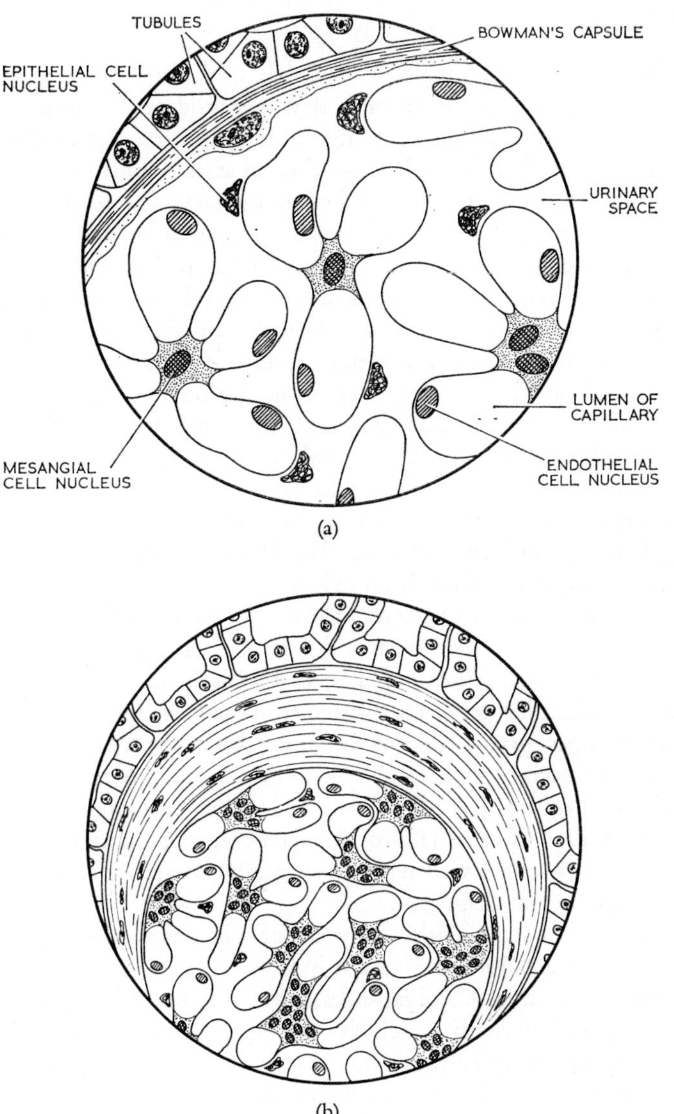

FIG. 21.3. (a) Normal. (b) Diffuse proliferative glomerular nephritis with crescents.

deposits. B_1C is also seen in coarse irregular deposits in the capillary walls and in the mesangial areas. IgA, IgG and IgM is found in various combinations in a coarse, irregular and globular pattern along the capillary wall, and in the mesangium. Occasionally IgG is found in a smooth intensely fluorescent line along the capillary wall.

Clinical features

Rapidly progressive glomerular nephritis often begins abruptly with an acute nephritic syndrome or it may develop insidiously. Some authorities state that it never follows an acute nephritic syndrome due to β haemolytic streptococcal infection. When it is a sequel to an acute nephritic syndrome there is often an initial diuresis and the signs of pulmonary oedema usually diminish or disappear, but the patient remains severely ill with lassitude, headache and malaise. Some oedema remains and there is much pallor. The blood pressure remains raised and tends to continue rising, the erythrocyte sedimentation rate is considerably raised and there is a persistent anaemia. Glomerular filtration rate and blood urea fluctuate, but both gradually deteriorate; the ability to concentrate is always grossly impaired from the beginning. Proteinuria may increase greatly and a nephrotic syndrome often develops after a few weeks. Urinary red cell excretion is always raised to extremely high levels. From time to time there may be macroscopical haematuria.

When the condition develops insidiously, the patient presents because of increasing lethargy, malaise and headache. The signs and symptoms are those just described except that there is no evidence of pulmonary oedema.

RELATIONSHIP BETWEEN CLINICAL AND STRUCTURAL FEATURES. Renal biopsy and autopsy findings have demonstrated that there is a fairly constant relationship between the clinical syndrome associated with the rapidly progressive form of persistent glomerular nephritis and the structural changes. Nevertheless, the glomerular changes give little information about the extent of functional impairment. For instance, it is impossible to distinguish those patients who have a nephrotic syndrome and a blood urea of less than 100 mg per 100 ml from those who have died of renal failure. On the other hand, extensive tubular and interstitial lesions correlate well with the creatinine clearance and gross inability to concentrate the urine (Fig. 3.9).

COURSE. Death occurs within 2 years of the onset of symptoms and is usually due to renal failure and severe hypertension.

DIFFERENTIAL DIAGNOSIS. Polyarteritis and disseminated lupus erythematosus are the two conditions with which the rapidly progressive form of persistent glomerular nephritis may be most often confused. Occasionally when the onset is gradual and the patient is middle-aged or older the condition may have to be distinguished from subacute endocarditis, amyloid disease or myelomatosis. A renal biopsy may be the only way to make certain of the diagnosis.

TREATMENT. There is no effective treatment. Prednisone usually makes things worse. In the past few years there have been certain claims that cytotoxic drugs can arrest the disease and even cause the proteinuria to disappear. It has also been claimed that treatment with heparin is beneficial. As there have been no satisfactory controls these claims have not been accepted, the criticism being that the good results are due to the inclusion of patients who were not primarily suffering from rapidly progressive glomerular nephritis.

Recurrent Macroscopic Haematuria Including Some Cases of Persistent Proteinuria with Microscopic Haematuria, and Others with Persistent Proteinuria without Haematuria

Pathology

This group is brought together by the histological appearances of focal proliferative glomerular nephritis (Fig. 21.4). The glomerular lesions are both focal and segmental, i.e. only some glomeruli are involved and often, only a portion of a glomerulus is affected. The lesions consist of mesangial cell prolifera-

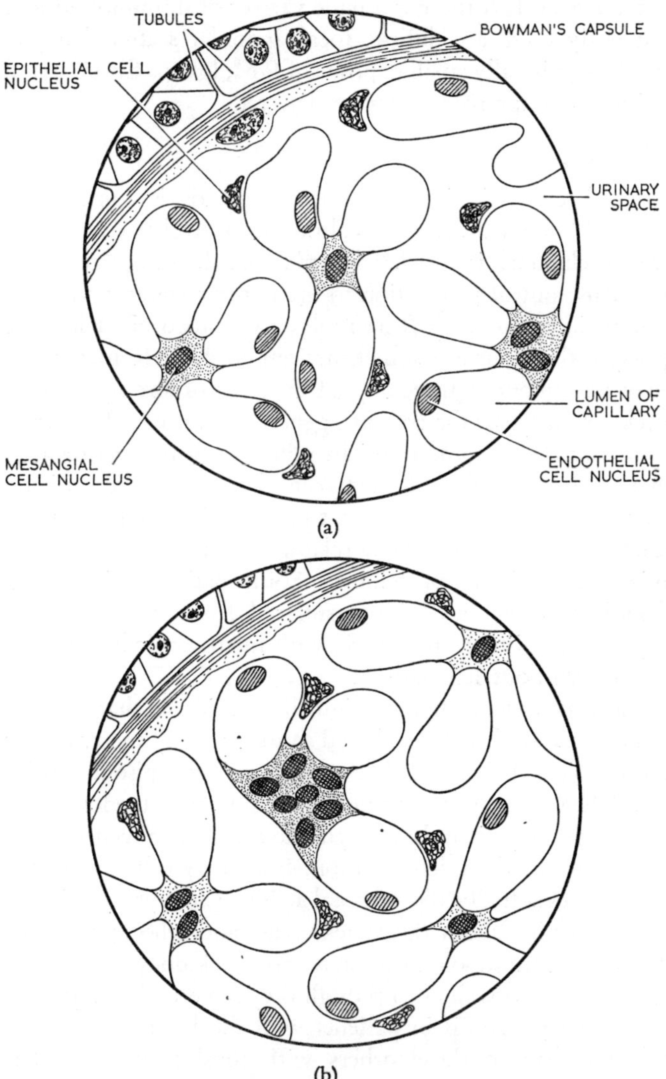

FIG. 21.4. (a) Normal. (b) Focal proliferative glomerular nephritis.

tion with intercapillary eosinophilic deposits, capsular adhesions, focal areas of glomerular fibrosis and very occasionally partial necrosis of the tuft.

The main immunodeposit is IgA. It is present in the mesangium but in striking contrast to the light microscopy appearances which are focal and segmental the mesangial IgA is in all the glomeruli and is scattered diffusely within each tuft. This is of the greatest interest for it demonstrates that immunoglobulin can be fixed to the capillary wall without producing a recognisable light microscopy change in the capillary wall. Sometimes the mesangium also contains small amounts of IgG, B_1C and fibrinogen.

When there is no IgA there is a wide variety of immunofluorescent appearances. Frequently there are diffuse, focal, granular scattered deposits of B_1C together with occasionally small deposits of IgM, IgG or fibrin. In a third of this group no immunofluorescence can be detected.

Clinical features

Recurrent haematuria in glomerular nephritis is sometimes known as recurrent "focal" nephritis. It occurs almost exclusively in young or adolescent males. Often each attack is associated with a sore throat or "cold" and a general feeling of malaise out of proportion to the upper respiratory symptoms. These are not due to infection with β haemolytic streptococci; it has been claimed, but not proven, that a virus is sometimes responsible. Haematuria begins at the same time or within one to three days of the onset of sore throat and it may last several weeks. As it settles the patient's general symptoms also improve. During the attack there may be some transient mild impairment of renal function but no oedema or hypertension. In between the attacks the patient feels well. Eventually most patients have persistent proteinuria though it may not become persistent until they have had several relapses. A raised urinary red cell excretion accompanies the persistent proteinuria. Some patients with the pathological lesions described above have never suffered from macroscopic haematuria. Either they have persistent proteinuria with microscopic haematuria or persistent proteinuria without haematuria.

COURSE AND PROGNOSIS. It was originally considered that when macroscopic haematuria and a sore throat developed simultaneously the renal condition was benign and transient. It is probable that with a single episode this is a justifiable conclusion. When there are recurrent attacks, however, the long-term prognosis is not so good. Some patients have been known to have recurrent attacks for 25 years without any marked deterioration. But many others with perhaps more frequent attacks eventually die of renal failure and hypertension. There is an unknown number in whom the attacks cease and who appear to make a full recovery. As in all immunological diseases of the kidney children have the best prognosis and often do well even though they have multiple attacks. There is a suspicion that the prognosis in patients with focal nephritis and IgA deposits is much better than in those others with focal nephritis and no IgA (see below).

Differential diagnosis. This syndrome is quite easily separated clinically and histologically from the rapidly progressive form of persistent glomerular nephritis or acute glomerular nephritis. The combination of recurrent painless haematuria and a sore throat should exclude local structural conditions of the kidney though the condition has been confused with recurrent pyelonephritis or renal stones. The first attack is the most difficult to distinguish with any certainty. It can easily be confused with the onset of polyarteritis nodosa, or some "bleeding" disorder including Henoch–Schonlein's purpura.

Treatment. There is no consistently effective treatment. It seems reasonable to keep the patient in bed until he feels better, and it is convenient that the duration of this period usually coincides with the duration of macroscopic haematuria. Some authorities give prophylactic oral penicillin to avoid a super-imposed β haemolytic streptococcal infection. In some patients prednisone may produce a quick remission, but in others it only makes things worse. A control trial of cytotoxic drugs, in those patients who have repeated attacks, is needed.

Nephrotic Syndrome, or Persistent Proteinuria with or without Haematuria, Associated with either no Light Microscopy Changes or with Equivocal Changes

This group of patients either have a nephrotic syndrome, which is indistinguishable from that which occurs with any other microscopical appearance. Or they may present with asymptomatic proteinuria, sometimes with microscopical haematuria.

Pathology

The light microscopy appearances are either normal (nil change) or the changes are difficult to interpret because they are so mild (minimal change). Electron microscopy, however, usually shows fusion of the epithelial foot processes and occasionally electron dense deposits in or near the glomerular basement membrane. Electron microscopy also demonstrates very small amounts of fibrin in the glomerular wall which are too small to be detected with immunofluorescence. Antisera specific for IgG, IgA, IgM, B_1C globulin and fibrinogen fail to demonstrate any fixation of these materials on the glomerulus.

Course and prognosis. These patients have an excellent prognosis and eventually have a complete remission of activity. They may remit permanently after the first attack of a nephrotic syndrome or they may have several relapses and remissions. Prednisone often hastens recovery, and cyclophosphamide may produce a long remission if the patient is prednisone dependent (p. 153).

Differential diagnosis. Persistent proteinuria, particularly with microscopic haematuria, associated with a normal renal biopsy on light microscopy should promote a thorough examination of the urinary tract for a neoplasm. A cystoscopy should be performed. The most difficult differential diagnosis is that of focal glomerular sclerosis (see below) which may be overlooked in the first biopsy because the early sclerotic lesions are small and few and far between, and, more important, they begin in the glomeruli which are near the medulla. It is also possible to miss an early extra-membranous glomerular nephritis if the biopsy is only examined with a light microscope, before the capillary walls have thickened. With silver stains and immunofluorescence however the distinction is easily made.

TREATMENT (see p. 148).

Patients with Persistent Proteinuria with and without Microscopical Haematuria, or a Nephrotic Syndrome or Chronic Renal Failure who do not Fit into the Four Groups Described Above

Pathology

The pathological findings in this group include all those histological changes that accompany glomerular nephritis, other than "nil change". Three have already been described. They are the varieties of diffuse proliferative and focal proliferative lesions which accompany the clinical syndromes of acute glomerular nephritis, rapidly progressive glomerular nephritis and recurrent macroscopic haematuria. These pathological changes are also found in some patients with persistent proteinuria with or without microscopical haematuria, or in others who have a nephrotic syndrome or chronic renal failure. These clinical syndromes are also accompanied by five additional pathological appearances in the glomeruli. They are: extra-membranous; membrano-proliferative; focal sclerosis, intramembranous; and advanced lesions, the origin of which is no longer distinguishable.

DIFFUSE PROLIFERATIVE WITH AND WITHOUT CRESCENTS. These appearances have been described earlier in conjunction with rapidly progressive glomerular nephritis. They may present with other clinical syndromes. The light microscopy and immunofluorescent patterns are the same whatever the clinical syndrome.

FOCAL PROLIFERATIVE. This appearance has also been described earlier in association with recurrent macroscopic haematuria, and with persistent proteinuria with or without microscopic haematuria. They may, however, also accompany a nephrotic syndrome or chronic renal failure. The light microscopy appearances are the same but the immunofluorescent pattern is different. There is no IgA deposition. B_1C is present sometimes diffusely, or occasionally it is focal and scattered. Small deposits of IgM and IgG also occur. Often there are no immunofluorescent deposits.

EXTRA-MEMBRANOUS. There is a diffuse even thickening of the capillary wall which electron microscopy demonstrates to be due to deposits located on the epithelial side of the glomerular basement membrane (Fig. 21.5). With haemotoxylin and eosin these deposits are faintly eosinophilic and indistinguishable

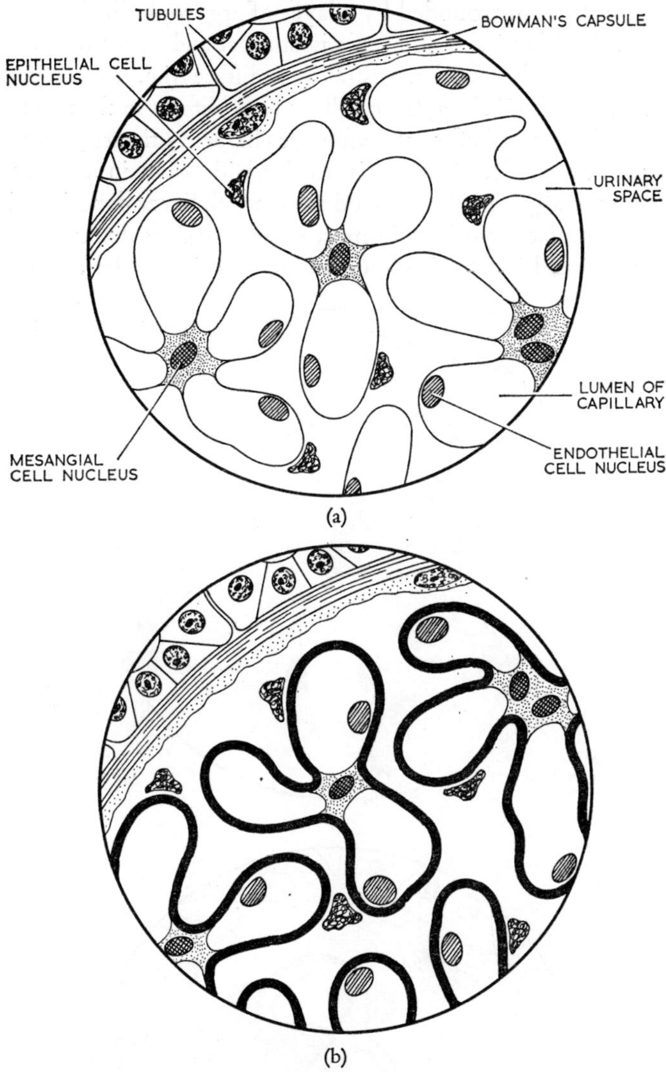

FIG. 21.5. (a) Normal. (b) Extra-membranous glomerular nephritis.

from the other components of the capillary wall. With silver strains, however, which pick out the basement membrane it is often possible to demonstrate that the basement membrane sends up spiky projections between the extra-membranous deposits. This gives the glomerular wall, when stained with silver, the appearance of a black stumpy, rather irregular comb (Fig. 3.3). At first before these argyrophyllic spikes have been formed the presence of the extra-membranous deposits may be overlooked by light microscopy. Conversely, at a later stage the deposits may become surrounded by fusion of the tips of the spikes so that the deposits are surrounded by a layer of argyrophyllic basement membrane material. Proliferation of the tufts is unusual and never more than mild. Immunofluorescence always demonstrates a diffuse (i.e. in all parts of all glomeruli) fixation of IgG along the capillary wall but not in the mesangial area. This appearance is present before and after the characteristic argyrophyllic spiky projections are discernible. The IgG is usually laid down in a finely granular pattern but occasionally it has been found as a smooth linear deposit (as in rapidly progressive glomerular nephritis). In most biopsies B_1C is detected in the same pattern as the IgG and in the same location, though in smaller amounts. Occa-

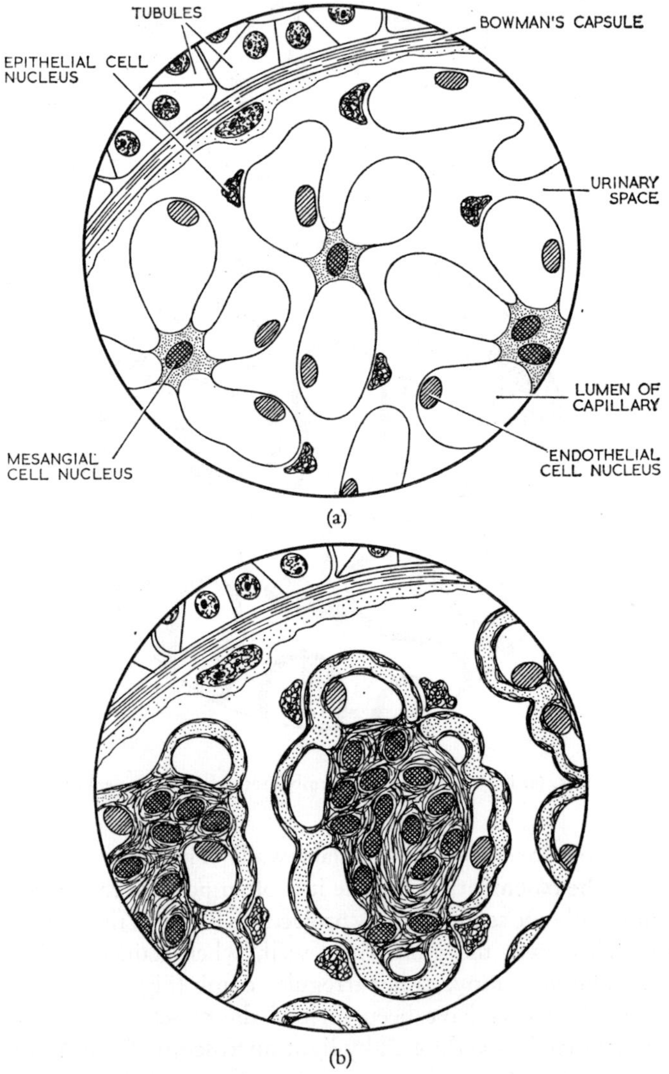

Fig. 21.6. (a) Normal. (b) Membrano-proliferative glomerular nephritis.

sionally small focal granular deposits of IgA, IgM and fibinogen can also be detected. When the light microscopy appearances are normal (see above) the finely granular fixation of the anti IgG in a regular manner in all parts of all glomeruli permits the lesion of extra membranous glomerular nephritis to be detected nevertheless.

MEMBRANO-PROLIFERATIVE GLOMERULITIS is characterised by a combination of mesangial cell proliferation, an increase in mesangial cell cytoplasm and matrix, and grossly irregular thickening of the capillary walls (Fig. 21.6). Electron microscopy demonstrates that the capillary wall thickening is due to extensions

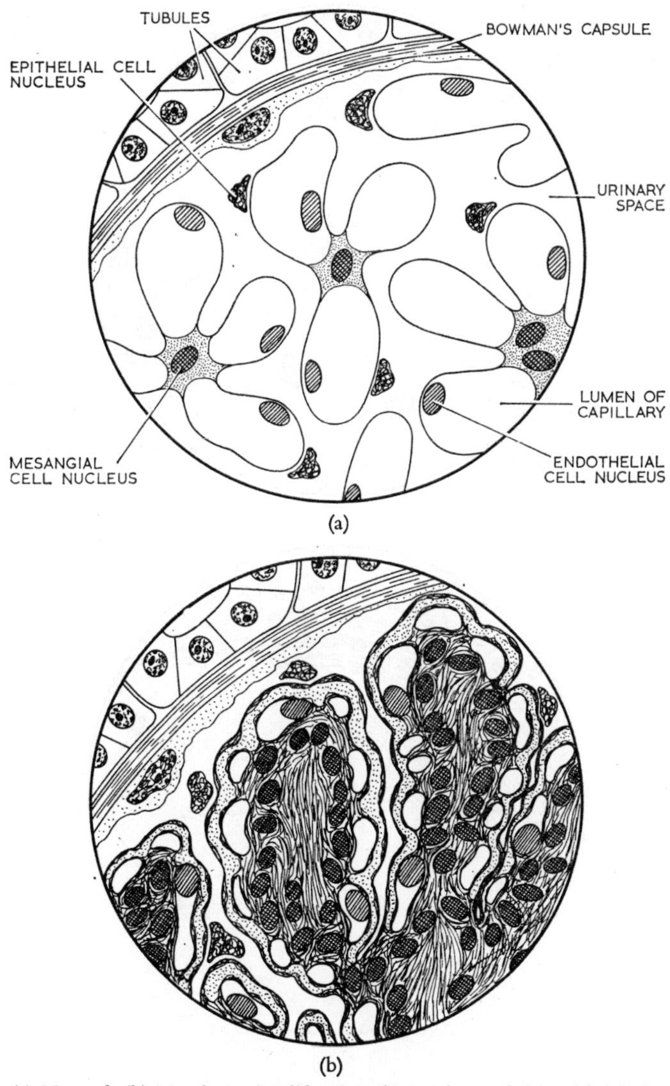

FIG. 21.7. (a) Normal. (b) Membrano-proliferative glomerular nephritis with lobular pattern.

of the mesangial cell cytoplasm penetrating between the glomerular basement membrane and the endothelium. With silver stains this gives the glomerular capillary wall, where this has happened, the appearance of two argyrophyllic parallel lines separated by an empty space (Fig. 3.1). The capillary wall may also be thickened by eosinophilic (non-argyrophyllic) deposits, on the endothelial side of the basement membrane. Sometimes the large accumulation of mesangial cytoplasm and matrix gives the glomerular tuft a lobular appearance (Fig. 21.7). Immunofluorescence demonstrates a coarse, irregular granular deposition of B_1C globulin, mainly in the capillary walls, and to a lesser extent in the mesan-

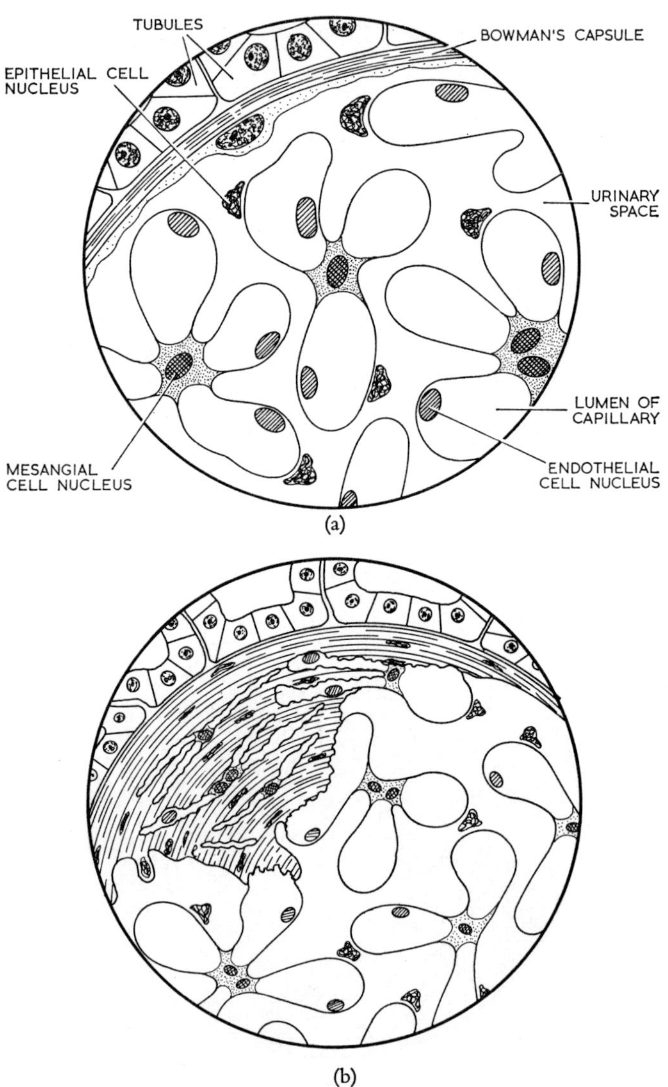

FIG. 21.8. (a) Normal. (b) Focal sclerosis glomerular nephritis.

gial areas. Sometimes this is diffuse, occasionally focal. Usually there are also focal coarse intramembranous deposits of IgM and fibrinogen, occasionally granular, irregular, diffuse deposits of IgG are found. IgA is not found. Very occasionally there is only B_1C unaccompanied by the presence of any immuno-globulin. In the biopsies showing a lobular appearance the B_1C is located only at the periphery of each lobule, never in the centre.

FOCAL SCLEROSIS is a focal (affects only some glomeruli) and segmental

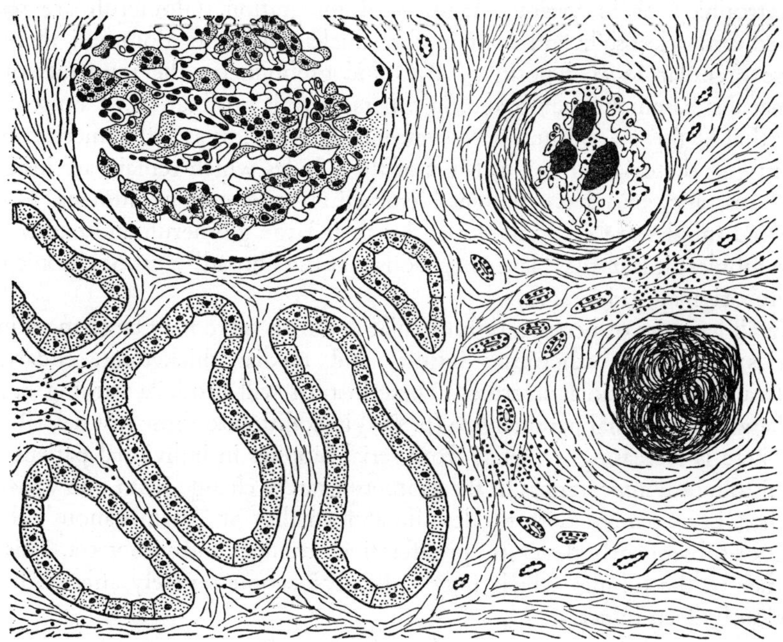

FIG. 21.9. Schema of persistent glomerular nephritis with chronic renal failure. The diagram emphasises the following points: the gross generalised disturbance with a hypertrophied glomerulus and tubule, surrounded by a matting of connective and fibrous tissue in which are embedded atrophic tubules, disintegrating glomeruli and some chronic inflammatory cells. One glomerulus is completely fibrosed (depicted as solid black) while the third shows a crescent and deposits of an eosin staining material in the tuft.

(affects only parts of a glomerulus) shrinkage of the glomerular tufts with capsular adhesions and occasional eosinophilic deposits on the endothelial side of the glomerular basement membrane (Fig. 21.8). The focal lesions characteristically contain fatty deposits. There is no cellular proliferation or mesangial deposits. In most biopsies focal collection of IgM and B_1C can be demonstrated with immunofluorescence only in the sclerosed areas. In about a third of patients there is no fixation of antisera in the biopsy.

INTRA-MEMBRANOUS GLOMERULITIS is a very rare lesion in which there is an infiltration of the glomerular basement membrane with dense deposits within the glomerular basement membrane. This substance also impregnates Bowman's capsule and the tubular basement membrane. There is usually an accompanying mesangial cell proliferation and some capsular crescents. By light microscopy, the appearance is that of a ribbon like eosinophilic deposit within the basement membrane. The deposits contain granular diffuse deposits of B_1C. Focal deposits of IgM are also found.

ADVANCED LESIONS. Beyond a certain stage the normal structural layout of the kidney is completely shattered and it becomes unrecognisable. There is a large amount of fibrous tissue interspersed with nephrons which are either hypertrophied or in various stages of disintegration. Glomeruli are scarce, scarred and sclerosed, and contain few nuclei. In some glomeruli there are coarse granular focal deposits of B_1C and globulin on the remnants of the glomerular basement membrane. In others there is no fixation of antisera. It is clear that at this stage immunofluorescence is as useless as light microscopy in identifying the original lesion. Most of the tubules which remain are insignificant, atrophic, and have flattened epithelium and narrow lumens. Hypertrophied tubules are easily identified by their large glomeruli and exceedingly wide tubules; it is in these large nephrons that the "broad" casts of chronic renal failure originate (Fig. 21.9).

In all varieties of persistent glomerular nephritis there may be changes in the arteries; including atheroma, intimal and medial thickening, endarteritis obliterans and arteriolar necroses. These in turn will produce varying degrees of change in the renal parenchyma (p. 125) in addition to those just described.

There is increasing evidence from serial biopsies in individual patients that the histological appearances in the glomeruli rarely change from one variety to another, i.e. a patient with no definite abnormality or "membranous" change will not subsequently develop "proliferative" changes and vice versa. This is in contrast to the tubules which may suddenly become severely affected having previously been intact.

Clinical Features

Persistent proteinuria

Persistent proteinuria as the only abnormal clinical feature may follow a clinically recognisable attack of acute glomerular nephritis, but more frequently it does not do so. It is usually discovered on routine investigation. At first it may be the only indication of the presence of glomerular nephritis. Later a nephrotic syndrome may develop, or chronic renal failure and hypertension, or there may be a sudden exacerbation with a superimposed acute nephritic syndrome. Often the proteinuria is accompanied by a fluctuating increase in red cell excretion.

RELATIONSHIP BETWEEN THE CLINICAL AND STRUCTURAL FEATURES. The most striking finding is that this symptomless proteinuria in an otherwise healthy person may be associated with any of the wide variety of those histological abnormalities which distinguish glomerular nephritis.

COURSE AND PROGNOSIS. These correlate best with the histological appearances. They are discussed below under Nephrotic syndrome.

DIFFERENTIAL DIAGNOSIS. As nearly all renal disease presents with proteinuria the differential diagnosis is a wide one. The first step is to exclude orthostatic proteinuria. Subsequently an extensive investigation is necessary, including an I.V.P., renal biopsy, urinary cell excretion rate, creatinine clearance, and the ability to concentrate and to acidify.

TREATMENT. This is discussed below with the treatment of the Nephrotic syndrome.

Nephrotic syndrome

The clinical features of a nephrotic syndrome have been described on p. 141. It is usual for the onset to be gradual, but a rapid onset sometimes occurs.

COURSE AND PROGNOSIS. Whether the patient presents with a nephrotic syndrome or persistent proteinuria the course and prognosis will vary according to the histological appearances. The good prognosis associated with "nil change" has been described above. The prognosis associated with all other forms of histological change is poor. Nearly all will die of chronic renal failure after one to 20 or more years. A few with diffuse proliferative and focal proliferative changes will survive. Patients with extra-membranous changes have a variable prognosis and may survive up to 20 years. Membrano-proliferative glomerular nephritis is often associated with abnormally low concentrations of plasma B_1C complement. Survival varies but often reaches 10–15 years in spite of the apparently very severe involvement of the glomeruli. Prognosis in patients with focal sclerosis is short; approximately five years. Before the introduction of antibiotics the commonest cause of death in patients with a nephrotic syndrome was infection. In such patients the oedema and heavy proteinuria may fluctuate with complete remissions interspersed with relapses. An exacerbation or relapse of oedema and proteinuria is sometimes heralded by the onset of an acute nephritic syndrome. As renal failure supervenes generalised oedema often persists even though proteinuria is less.

As death is due either to renal failure or hypertension it is clear that as long as there is no evidence of either, the immediate and short-term prognosis is good. But even when these ominous signs do appear the prognosis is not necessarily poor, for sometimes, after an anxious few weeks, renal function may improve, haematuria cease, and the blood pressure return to normal. Occasionally the glomerular filtration rate may remain around 40–60 ml/min and the blood urea 50–70 mg per 100 ml for many years even though there may be intermittent periods of transient deterioration (in two cases up to 20 years). In some instances the blood pressure rises gradually but there is no marked deterioration in renal function.

The earlier in the disease that hypertension and renal failure occur the worse the prognosis, particularly in children; it is also a bad sign when the extent of the oedema is massive and is difficult to remove.

DIFFERENTIAL DIAGNOSIS. Some of the other conditions in which the nephrotic syndrome may appear are given on p. 141. Cases due to myelomatosis, diabetes, anaphylactoid purpura or irradiation of the kidneys are easy to distinguish. An important cause which must always be kept in mind is the administration of troxidone. Amyloid disease of the kidney may be inferred from the clinical history and confirmed by biopsy; occasionally a renal biopsy shows amyloidosis when the clinical history is unhelpful or misleading and a liver biopsy negative. Thrombosis of the renal vein is suspected if there is evidence of inferior vena caval thrombosis, recurrent pulmonary emboli from the unknown site, or the patient is known to have only one kidney, or amyloidosis.

There remain polyarteritis and disseminated lupus erythematosus (D.L.E.). Polyarteritis as a cause of the nephrotic syndrome is unusual; at the onset it may be very difficult to distinguish from glomerular nephritis; renal biopsy is rarely helpful. The diagnosis is made when some more characteristic features of polyarteritis nodosa become evident (peripheral neuritis, fever, tachycardia, muscle pains, etc.) and is confirmed by muscle biopsy. D.L.E. is the most difficult condition to distinguish from glomerular nephritis, for sometimes there are no firm clinical reasons for suspecting the diagnosis. And the histological changes in D.L.E. are, for all practical purposes, the same as in glomerular nephritis. The distinction between the two diseases has to be made on the presence of the clinical features of D.L.E. cells in the peripheral blood or bone marrow, and antinuclear factor in the peripheral blood.

TREATMENT. Treatment is either symptomatic or attempts to be curative. Persistent proteinuria does not need symptomatic treatment and the symptomatic treatment of the nephrotic syndrome is described on p. 148. Prednisone and cytotoxic drugs have no effect on the course of glomerular nephritis when it is accompanied by any of the light microscopy changes described. There is some evidence that, on the contrary, the use of prednisone or cytotoxic drugs in such patients, particularly adults, may shorten survival because of their serious side effects.

Chronic renal failure

The clinical features of chronic renal failure have been described (p. 180). This is the final stage through which pass most patients who eventually succumb to persistent glomerular nephritis. In a few cases it is already known that the patient suffers from persistent glomerular nephritis. In the majority the symptoms of advanced chronic renal failure, or hypertensive cardiac failure, or malignant hypertension are the first indication of its presence.

RELATIONSHIP BETWEEN THE HISTOLOGICAL AND STRUCTURAL FEATURES. The individual lesions are the same as those described in patients with persistent proteinuria, recurrent haematuria or the nephrotic syndrome. The main difference is that the lesions are now more extensive, particularly those involving the tubules and interstitial spaces.

Renal function and the duration of survival are only poorly correlated with the extent of the histological findings.

COURSE AND PROGNOSIS. The rate of renal destruction varies very greatly;

it may fluctuate with quiescent periods and acute exacerbations. The duration of
the disease, from beginning to end, may extend to 30 years, but, once the
glomerular filtration rate has begun to fall and the blood urea to rise, there is a
tendency for the advance of chronic renal failure to be fairly rapid and inexorable.
As a very rough approximation once the blood urea is greater than 100 mg per
100 ml the prognosis is not likely to be greater than 2–3 years, and when it
is over 200 mg per 100 ml it is less than 1–2 years. These figures relate to the
concentration of blood urea when the patient is on an unrestricted diet, has
not had a recent haemorrhage or attack of diarrhoea and vomiting, is free
from cardiac failure, and is not suffering from an acute exacerbation of the
disease process as evidenced by the development of an acute nephritic syndrome
or haematuria. It has already been stressed repeatedly how circulatory insufficiency exacerbates renal failure and tends to give an erroneous impression of
the extent of any underlying renal structural damage. Such an exacerbation
may cause death from acute renal failure at a time when there is only a moderate
amount of renal structural damage.

Hypertension shortens the duration of survival, particularly if it is difficult
to treat.

DIFFERENTIAL DIAGNOSIS. Unless there is a suggestive past history, it is almost
impossible to confirm a diagnosis of persistent glomerular nephritis as a cause of
chronic renal failure without a renal biopsy.

Persistent glomerular nephritis has to be distinguished from the other causes
of chronic renal failure (p. 180). It is important that there should be no confusion
with chronic renal failure due to *chronic urinary obstruction*; the distinction is not
particularly difficult.

The most common causes of confusion are phenacetin nephropathy, and
nephrosclerosis (i.e. renal destruction directly due to hypertension (p. 124)).

With phenacetin nephropathy there are, in addition to persistent proteinuria,
chronic renal failure and hypertension, the following signs and symptoms:
(1) The urine usually contains an excess of white cells whether or not it is
infected; (2) judicious enquiry will reveal that there is, and has been an excess
ingestion of phenacetin (p. 322); (3) an intravenous pyelogram shows the
characteristic radiological lesions.

The distinction between persistent glomerular nephritis and nephrosclerosis
is often impossible without a renal biopsy. Statistically the more severe the renal
failure the more certain the diagnosis of persistent glomerular nephritis becomes,
"non-malignant" hypertension only rarely causes advanced renal failure.
Again, if a patient is found to have malignant hypertension and there is no
previous history of renal disease, it may be impossible to determine whether
there exists an underlying chronic structural lesion such as persistent glomerular
nephritis. Malignant hypertension is more likely to be a complication of pre-
existing renal disease if the kidneys are small (straight X-ray of the abdomen or
I.V.P.), or the renal failure is advanced when the diagnosis is first made.

TREATMENT is that of chronic renal failure. It aims at minimising or con-

K

trolling certain functional impairments. It is doubtful if any method slows the rate of renal structural disintegration, except the control of hypertension.

RENAL POLYARTERITIS NODOSA

This disease produces generalised disturbances (such as fever), and focal vascular lesions; in about 80 per cent of cases the kidneys are involved, either alone or in combination with other organs.

Pathology

The characteristic vascular lesions in the kidney may occur in the glomerular capillaries, the arterioles, or the small and medium sized arteries. In renal biopsies, however, the overall changes are difficult to distinguish from those of glomerular nephritis. The arterial lesions are scattered and difficult to find.

The characteristic glomerular lesion is a focal necrotising capillaritis in the midst of an acute inflammatory reaction; occasionally the entire glomerulus is necrosed (Fig. 21.10). The arterioles may either show arteriolar necrosis with

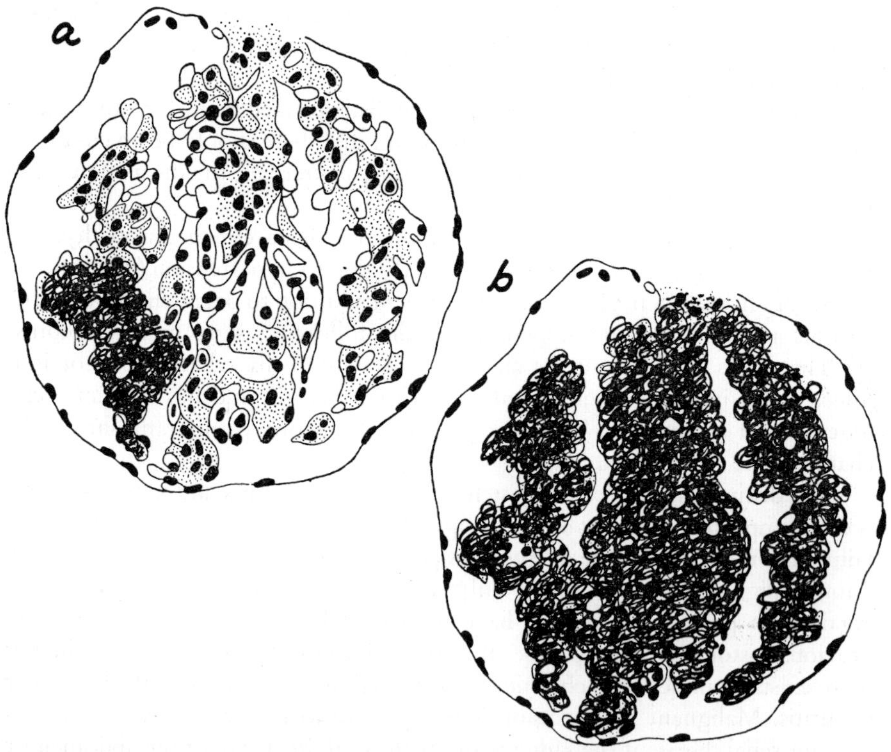

Fig. 21.10. Polyarteritis nodosa. Schema of two glomeruli; one (*a*) illustrates that the necrotic lesions may be focal while the other (*b*) shows that the whole glomerulus may become necrosed.

perivascular inflammatory cell reaction, or endarteritis obliterans (i.e. the same lesions as in malignant hypertension, except for the perivascular inflammation). The medium and small sized arteries show the diagnostic lesion of polyarteritis nodosa; that is focal areas of acute segmental necrosis of a part or the whole of the arterial wall, together with an acute inflammatory reaction which invades and surrounds the necrotic area.

All these lesions occlude the lumen of the affected vessels and therefore the changes in the renal parenchyma (and the clinical features) largely depend on which vessels are involved. When the glomerular capillaries and the arterioles are affected the glomeruli show exudative and proliferative changes.

When the small and medium sized arteries are affected there will be wedge-shaped areas of infarction in which the glomeruli will at first only appear "coagulated" or "clumped" and then become fibrosed and structureless, while the tubules, particularly the proximal tubules, become atrophied at an early stage; relatively normal renal tissue may surround the infarcts.

Sometimes when the larger vessels are affected, the glomeruli may appear relatively normal but there are widespread tubular changes throughout the renal parenchyma, including tubular separation, changes in the nuclei, flattening of the tubular cells, and increase in size of their lumens. It is possible that these lesions are due to partial occlusions of the arcuate arteries.

Immunofluorescence demonstrates the presence of large amounts of fibrin deposits. These are focal in the glomeruli and in some vessels.

When the vascular lesions heal there are focal areas of marked intimal fibrosis which contain capillaries (the sites of recanalised thrombi); focal ruptures of the internal elastic lamina; and areas of focal fibrosis of the arterial walls extending into the surrounding tissues.

Clinical features

The wide variety of pathological changes accounts for the extensive range of clinical features. Renal polyarteritis nodosa may present as acute renal failure, chronic renal failure, an acute nephritic syndrome, or a nephrotic syndrome; the predominant abnormality may be proteinuria or severe haematuria, or tubular inability to control electrolyte excretion. The blood pressure tends to rise after the renal symptoms have appeared, and may continue to rise until there is malignant hypertension. The disease is more common in men than women and is more easily diagnosed in the young than in the elderly.

Acute renal failure occurs if there are extensive necrotic lesions in the glomeruli, while proteinuria, chronic renal failure and severe hypertension are more likely if the lesions are in the small and medium sized arteries and there are multiple infarcts.

One of the most frequent ways in which renal polyarteritis presents is as an acute nephritic syndrome. For a few weeks the diagnosis is usually confused with acute glomerular nephritis, but eventually the slow rate of recovery, or the stormy course of the syndrome, together with the appearance of some other non-renal clinical feature of polyarteritis nodosa, suggests the proper diagnosis. There may be attacks of severe unexplained central abdominal pain, fever, tachycardia, leucocytosis and eosinophilia, peripheral neuritis, pulmonary symptoms and radiological opacities in the lungs, skin rashes and nodules, or muscle pains and tenderness. The most characteristic features of active renal polyarteritis are (1) recurrent, irregularly spaced, sharp attacks, of unremitting, unilateral loin pain of sudden onset, usually lasting for less than an hour, and followed by an increased rate of red cell excretion in the urine; these probably occur at the moment of, or shortly after, the formation of small renal infarcts; occasionally the pain radiates to, or may be situated entirely in, the flanks and front of the abdomen; and (2) long continued excretion of fluctuating quantities of *macroscopic* haematuria. (3) Selective renal arteriogram may reveal a very characteristic appearance. This consists of small rounded opacities less than 1 mm diameter lying irregularly in the cortex. Finally the ability of the kidney to concentrate the urine is often impaired to a far greater extent than is the glomerular filtration rate.

Course and prognosis

Before the use of cortisone the majority of cases of renal polyarteritis nodosa died of renal failure or hypertensive cardiac failure within one or two years of the onset of the disease. The prognosis today is better.

The natural clinical course is often one of remissions and relapses, and occasionally evidence of such fluctuations can be found at autopsy, when both healed and active lesions of polyarteritis are seen. At any moment acute activity may cease. Ultimate recovery then depends on the extent of the vascular lesions, for healed lesions may continue to produce harmful effects, such as malignant hypertension or chronic renal failure.

Death may occur from lesions in other sites, but renal failure is the commonest cause of death in polyarteritis. Many cases develop renal failure fairly rapidly and die within a few months; those who begin with acute renal failure die within a few days.

Nevertheless some cases do recover; their number is not known, for unless there is positive histological evidence the diagnosis is uncertain, and it is obvious that such evidence is obtained less often in those patients who recover than in those who succumb.

Differential diagnosis

The renal disturbance caused by polyarteritis may suggest almost any form of renal disease. A renal biopsy is of some help in diagnosis, but unless a necrosed arteriole or artery is seen, surrounded by an intense inflammatory reaction, the diagnosis remains in doubt; and the chance of finding such a lesion in the small amount of tissue removed by biopsy is remote. The other renal histological features of polyarteritis may also appear in glomerular nephritis, lupus erythematosus, "embolic nephritis", and malignant hypertension. Immunofluorescent studies, however, make it relatively easy to distinguish the renal lesions of disseminated lupus erythematosus and most cases of glomerular nephritis.

A useful clinical point in difficult cases is the presence of fever, however mild it may be. If blood cultures are negative, there are no lupus erythematosus cells or antinuclear factor in the peripheral blood, and the urine is sterile, renal disease associated with a pyrexia is due to polyarteritis nodosa until it is proved to the contrary. When polyarteritis is responsible for a nephrotic syndrome it is characteristic that the 24-hour urinary excretion of protein and the decrease in plasma proteins is more moderate than the extent of the oedema would suggest. Intermittent cardiac failure of uncertain origin and associated with only mild hypertension is another tenuous indication of polyarteritis.

Treatment

Adrenal steroids and ACTH are the only effective means of treatment. They often produce a remarkable and immediate remission of the acute symptoms, and in some cases they indubitably prolong life. The dose should be large (e.g. 40–100 mg prednisone per day), and it is essential that once a favourable effect has been produced the quantity should be continued uninterruptedly at a high level for several weeks. If the dose of adrenal steroids is lowered too rapidly there is often a relapse of symptoms, which for some inexplicable reason then no longer respond to adrenal steroids, or only do so when they are given in very large and potentially dangerous amounts (150 mg of prednisone per day). Treatment with adrenal steroids should be continued for at least a year, the dose eventually being lowered very gradually at monthly intervals during that time (e.g. by 1–2 mg each month). If signs of activity persist or recur (e.g. raised ESR) treatment should be continued for longer.

The complications of adrenal steroid therapy have been mentioned (p. 152). The most important risk in the treatment of polyarteritis nodosa is retention and accumulation of salt and water, which may precipitate pulmonary oedema or a further rise in blood pressure. Initially therefore it is essential to measure the patient's weight and blood pressure and observe his jugular venous pressure each day. If necessary salt and water retention can be controlled by diuretics, and if the blood pressure begins to rise, it should be lowered by hypotensive drugs. In some cases in which the blood pressure is very high at the onset it may be advisable for it to be lowered before beginning treatment with adrenal steroids.

RENAL LUPUS ERYTHEMATOSUS

Systemic lupus erythematosus (S.L.E.) resembles polyarteritis nodosa in that it also produces generalised disturbances and affects a wide variety of organs. The aetiology is not understood. Nuclear material is released into the plasma. Antibodies to DNA are then produced which attach themselves on to the circulating DNA to form immune complexes which fix on to capillary walls where they activate complement and give rise to inflammation. The disease in man resembles very closely a similar disturbance which affects a certain strain of New Zealand mice which are infected *in utero* with chorio-meningitis virus. The virus destroys the cells and releases the DNA into the circulation. Many attempts have been and are being made to find a similar virus aetiology for systemic lupus erythematosus.

Pathology

Systemic lupus erythematosus may occur without any structural abnormality evident in the kidneys. Patients with renal lesions may be divided into two groups, some who only have mild focal glomerular lesions, and the others who have more extensive glomerular lesions together with changes in the interstitial spaces and the tubules.

The glomerular lesions include "nil change" (approx. 30 per cent), extra-membranous (approx. 15 per cent), focal proliferative (approx. 25 per cent) and diffuse proliferative changes (approx. 30 per cent). The characteristics of all four are similar to those found in glomerular nephritis; with a few rare exceptions. For instance when there are no histological changes immunofluorescent staining will sometimes show some mild fixation of IgG globulin both along the capillary wall and in the mesangium. Occasionally IgM, IgA and B_1C globulin are found. Extra-membranous changes appear to be identical to those found in glomerular nephritis. Focal proliferative changes are associated with much focal nuclear disruption and extremely rarely with structureless haematoxylin "bodies". These are aggregations of breakdown products of disintegrating nuclei circulating in the peripheral blood which become trapped in the glomerular capillaries. There are also focal areas of voluminous deposits lying between the endothelial cell cytoplasm and the basement membrane. They have the appearance of eosinophilic fibrinoid areas and are responsible for the classical "wire-loop" lesions of lupus nephritis. There are also smaller extra membranous deposits. Finally, focal glomerular changes in lupus are associated with multiple small foci of necrosis in the glomerular tufts. Immunofluorescence shows mainly deposits of IgG laid out in a granular pattern along the walls of the capillaries. The histological appearances of diffuse glomerular changes are the same as those found with focal changes except that the lesions are widespread. Focal and diffuse changes are associated with varying involvement of the tubules with collections of interstitial inflammatory cells.

Death from renal failure may take place before there has been much disintegration and absorption of nephrons. In such cases the kidneys macroscopically are of normal size, or enlarged, while histologically there is a striking proliferation of both the glomerular capsule and the tufts, thickening and granularity of the capillary walls, exudates, haemorrhages, and even necrosis in the tufts. If, on the other hand, the changes have occurred more slowly, particularly when they have been retarded by prednisone, the kidneys will be smaller and the histological changes will resemble more closely those of advanced glomerular nephritis.

Vascular changes may not be particularly pronounced, though sometimes the lesions of polyarteritis nodosa, or fibrinoid necrosis of arterioles, may be present.

Clinical features

Renal lupus erythematosus presents as proteinuria, a nephrotic syndrome, chronic renal failure or occasionally as an acute nephritic syndrome.

Proteinuria and a nephrotic syndrome are the two most frequent presentations. Usually the correct diagnosis is not made until some other more characteristic features of lupus erythematosus become manifest, e.g. skin lesions, fever, pleural effusion, pericarditis, arthritis, leucopenia, high erythrocyte sedimentation rate, and "L.E." cells in the blood or bone marrow, or antinuclear factor in the blood. Sometimes a patient may develop a nephrotic syndrome without a raised blood cholesterol.

By the time chronic renal failure occurs the diagnosis is usually less difficult. It is characteristic that the blood pressure rises less frequently and much later than in other causes of renal failure, and that malignant hypertension is exceptional.

The disease is more common in women than in men.

Relation between the clinical and structural features

In keeping with most other renal diseases there is little correlation between the clinical picture and the histological changes, except that when there is some degree of renal failure there are lesions in the interstitium and tubules as well as in the glomeruli. But in the absence of renal failure, proteinuria may be present with either no histological abnormality, or with well-defined lesions in both the glomeruli, and the interstitial space and the tubules.

Course and prognosis

Follow-up studies with serial renal biopsies have shown that it is most unusual for patients with systemic lupus erythematosus who initially have no renal lesions to develop such lesions at a later date. Similarly, it is uncommon for a patient whose renal lesions are confined to the glomeruli to develop tubular and interstitial lesions subsequently, though it can happen.

The prognosis is related to the histological appearances. Patients with nil change, membranous and focal changes tend to live 10–20 years before there is any deterioration of renal function. Whereas patients with diffuse glomerular changes die of renal failure within a few years. Persistent hypertension or renal failure with blood ureas greater than 100 mg/100 ml also carry a poor prognosis death occurring within a few years. Transient rises in blood pressure, however, during acute exacerbations of S.L.E. are not important.

In the absence of hypertension or renal failure, pregnancy does not appear to influence the progress of the disease.

Differential diagnosis

The most diagnostic features of lupus erythematosus are the skin lesions, the presence of "L.E." cells in the blood and bone marrow and the presence of antinuclear factor in the blood. Without these it may be impossible to distinguish with certainty renal lupus erythematosus from other causes of renal disorders such as glomerular nephritis, renal polyarteritis nodosa and the renal lesions which accompany sub-acute bacterial endocarditis.

Treatment

In diffuse proliferative glomerulitis with lesions in the tubules and the interstitial space and deteriorating renal function it is essential to give large quantities of steroids over a prolonged period, e.g. 40–60 mg/day for six months gradually reducing to 15 mg/day thereafter. This will increase survival and reverse the structural lesions. It is problematical whether any treatment affects the other forms of lupus nephritis and whether, in view of their good prognosis, any known form of treatment is justified. The administration of prednisone causes the disappearance of the IgG deposits in the glomeruli.

It is important in all patients with S.L.E. to try to avoid factors which may cause an acute exacerbation of the process, e.g. sunbathing, drugs such as penicillin, certain cosmetics, hair dyes and certain household and garden chemicals.

RENAL DISTURBANCES IN SUB-ACUTE BACTERIAL ENDOCARDITIS

Renal disease due to sub-acute bacterial endocarditis used to be known as "embolic" nephritis, on the assumption that the disturbance is due to multiple renal emboli. There is, however, considerable doubt about this assumption, for:

1. The lesions are rarely seen until the infection has been present for at least six weeks.
2. Bacteria are almost never found in the kidney.
3. When they are found it can be seen that the lesions they have provoked do not resemble the majority of the lesions which are present and which do not contain bacteria.
4. In some instances there are large numbers of lesions in the kidney, and few in other parts of the body.
5. The typical renal lesions can be produced experimentally as a feature of an abnormal antigen–antibody response.
6. Foreign particles injected into the circulation may embolise in the kidney but do not produce the characteristic lesions found in sub-acute bacterial endocarditis.

These points suggest that the renal lesions in sub-acute bacterial endocarditis may be due principally to an abnormal antigen–antibody response to the organism responsible for the infection in the heart.

Pathology

Macroscopically the kidney may appear normal, but if a considerable number of glomeruli are undergoing acute changes it may be swollen and covered with numerous petechial haemorrhages, as in acute glomerular nephritis, malignant hypertension and diffuse lupus erythematosus.

The characteristic microscopical lesion is an area of acute necrosis of a part (Fig. 21.10a) or the whole of a glomerulus, surrounded by varying quantities of acute inflammatory cells, and in the midst of which there may be intracapillary thrombi. Immunofluorescence microscopy demonstrates the presence of IgG and complement on the basement membrane of the glomerular capillaries. In one patient with staphylococcal septicaemia a staphylococcal antigen was also found bound to the capillary wall. Occasionally there may also be arteriolar necrosis of afferent arterioles. These lesions are usually scattered in widely separated glomeruli, but they are sometimes present in the majority. They are identical to the changes seen in the glomeruli and afferent arterioles in polyarteritis nodosa; the difference between the two conditions being that in bacterial endocarditis the small and medium-sized arteries are not affected.

Following this acute stage the glomerular lesions become round structureless masses of eosin staining material and eventually become fibrosed. Characteristically these circular collections can be seen within otherwise normal glomeruli.

Patients who have died from renal failure usually show, in addition, widespread proliferative lesions.

Clinical features

Frequently the patient is thought, or known to be suffering from sub-acute bacterial endocarditis, and routine examination of the urine shows occasional showers of red cells, or frank haematuria; such findings then help to establish the correct diagnosis.

Sometimes the diagnosis of endocarditis has not been considered or has been rejected because pyrexia and cardiac murmurs have been absent, and repeated blood cultures have been sterile. In these patients the significance of the proteinuria and the excretion of a few red cells may not be properly appreciated. This occurs particularly in the elderly, who may then die of renal failure.

In early cases treatment successfully prevents the further development of renal disturbances, but in cases with advanced renal failure treatment is unlikely to save life.

Diagnosis

A positive blood culture settles the diagnosis.
When blood cultures are sterile, a renal biopsy may be helpful.

Treatment

This consists in identifying the organism, determining its sensitivity to various antibiotics, and then giving the appropriate one in suitable doses for a

K§

period of six weeks or longer, depending on when the blood cultures become sterile. The treatment of the renal failure which may accompany the immunological renal disturbance is to give large doses of prednisone. This usually produces a rapid improvement.

SHUNT NEPHRITIS

A membrano-proliferative glomerular nephritis which occurs in children with an infected ventriculo-atrial shunt for hydrocephalus. Complement and IgM are found along the capillary walls. When the shunt is removed the renal lesions rapidly resolve and disappear.

RENAL DISTURBANCES IN ANAPHYLACTOID PURPURA

Anaphylactoid purpura (the Schönlein–Henoch syndrome) is characterised by a purpuric rash, abdominal pains, polyarthritis and haematuria; these usually occur in the young and follow a well-recognised infection such as tonsillitis, or occasionally they may be precipitated by the ingestion or administration of some substance to which the patient is subsequently found to be sensitive, e.g. tomatoes.

The aetiology of this syndrome is considered to be an abnormal antigen–antibody response.

Pathology

There does not appear to be any characteristic lesion. There are either focal or diffuse proliferative glomerular changes, the latter is sometimes accompanied by crescents. Immunofluorescence reveals diffuse substantial deposits of IgA, IgG and B_1C complement in both the capillary walls and the mesangial areas. There are even thicker deposits of fibrin diffusely distributed in all glomeruli, particularly in the mesangial areas and also in the capillary walls. There are focal collections of chronic inflammatory cells in the interstitial tissues, particularly around abnormal glomeruli, and glomerular fibrosis and tubular atrophy.

Clinical features

About 10–20 per cent of all cases of anaphylactoid purpura have haematuria and proteinuria; an acute nephritic syndrome may also be present. In the majority of patients there is subsequently a rapid and complete recovery, while a few continue to excrete protein and red cells. In most of these proteinuria eventually disappears, but in the remainder it persists, chronic renal failure develops, and death occurs in one to five years. Recurrent attacks of macroscopical haematuria are a characteristic feature of this last group; they may also develop transient acute nephritic syndromes, and on occasion a nephrotic syndrome.

Approximately 10 per cent of adults who have haematuria and proteinuria at the onset of an attack of anaphylactoid purpura die of chronic renal failure subsequently. The prognosis is much better in children.

Treatment

It is doubtful if any treatment influences the course of the renal lesions; nevertheless, it is reasonable in the acute attack to treat any residual infection with antibiotics. In some instances it may be necessary to give prophylactic penicillin when there are recurrent relapses due to β-haemolytic streptococcal infections.

Treatment of the advanced renal disturbances is unrewarding, though occasionally a patient may respond dramaticaly to ACTH or adrenal steroids; there are even some reports of complete cure. More often, however, adrenal steroids only produce a rapid rise in blood pressure, jugular venous pressure and blood urea, and treatment must be discontinued.

There have been claims, particularly by paediatricians, that the administration of cytotoxic drugs is beneficial and life saving. Again these observations are uncontrolled.

LUNG PURPURA WITH NEPHRITIS
(Goodpasture's Syndrome)

This devastating and rare condition occurs particularly in young men between the ages of 18 and 26 years, and is most often seen during an influenzal pandemic. Following an upper respiratory or gastric type of influenzal illness there is a sudden onset of profuse haemoptysis which lowers the haemoglobin within a few days. Serial chest X-rays demonstrate the presence of fluctuating pulmonary shadows due to blood in the pulmonary alveoli. The presence of glomerular nephritis is usually detected a few days after the onset of the haemoptysis. There is proteinuria, haematuria, and renal failure. Death usually occurs within a few months from renal failure; occasionally there is acute renal failure.

Histologically the lesion is one of diffuse proliferative glomerular nephritis. IgG and B_1C are laid down in a smooth continuous pattern on the inner surface of the basement membrane of the glomerular capillaries (Fig. 3.7). The pattern is the same as that of experimentally induced anti-glomerular basement disease (p. 254). In the blood of some patients it is possible to detect anti-glomerular basement antibodies, particularly after bilateral nephrectomy. The lungs contain collections of haemosiderin in the alveoli and alveolar walls, with many histiocytes; both these changes are presumably consequent upon the haemorrhage. IgG and B_1C are present in smooth linear pattern in the basement membrane of the alveoli. Some patients have survived after being placed upon maintenance haemodialysis. If they are given a renal transplant the circulating anti-glomerular basement antibodies may rapidly destroy the graft.

HAEMOLYTIC URAEMIC SYNDROME

This is a rare condition occurring often in minor epidemics which suggests that it is triggered off by an infection. It is unusual in adults but it is probable that the diagnosis is often missed. It is then accompanied by malignant hypertension, or associated with childbirth. The overt clinical and histological manifestations are probably due to rapid intravascular coagulation. There is usually a preceding attack of diarrhoea and vomiting followed by a rapid onset of pallor with bruising or petechiae. Oliguria is common and occasionally hypertension develops. The peripheral blood picture is one of severe anaemia with bizarre, distorted and fragmented red blood cells with thrombocytopenia. There is renal failure of varying severity with microscopic haematuria and proteinuria.

The renal lesions consist of bilateral cortical necrosis, or focal, or diffuse necrosis of the glomeruli only, with fibrinoid necrosis of the arterioles. There may also be diffuse proliferative glomerular changes. There are often microthrombi in glomerular capillaries and most capillary lumens contain laminated deposits of fibrin. There is little correlation between the intensity of the initial renal failure and the histological lesions. Treatment consists of blood transfusions and dialysis until renal function recovers. Whether heparin should also be given is problematical, its administration often causes bleeding and complicates treatment. The administration of steroids sometimes produces a remarkably clear-cut improvement. Mortality before the introduction of haemodialysis was about 50 per cent.

RENAL DISTURBANCES IN QUARTAN MALARIA

Large numbers of children infected with quartan malaria, particularly in East Africa, develop a nephrotic syndrome or sometimes an acute nephritic syndrome. The renal lesions consist of focal and segmental glomerular proliferation. Glomerular capsular crescents, and interstitial and tubular changes are rare. IgG, IgA and IgM and B_1C can be demonstrated in a granular pattern mainly distributed along the walls of the capillaries. Occasionally the fluorescence can be smooth and linear. Malarial antigens have also been demonstrated both in the serum and fixed on to the glomerular capillaries. Treatment with cyclophosphamide in a control trial has been found to diminish the proteinuria. Otherwise intensive treatment of the malaria gradually eradicates the disease.

RENAL DISTURBANCES IN MALIGNANT DISEASE

Occasionally a patient with a carcinoma or a lymphoma may develop a nephrotic syndrome. Granular deposits of immunoglobulins and complement can be demonstrated in the glomerular capillary walls. In one patient the immunoglobulins eluted from the glomeruli reacted specifically with the surface plasma membranes of the neoplastic tumour cells. Removal of a tumour may cause a rapid diminution of proteinuria and temporary recovery.

RENAL LESIONS IN LIVER DISEASE

A mild impairment of renal function in cirrhosis of the liver is well recognised. It is often overlooked because the diminished dietary intake of protein of alcoholism, or the diminished urea production in liver failure causes the plasma urea level to remain normal in spite of a diminution of glomerular filtration rate. Occasionally there may be a nephrotic syndrome, or only proteinuria. The outstanding lesion histologically is an intercapillary thickening associated with lumpy mesangial deposits of IgG, IgA and complement. Occasionally there is focal mesangial proliferation. The glomerular capillary walls are unaffected. There is no correlation between the severity of the renal lesion and the severity of the liver disease but there may be some relation between the accumulation of mesangial immunoglobulins and the raised plasma gammaglobulin.

BIBLIOGRAPHY

Aetiological mechanisms in immunological renal diseases
CARPENTER, C. B. (1970). "Immunologic aspects of renal disease." *Annual Review of Medicine*, **21**, 1.
DIXON, F. J. (1958). Editorial "The pathogenesis of glomerulonephritis." *Amer. J. Med.*, **44**, 493.
FREEDMAN, P., MEISTER, H. P., LEE, H. J., SMITH, E. C., CO, B. S., and NIDUS, B. D. (1970). "The renal response to streptococcal infection." *Medicine*, **49**, 433.
GLYNN, L. E., and HOLBOROW, E. J. (1952). "Conversion of tissue polysaccharides to auto-antigens by group-A Beta-haemolytic streptococci." *Lancet*, **2**, 449.
GOOD, R. A., and FISHER, D. W. (1971). "Immunobiology." Sinaver Associates, Inc., Stamford, Connecticut, U.S.A.
HARDWICKE, J. (1971). "Immunological mechanisms in glomerulonephritis." *J. Roy. Coll. Physcns.*, **5**, 140.
IMMUNE COMPLEXES AND DISEASE (1971). Proceedings of a Symposium. *J. Exp. Med.*, **134**.
McCLUSKEY, R. T., VASSALI, P., GELLO, G., and BALDWIN, D. S. (1966). "An immunofluorescent study of pathogenic mechanisms in renal disease." *New Eng. J. Med.*, **274** 695.
RAMMELKAMP, C. H. (1967). Aetiology of glomerulonephritis in renal disease. In "Renal Disease", edited by D. A. K. Black. Blackwell Scientific Pubs., Oxford, 209.
UNANUE, E. R., and DIXON, F. J. (1967). "Experimental glomerulonephritis: Immunological events and pathogenetic mechanisms." *Advances in Immunology*, **6**, 1.
VASSALI, P., and McCLUSKEY, R. T. (1966). "The coagulation process and glomerular disease." *Amer. J. Med.*, **39**, 179.
ZABRISKIE, J. B. (1971). "The role of streptococci in human glomerulonephritis." *J. Exp. Med.*, **134**, 180.

Glomerular nephritis
ADDIS, T. (1949). "Glomerular Nephritis. Diagnosis and Treatment." The Macmillan Co., New York.
AKERREN, Y., and LINDGREN, M. (1955). "Investigation concerning early rising in acute haemorrhagic nephritis." *Acta med. scand.*, **151**, 419.
BERGER, J. (1969). "Glomerular deposits in renal disease." *Transplant Proc.*, **I**, 939.

BERGER, J., YANEVA, H., and ANTOINE, B. "Applications de l'immunofluorescence à la pathologie rénale. Études immunoclinique des lésions glomerulaires." *J. Urol. Nephrol. (Paris)*, **75**, 268.

BERGER, J., DE MONTERA, H., and HINGLAIS, N. (1966). "Comment évoluent les lésions rénales des malades atteints de syndrome néphrotique." Actualités Néphrologiques de l'Hopital Necker, Éditions Médicales Flammarion, Paris.

BLACK, D. A. K. (1970). "Immunosuppressive agents in protein-losing nephritis." *Sci. Basis of Med. Ann. Reviews*, p. 114.

BLACK, D. A. K., ROSE, G., and BREWER, D. B. (1970). "Controlled trial of Prednisone in adult patients with the nephrotic syndrome." *Brit. med. J.*, **2**, 239.

BRIGHT, R. (1836). "Cases and observations, illustrative of renal disease accompanied with the secretion of albuminous urine." *Guy's Hosp. Rep.*, **1**, 338.

CAMERON, J. S. (1971). "Immunosuppressant agents in the treatment of glomerular nephritis. Part 1. Corticosteroid drugs. Part 2. Cytotoxic drugs." *J. Roy. Coll. Phycns. Lond.*, **5**, 282 and 301.

CHAMBERLAIN, M. S., PRINGLE, A., and WRONG, O. M. (1966). "Oliguric renal failure in the nephrotic syndrome." *Quart. J. Med.*, **35**, 215.

CLARKSON, A. R., MACDONALD, M. K., PETRIE, J. J. B., CASH, J. D., and ROBSON, J. S. (1971). "Serum and urinary fibrin of fibrinogen degradation products in glomerulo-nephritis." *Brit. med. J.*, **1**, 447.

CONTROLLED TRIAL OF AZATHIOPRINE AND PREDNISONE IN CHRONIC RENAL DISEASE (1971). Report by Medical Research Council Working Party. *Brit. med. J.*, **2**, 239.

HABIB, R. (1970). "Classification anatomique des néphropathies glomerulaires." *Pädiat. Fortbild. Prax.* (Karger Ed.), **28**, 3.

HUTT, M. S. R., PINNIGER, J., and DE WARDENER, H. E. (1958). "The relationship between the histological and clinical features in acute glomerular nephritis based on a study of renal biopsy material." *Quart. J. Med.*, N.S. **27**, 265.

KASSIRER, J. P., and SCHWARTZ, W. B. (1961). "Acute glomerular-nephritis." *New Eng. J. Med.*, **265**, 686.

KINCAID-SMITH, P., SAKER, B. M., and FAIRLEY, K. F. (1968). "Anticoagulants in irreversible acute renal failure." *Lancet*, **2**, 1360.

LEONARD, C. D., NAGLE, R. B., STRIKER, G. E., CUTLER, R. E., and SCRIBNER, B. H. (1970). "Acute glomerulonephritis with prolonged oliguria. An analysis of 29 cases." *Ann. of Int. Medicine*, **73**, 703.

LEWIS, E. J., CAVALLO, T., HARRINGTON, J. T., and COTRAN, R. S. (1971). "An immuno-pathologic study of rapidly progressive glomerulonephritis in the adult." *Human Pathology*, **2**, 185.

MICHAEL, A. F., HERDMAN, R. C., FISCH, A. J., PICKERING, R. J., and VERNIER, R. C. (1969). "Chronic membrano-proliferative glomerulonephritis with hypocomplementinaemia." *Transplant Proc.*, **1**, 925.

MOREL-MAROGER, L., LEATHEM, A., and RICHET, G. (1972). "Glomerular abnormalities in non-systemic disease: Relationship between light microscopy and immunofluores-cence in 433 renal biopsies." *Amer. J. Med.*, **53**, 170.

MORTENSON, V. (1947). "Treatment of acute glomerulo-nephritis with high protein diet." *Acta med. scand.*, **129**, 321.

M.R.C. (1970). "Report of a multi-centre controlled trial of prednisone in adult patients with the nephrotic syndrome." *Brit. Med. J.*, **3**, 425.

RICH, A. R. (1946–47). "Hypersensitivity in disease." *Harvey Lect.*, **42**, 106.

ROSS, J. H. (1960). "Recurrent focal nephritis." *Quart. J. Med.*, N.S. **29**, 391.

STICKLER, G. A., HAYLES, A. B., POWER, M. H., and ULRICH, J. A. (1960). "Renal tubular dysfunction complicating the nephrotic syndrome." *Paediatrics*, **26**, 75.

Polyarteritis nodosa
AHLSTROM, C. G., LIEDHOLM, K., and TRUEDSSON, E. (1953). "Respirato-renal type of polyarteritis nodosa." *Acta med. scand.*, **144**, 323.

DAVSON, J., BALL, J., and PLATT, R. (1948). "Kidney in periarteritis nodosa." *Quart. J. Med.*, N.S. **17**, 175.

DARMADY, E. M., GRIFFITHS, W. J., MATTINGLY, D., SPENCER, H., STRANAK, F., and DE WARDENER, H. E. (1955). "Renal tubular failure associated with polyarteritis nodosa." *Lancet*, **1**, 378.

GRANT, R. T. (1940). "Observations on periarteritis nodosa." *Clin. Sci.*, **4**, 245.

RALSTON, D. E., and KVALE, W. F. (1949). "Renal lesions of periarteritis nodosa." *Proc. Mayo Clin.*, **24**, 18.

SPENCER, H., and ROSE, G. A. (1957). "Polyarteritis nodosa." *Quart. J. Med.*, N.S. **26**, 43.

WAINWRIGHT, J., and DAVSON, J. (1950). "Renal appearances in microscopic form of periarteritis nodosa." *J. Path. Bact.*, **62**, 189.

Systemic lupus erythematosus

COMERFORD, F. R., COHEN, A. S., and DESAN, R. G. (1968). "The evolution of the glomerular lesion in NZB mice. A light and electron microscopic study." *Lab. Invest.*, **19**, 643

EVANS, A. S., ROTHFIELD, N. F., and NIEDERMAN, J. C. (1971). "Raised titres to E.B. virus in systemic lupus erythematosus." *Lancet*, **1**, 167.

LAMBERT, P. H., and DIXON, F. J. (1968). "Pathogenesis of the glomerulo-nephritis of NZB/W mice." *J. exp. Med.*, **127**, 507.

POLLAK, V. E., and PIRANI, C. L. (1966). Pathology of the kidney in systemic lupus erythematosus: serial renal biopsy studies and the effects of therapy on kidney lesions in E. L. Dubois, "Lupus Erythematosus", I Vol. McGraw-Hill, New York, ed., p. 54.

SIMENKOFF, M. L., and MERRILL, J. P. (1964). "The spectrum of lupus nephritis." *Nephron*, **1**, 348.

Sub-acute bacterial endocarditis

ALLEN, A. C. (1951). "The Kidney, Medical and Surgical Diseases." J. & A. Churchill, London.

BAEHR, G. (1912). "Glomerular lesions of subacute bacterial endocarditis." *J. exp. Med.*, **15**, 330.

BELL, E. T. (1932). "Glomerular lesions associated with endocarditis." *Amer. J. Path.*, **8**, 639.

LITTMAN, D., and SCHAAF, R. S. (1950). "Therapeutic experiences with subacute bacterial endocarditis with special reference to the failures." *New Engl. J. Med.*, **243**, 248.

Anaphylactoid purpura

BURKE, E. C., MILLS, S. D., and STICKLER, G. B. (1960). "Nephritis associated with anaphylactoid purpura in childhood; clinical observations and prognosis." *Proc. Mayo Clin.*, **35**, 641.

BYWATERS, E. G. L., ISDALE, I., and KEMPTON, J. J. (1957). "Schönlein–Henoch purpura." *Quart. J. Med.*, N.S. **26**, 161.

CREAM, J. J., GUMPEL, J. M., and PEACHEY, R. D. G. (1970). "Anaphylactoid purpura in adults." *Quart. J. Med.*, **39**, 461.

FILLASTRE, J. P., MOREL-MAROGER, L., and RICHET, G. (1971). "Schönlein–Henoch purpura in adults." Letter in *Lancet*, **1**, 1243.

Lung purpura with nephritis

BENOIT, F. L., RULSON, D. B., THEIL, G. B., DOOLEN, P. D., and WATTEN, R. H. (1964). "Goodpasture's syndrome." *Amer. J. Med.*, **37**, 424.

CANFIELD, C. J., DAVIS, T. E., and HERMAN, R. H. (1963). "Haemorrhagic pulmonary-renal syndrome." *New Eng. J. Med.*, **268**, 230.

McPHAUL, J. J., and DIXON, F. J. (1970). "Characterization of human anti-glomerular basement membrane antibodies eluted from glomerulonephritic kidneys." *J. clin. Invest.*, **49**, 308.

LLOYD RUSBY, N., and WILSON, C. (1965). "Lung purpura with nephritis." *Ann. Rev. Med.*, **16**, 301.

Shunt nephritis

STICKLER, G. B., SHIN, M. H., BURKE, E. C., HOLLEY, K. E., MILLER, R. H., and SEGAR, W. E. (1968). "Diffuse glomerulonephritis associated with infected ventriculoarterial shunt." *New Eng. J. Med.*, **279**, 1077.

Haemolytic uraemic syndrome
CLARKSON, A. R., LAWRENCE, J. R., MEADOWS, R., and SEYMOUR, A. E. (1970). "The haemolytic uraemic syndrome in adults." *Quart. J. Med.*, **39**, 227.
HABIB, R., MATHIEU, H., and ROYER, P. (1967). "Le syndrome hémolytique et urémique de l'enfant." *Nephron*, **4**, 139.
LIEBERMAN, E., HEUSSER, E., DONNEL, G. N., LANDING, B. H., and HAMMOND, G. D. (1966). "Hemolytic-uremic syndrome. Clinical and pathological considerations." *New Eng. J. Med.*, **275**, 227.
SHARPSTONE, P., EVANS, R. G., O'SHEA, M., ALEXANDER, L., and LEE, H. A. (1968). "Haemolytic-uraemic syndrome: survival after prolonged oliguria." *Arch. dis. Childh.*, **43**, 711.

Renal disturbances in quartan malaria
ALLISON, A. L., HENDRICKSE, R. G., EDINGTON, G. M., HOUBA, V., PETRIS, D. E., and ADENIYI (1969). "Immune complexes in the nephrotic syndrome of African children." *Lancet*, **1**, 1232.
WARD, P. A., and KIBUKAMUSOKE, J. W. (1969). "Evidence for soluble immune complexes in the pathogenesis of glomerular nephritis in quartan malaria." *Lancet*, **1**, 283.
VOLLER, A., DRAPER, C. C., TIN SHWE, and HUTT, M. S. R. (1971). "Nephrotic syndrome in monkey injected with human quartan malaria." *Brit. Med. J.*, **4**, 208.

Renal disturbances in malignant disease
CANTRELL, E. G. (1969). "Nephrotic syndrome cured by removal of gastric carcinoma." *Brit. Med. J.*, **2**, 739.
GHOSH, L., and MUEHRCKE, R. C. (1970). "The nephrotic syndrome. A prodrome to lymphoma." *Ann. intern. Med.*, **72**, 379.
LEWIS, M. G., LOUGHRIDGE, L. W., and PHILLIPS, T. M. (1971). "Immunological studies in nephrotic syndrome associated with extrarenal malignant disease." *Lancet*, **2**, 134.
LOUGHRIDGE, L., and LEWIS, M. G. (1971). "Nephrotic syndrome in malignant disease of non-renal origin." *Lancet*, **1**, 256.

Immunological renal disturbances in liver disease
FISHER, E. R., and PEREZ-STABLE, E. (1968). "Cirrhotic lobular glomerulonephritis. Correlation of ultrastructural and clinical factors." *Amer. J. Pathol.*, **52**, 869.
MANIGAND, G., MOREL-MAROGER, L., SIMON, J., and DEPARIS, M. (1970). "Lésions rénales glomérulaires et cirrhose du foie." *Rev. Europ. Clin. et Biol.*, **15**, 989.
SAKAGUCHI, H., DACHS, G., GRISHMAN, E., PARONETTO, F., SALOMON, M., and CHURG, J. (1965). "Hepatic glomerulosclerosis. An electronic microscopic study of renal biopsies in liver diseases." *Lab. Invest.*, **14**, 533.

22

Orthostatic Proteinuria

This benign condition is also called postural proteinuria. It consists of the excretion of protein in the urine only when the patient is in certain positions.

Aetiology

Proteinuria can be produced in 75 per cent of youths if they are placed in extreme lordosis; with increasing age the proportion gradually dwindles and, of men over 50, only 10 per cent will have proteinuria in this position.

It has been demonstrated that in the lordotic position the liver in these persons rotates forwards and downwards thus kinking the inferior vena cava. As a result there is a rise in the pressure within the inferior vena cava and renal veins, and protein appears in the urine.

If, however, the patients stands in the lordotic position but the liver is prevented from sliding forward by firm digital restraint under the right costal margin, the inferior vena caval pressure does not rise and there is no proteinuria. In bed, the lordosis of the upright position disappears and again there is no proteinuria, though it can be made to reappear by purposely assuming the lordotic position. Conversely, proteinuria will not appear in the upright posture if the patient remains bent forward.

Renal function

Excluding the proteinuria renal function is normal.

Clinical features

Orthostatic proteinuria occurs most frequently in children, adolescents and young adults. It has been reported in 12–40 per cent of children aged 10–16 years; and it is claimed that this proportion is greater if the urine is examined at frequent intervals. Orthostatic proteinuria occurs in about 5 per cent of young adults.

The presence of protein in the urine is usually detected during a routine examination on going to school or university, or on entering the services. Occasionally it is noted as an incidental finding during an illness which is unrelated to the kidney. If many urine samples are tested it is found that protein is present throughout the day, except in the first sample passed in the morning. The concentration of protein rarely exceeds + + and is usually + or less; the daily excretion is seldom more than 2–3 g. It is not unusual to find protein on some days and not on others. Orthostatic proteinuria is of no importance; it does not influence the patient's health or the functional capacity of his kidneys. The majority of patients lose their proteinuria as they become older though it may continue for 10–30 years.

For routine purposes orthostatic proteinuria is distinguished from persistent proteinuria by asking the patient to empty his bladder just before going to bed, and to keep for examination the urine he passes next morning immediately he gets up. If necessary this test can be combined with a 16- to 24-hour fluid deprivation test, when the ability to concentrate can be tested simultaneously.

Differential diagnosis

If proteinuria can be made to disappear with a change in posture it is almost certain that there is no renal disease. Nevertheless it is also characteristic of the proteinuria of renal disease that it is greater when the patient is up and about, and diminishes upon lying down. On very rare occasions the proteinuria of renal disease may be altogether absent from the urine formed during the night, when it is then indistinguishable from benign orthostatic proteinuria. These confusing cases usually declare themselves eventually; sometimes they can be differentiated earlier by an examination of the urinary deposit, or a renal biopsy. It is a paradox that orthostatic proteinuria like that which occurs with fever and exercise demonstrates a pattern of unselective glomerular permeability (p. 145) though the glomeruli show no histological changes. Orthostatic proteinuria should not be dismissed too lightly when it occurs in a patient over 30 years old.

Treatment

No treatment is necessary.

Proteinuria from Non-gonococcal Urethritis

Superficially, this appears to be a variant of orthostatic proteinuria, but in fact it has no direct relation to posture. It is an important diagnostic trap. The proteinuria is present in the *morning* and disappears during the course of the day. The condition is most commonly seen in young men. Urethral massage in the morning, before any urine has been excreted, and examination of the contents of the urethra establishes the diagnosis. The two glass test is also a useful screening test.

BIBLIOGRAPHY

BULL, G. M. (1948–49). "Postural proteinuria." *Clin. Sci.*, **7**, 77.
KING, S. E. (1955). "Patterns of protein excretion by the kidneys." *Ann. intern. Med.*, **42**, 296.
KING, S. E. (1957). "Postural adjustments and protein excretion by the kidney in renal disease." *Ann. intern. Med.*, **46**, 360.
LOWGREN, E. (1955). "Studies on benign proteinuria (with special reference to the renal lymphatic system)." *Acta med. scand.*, suppl. 300.
LYALL, A. (1941). "Classification of cases of albuminuria." *Brit. med. J.*, **2**, 113.

23

Renal Infections

INFECTIONS of the kidney can be divided into those due to the tubercle bacillus and those due to other organisms; only the latter are described below. The outstanding features about renal infections are their diagnostic difficulties, the lack of precise knowledge of their natural history, and how they should be treated.

INTERSTITIAL NEPHRITIS, RENAL INFECTIONS AND PHENACETIN NEPHROPATHY

Interstitial nephritis means inflammation of the interstitial spaces. It is a structural abnormality which accompanies most renal diseases. Unfortunately, the words involved in describing this disturbance, and the disturbance itself have been the cause of much confusion. It is obvious that inflammation of the interstitial spaces must be due to some cause. The semantic tradition which lingers on however, reserves the term interstitial nephritis mainly for those kidneys in which the cause of the inflammation is not known. For instance, though the immunological diseases of the kidney are usually associated with inflammation of the interstitial spaces the characteristic changes in the glomeruli permit the overall changes to be defined as those due most probably to an immunological disturbance. The interstitial changes are then either not mentioned specifically or referred to as an accompanying "inflammation of the interstitial spaces". In the same way the term interstitial nephritis is not used if an inflammation of the interstitial spaces is found in association with widespread deposits of calcium or collections of urate crystals, when the appearances are described as those of nephrocalcinosis and gouty nephropathy respectively. Additional causes of inflammation of the interstitial spaces include viral, bacterial and spirochaetal infections, partial occlusions of the renal vasculature with or without hypertension, prolonged phenacetin administration, radiation nephritis, oxalosis, potassium deficiency, back pressure from obstruction to urine flow and lead poisoning. Many of these, particularly if only a biopsy sample is available often show changes which are simply those of inflammation of the interstitial spaces and they cannot be distinguished one from another histologically.

That inflammation of the interstitial spaces must be due to some underlying cause, even when it cannot be discerned, preys heavily upon those who examine the structural appearances of the kidneys. They are inevitably tempted to ascribe causes when none are evident histologically. Their choice is then influenced by the clinical history, the blood pressure, the biochemical findings, the urine culture, etc. Instead of reporting simply that the histological appearances are those of inflammation of the interstitial spaces of unknown cause, the histological changes are said to be due to ischaemia, infection, gout, etc., whichever seems to suit the *ante-mortem* information most closely. This has inevitably given rise to the false impression that the various causes of interstitial inflammation *can* easily be differentiated histologically from each other, and that interstitial nephritis, i.e. inflammation of the interstitial space of unknown cause, is a most unusual condition. This self deception has been particularly prominent in English speaking countries where some authorities used to equate "interstitial nephritis", i.e. inflammation of the interstitial spaces of unknown cause, with pyelonephritis, i.e. inflammation of the interstitial spaces due to infection. This manoeuvre neatly avoided the term interstitial nephritis and its connotation that the histologist can sometimes be baffled. It has been responsible for the ludicrous disparity between the various estimates of the incidence of renal infection in kidneys examined at autopsy (from 10 to 80 per cent!).

The following section is concerned with renal infection, and the renal destruction which follows excess ingestion of phenacetin, two causes of inflammation of the interstitial spaces which are often particularly difficult to distinguish histologically from other conditions which produce inflammatory changes in the interstitium.

PYELONEPHRITIS

Aetiology

A wide variety of organisms may cause pyelonephritis; those found most frequently are *Escherichia coli*, coagulase negative *Staphylococcus albus*, coagulase positive *Staphylococcus aureus*, *Klebsiella pneumoniae*, *Pseudomonas pyocyanea*, *Proteus vulgaris* and *Streptococcus faecalis*.

Many infections are associated with uretric reflux, obstruction, or deformation of the urinary tract; these cause a rise in pressure, and possibly a slowing in the rate of urine flow in those parts which lie proximal to the obstruction. Most infections, however, occur in kidneys with normal urinary tracts, nearly always in women. A few infections occur during a widespread and easily recognised dissemination of organisms from a primary focus, such as malignant endocarditis, osteomyelitis, empyema, etc. The renal lesion thus caused is sometimes known as a "pyaemic kidney" but, as it is indistinguishable from severe acute pyelonephritis from other causes, it is included here. One of the commonest causes for such a bacteraemia is the introduction of a catheter, or cystoscope, into a bladder containing infected urine.

Lesions which obstruct the urinary tract include certain abnormalities of the renal parenchyma which deform the calcyes, such as hypoplasia, polycystic kidneys, and scarring from previous infections (including tuberculosis). Other causes are congenital abnormalities of the pelvis, ureter and urethra; aberrant renal arteries; renal and ureteric calculi; pregnancy; "neurogenic bladders"; pelvic tumours; prostatic enlargement and urethral strictures. Calculi and pregnancy are the two most frequent causes of obstruction.

Infections frequently complicate other parenchymal renal diseases; for instance, acute pyelonephritis may develop in a patient known to be suffering from renal polyarteritis nodosa. In this connection it is interesting to note that animal experiments have shown that the intravenous administration of large numbers of Gram-negative organisms only causes acute pyelonephritis if the ureters are temporarily occluded or the kidneys are already scarred from previous infections. It has also been shown, in animals, that an increased susceptibility to infection can be produced by a period of potassium deficiency or hypertension. The relation to hypertension is of immense potential significance.

The infecting organism may be conveyed to the kidney in (1) the blood stream, (2) the urine, from the bladder up to the lumen of the ureters, or (3) the lymphatics alongside the ureters. Observations in human infection suggest that the organisms nearly always travel up the ureters. Acute upper urinary infections in previously normal kidneys occur predominantly in women whose urine has contained large numbers of organisms for some time before the onset of symptoms. There is no doubt, however, that a transient bacteraemia can also cause pyelonephritis. Occasionally (e.g. after routine catheterisation) the two mechanisms occur together; the bladder urine is first infected by the catheter, the organisms then multiply in the bladder and after an interval there is a simultaneous bacteraemia and acute pyelonephritis. In animal experiments organisms have been introduced into the bladder after tying one ureter. It has been found that the kidney with a patent ureter becomes infected while the other kidney remains intact, unless there is an associated bacteraemia. The lesions in both human and animal infections are often most pronounced in the

Linnaean and other Names of some of the Organisms which cause Urinary Infections

Linnaean name	Other names	Comment
Escherichia coli . .	B. coli	The most frequent cause of acute urinary infections.
Staphylococcus albus . (Coag − ve)		Causes up to 25 per cent of all urinary infections.
Staphylococcus aureus . (Coag + ve)	*Staph. pyogenes*	Occasionally found in structurally abnormal urinary tracts
Klebsiella pneumoniae .	Friedlander's bacillus *Aerobacter aerogenes*	Usually in mixed infections and when there are structural deformities of the urinary tract.
Pseudomonas pyocyanea .	B. pyocyaneus Ps. aeruginosa	Frequently after antibiotic therapy and an indwelling catheter.
Proteus vulgaris . .	B. proteus	
Streptococcus faecalis .	Enterococci	Often follows catheterisation in women.
Haemophilus influenzae .	B. influenzae Pfeiffer's bacillus	Rarely found.

medulla. In animals it has been shown that the medulla's ability to restrain bacterial growth is relatively poor. This is due to the hypertonicity of the medulla which inhibits (i) the natural bactericidal activity of plasma, (ii) the mobilisation of white cells towards an injured area, and (iii) the phagocytic capacity of the white cells.

There is increasing evidence that the strains of organisms that cause acute infections of the upper urinary tract are often specifically adapted to do so. Either they are immune to the bactericidal activity of plasma or they have some other particular property that distinguishes them from other strains, e.g. they haemolyse red blood cells. In a large proportion of cases the bacteria having ascended the ureter and invaded the highly vascular parenchyma, then spill into the blood and cause a septicaemia. In some instances the bacterial invasion of the renal parenchyma is associated with a rise in serum antibody titre to the infecting organism.

Examination of the Urine for Evidence of Infection and Inflammation

The urine is cultured (see below) and examined microscopically for the presence of excess numbers of white cells. It is important to realise that a positive culture is evidence of infection, but not of inflammation, whereas an increased number of white cells is evidence of inflammation but not of infection. The two investigations are therefore complementary.

Examination of the urine for infection

Because of the risk of infection it is no longer justifiable to catheterise the bladder to obtain urine for culture. Urine is therefore obtained either by a mid stream sample (M.S.U.) or by suprapubic aspiration.

M.S.U. Using this technique the urine sample is often contaminated by organisms which reside in the urethra and the vulva. It is imperative therefore that cultures from mid stream samples of urine should be quantitated. It is then possible to distinguish whether the organisms found in the urine are likely to be contaminants or whether they were present and multiplying in the bladder before micturition. If the urine is carefully collected (see below) and either cultured immediately or kept cold until it is cultured, then a bacterial count greater than 100,000/ml has an 85 per cent probability of being due to true infection of the urine; a count of less than 10,000/ml is due to contamination. Two consecutive cultures with counts greater than 100,000/ml increase the probability that there is an infection to 99 per cent. In a well run establishment counts between 10,000/ml and 100,000/ml should occur in less than 10 per cent of all urine cultures. If they occur more frequently the urine is not being collected with sufficient care. When the count is between 10,000/ml and 100,000/ml it should be repeated. Pure cultures with only one type of organism support the probability that the organisms are multiplying in the bladder. These interpretations of the significance of quantitative bacterial cultures do not hold if the patient is on antibiotics. The uselessness of culturing an M.S.U. in a non-quantitative manner is well illustrated in Fig. 23.1 where a non-quantitative and a quantitative technique are compared. It can be seen that a report of "growth" from a non-quantitative culture gives no indication whether the urine is infected or contaminated.

Urine is collected from a woman after swabbing the perineum with soap and water, rinsing with sterile water and drying with a sterile swab. It is unwise to use a disinfectant for a drop may fall into the urine and sterilise it. The labia

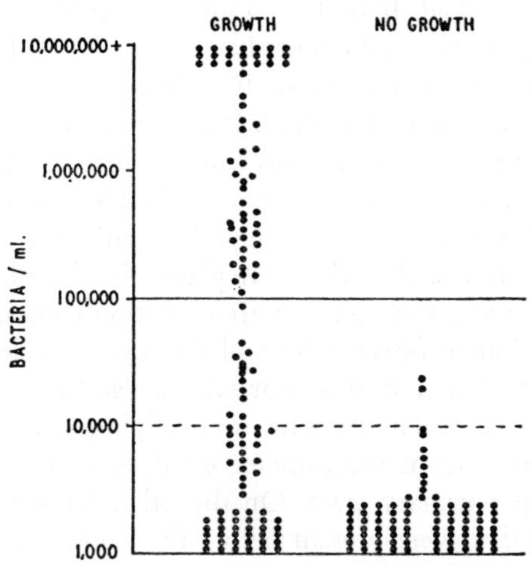

Fig. 23.1. Routine urine culture report of "growth" and "no growth" compared with the number of organisms found on quantitative culture. Each dot represents one urine. The interrupted horizontal line at 10,000 organisms/ml and the continuous horizontal line at 10,000/ml. The block of dots at the bottom of the figure represent counts of from less than 100/ml to 2,000/ml and at the top of the figure the block indicates counts greater than 10,000,000/ml. (Bradley and Little, 1963, *Brit. med. J.*)

are then held open and the patient is asked to micturate. The whole volume of urine is collected, the first 10–50 ml into one container and the remainder into a wide-mouthed autoclaved honey jar. Urine is obtained from a man in a similar way, after cleaning the urethral meatus with benzalkonium chloride 1/1,000. The urine in the autoclaved jar is cultured. There are a variety of ways to perform quantitative cultures. For routine purposes it is only necessary to distinguish whether the count is greater than 100,000/ml or less than 10,000/ml. Culturing the urine not only establishes whether or not the urine is infected but it also permits the sensitivity of the organism to various antibiotics to be established.

Suprapubic aspiration. The bladder is allowed to fill either after the administration of several glasses of water or after the administration of 20 mg of frusemide. When the bladder is palpable, **and not before**, a sample of urine is obtained by inserting into the bladder a number 1 needle in the mid line of the anterior surface of the abdomen 1 in. above the symphysi pubis. A local anaesthetic is unnecessary. The procedure is much less painful and no more dangerous than the insertion of an intravenous needle in the antecubital fossa but it is considerably more alarming to witness. It is best therefore if the patient cannot see what is going on. **Any infection in urine obtained in this way represents a true infection however small the number of colonies.** The technique is gradually being used more widely. It has enormous advantages in reliability and speed of execution over a mid stream sample of urine. It is particularly useful when the patient is obese, dirty or cannot easily cooperate and pass water when asked. It is also useful when mid stream samples from a patient repeatedly give bacterial counts between 10,000/ml and 100,000/ml.

Localisation of urinary tract infection. It is important to know whether the urinary organisms are confined to the bladder or whether they are also multiplying in the upper urinary tract. This can be ascertained either by inserting ureteric catheters, which can occupy much valuable "urological" time, or by an ingenious technique devised by Fairley. The patient is encouraged to drink a large quantity of fluids. A catheter is placed in the bladder. The urine is collected and the bladder then filled with a solution containing neomycin and "elase" (a combination of fibrinolysin and desoxyribonuclease). After an hour the bladder is emptied and washed out with several litres of sterile water to remove all the neomycin. The catheter is now lying in a sterile bladder and if the urine that emerges from the catheter is infected then the organisms have come from the upper urinary tract. On the other hand if the urine is sterile then the organisms that were present before the bladder was washed out were confined to the lower urinary tract.

Examination of the urine for inflammation

The presence of an area of inflammation contiguous with the renal tract may be made manifest by the release of leucocytes into the urine. The methods used to determine the white cell content of the urine accurately are described on p. 43. It is necessary to mention that some reactionary routine laboratories refuse to culture a urine unless it contains more than a normal number of white cells. Conversely some clinicians are apt to ignore a positive urine culture if the number of white cells in the urine is not raised. Both practices are to be deplored. It is well established that the urine may be heavily infected without its content of white cells being raised, particularly in patients with chronic pyelonephritis and symptomless bacteruria. In addition it cannot be stressed too often that the presence of an excess number of white cells in the urine is only evidence of inflammation. It does not follow automatically that this inflammation is due to infection with pyogenic organisms. "Sterile" pyuria classically occurs in renal tuberculosis when it is strictly inaccurate to say that the urine is sterile. It also occurs in many other conditions including phenacetin nephropathy, acute glomerular nephritis and renal stones. Of course sterile pyuria can also occur following an active renal infection with pyogenic organisms, for instance during recovery from an attack of acute pyelonephritis treated with antibiotics.

Sometimes the presence of an active inflammatory focus in the renal tract is *not* accompanied by an excess number of white cells in the urine. If, nevertheless, it is suspected that such a focus exists, its presence may be revealed by giving the patient 40 mg of prednisolone phosphate intravenously, when there may be a prompt increase in the number of white cells in the urine. This test is particularly useful in investigating patients who have been given antibiotics for

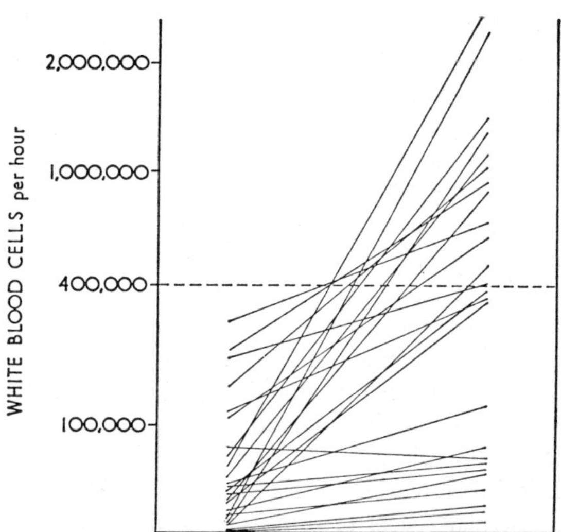

FIG. 23.2. White cell excretion rate before and after the administration of 40 mg prednisolone phosphate intravenously to 25 patients with radiological evidence of "chronic pyelonephritis", but in whom the urine was uninfected and the white cell content of the urine was normal. In about half of the patients there was a brisk rise in white cell excretion to a rate above 400,000/hr indicating that though these patients' urine was normal before the prenisone injection an active focus of inflammation was still present adjoining the lumen of the renal tract. (Little, 1965, *J. clin. Path.*)

an alleged attack of acute pyelonephritis before the urine has been examined. Later when the patient feels better and the urine is sterile, and contains a normal number of white cells the diagnosis of a recent urinary infection may be difficult to uphold. The prednisolone test is also useful in patients with chronic renal infections who appear to be in an inactive stage (Fig. 23.2). It is not known how prenisolone produces this effect. If the white cell excretion rate is raised without giving prednisolone there is clearly little point in doing a prednisolone test.

ACUTE PYELITIS, ACUTE PYELONEPHRITIS AND ACUTE NECROTISING PAPILLITIS

Pathology

The appearances of the kidneys depend largely on whether any underlying renal deformity was present before the onset of the acute infection. The following descriptions only refer to changes produced by infection. They are divided into three groups depending on their severity: (1) acute pyelitis; (2) acute pyelonephritis; and (3) acute necrotising papillitis.

ACUTE PYELITIS. This is the term which pathologists give to an acute infection confined to the lining membrane of the renal pelvis, that is an infection which does not involve the renal parenchyma. At *post-mortem* such a limited distribution is found extremely rarely; it does not follow that it is equally infrequent in life. It is usually bilateral.

ACUTE PYELONEPHRITIS. This is nearly always bilateral. Macroscopically the kidneys are usually enlarged and occasionally small abscesses show through the capsule. The surface may be discoloured by areas of pallor and congestion. On section, greyish wedge-shaped areas can be seen extending upwards from the pyramids into the cortex; there are also yellow streaks radiating from the medulla. The pelvis is red and covered with pus.

The pelvis microscopically is covered with an inflammatory exudate which penetrates within the pelvic wall; sometimes there are also areas of superficial necrosis. The renal parenchymatous lesions are more numerous in the pyramids and medulla. The tubules contain and are surrounded by leucocytes, though occasionally these are confined to the interstitial tissues. There are similar collections of neutrophils in the interstitial tissues of the cortex, in addition, some glomeruli become selectively invested by a thick concentration of acute inflammatory cells. In a few, the capsule is breached and leucocytes can be seen invading the glomerular space. In some sites an inflammatory destruction of tubules may cause a crowding together of glomeruli which are then separated only by granulation tissue. A varying number of small abscesses may be disseminated throughout the renal parenchyma and, before the use of antibiotics, bacteria were also found in large numbers.

The vascular lesions are of particular importance, and in this connection it should be recalled that the renal pelvis extends as far upwards as the corticomedullary junction. It is not surprising, therefore, to find that sometimes the acute inflammatory process involves some of the larger arteries and veins. Dense infiltrations with leucocytes may be localised in the arterial wall, leading to destruction of the muscle and elastic tissues; occasionally this process leads to occlusion of the lumen by a thrombus, and complete infarction of wedge-shaped areas of cortex. Other large arteries may show moderate degrees of narrowing of the arterial lumen by endarteritis. In the areas of acute inflammation thrombosis of arterioles is relatively frequent.

ACUTE NECROTISING PAPILLITIS. This consists of an acute pyelonephritis of such severity that there is focal suppurative necrosis of one or more renal pyramids. The process begins at the apices of the pyramids and extends upwards into the medulla, but does not involve the cortex. Microscopically there is a dense purulent exudate throughout the affected area which is sharply demarcated from the viable parenchyma.

Clinical Features

The most important paradox to remember is that many patients with acute pyelonephritis have severe constitutional symptoms such as fever and rigors and feel extremely ill without having any localising symptoms or signs either in the loins, abdomen or bladder, i.e. they do not have loin pain, abdominal tenderness, frequency or dysuria. Others do have tender loins and flanks, and have lower urinary symptoms. Frequently there is much nausea and vomiting particularly in pregnancy. The urine always contains a large number of white cells and bacteria, and sometimes there is gross macroscopical haematuria; proteinuria is rarely greater than +. The clinical features give no clue to the identity of the infecting organism.

As it is clinically difficult, particularly at the onset, to differentiate between acute pyelitis and pyelonephritis, and as a substantial number of clinically mild cases may show inflammatory lesions in the cortex (renal biopsy), it is best to consider that all upper urinary infections involve the renal parenchyma, i.e. that all such infections are due to acute pyelonephritis.

The extent of the parenchymatous involvement depends mainly on the presence of urinary tract obstruction or reflux; the greater the obstruction or reflux the more extensive the infection. Obstructions are often found in patients of either sex who have recurrent infection; they underlie most upper urinary infections that occur in men, whereas women mostly have recurrent infections without any abnormality of the urinary tract.

Renal function in upper urinary infections may be unaffected, or it may be so severely impaired that the patient dies from acute renal failure. Characteristically renal function returns to its previous level as the infection subsides. The magnitude of this transient impairment is probably of some value in assessing the amount of parenchyma that has been invaded in the acute inflammatory process. Proper appraisal may be difficult if some degree of renal failure preceded the infection; at such times renal function should be re-examined a few weeks after the infection has been controlled.

ACUTE NECROTISING PAPILLITIS. This occurs most often in elderly diabetics, most of whom have suffered from previous upper urinary infections. In addition to the usual features of a severe acute upper urinary infection, haematuria occurs frequently and, if the lesion is bilateral, there is a sudden reduction in urine flow, and the onset of acute renal failure. Sometimes pieces of necrosed papillae appear in the urine. If the patient recovers, the loss of part of one or more papillae may be defined in an I.V.P. or a retrograde pyelogram.

Aseptic necrosis of papillae occurs in phenacetin nephropathy (p. 322) and sickle cell anaemia. There have also been reports of patients on continuous sulphonamide therapy for chronic urinary infection who have developed renal colic or ureteric obstruction due to the necrosis of a papilla without any evidence of an associated acute infection.

Relationship between clinical and structural features

Renal biopsy studies have shown that in acute pyelonephritis there is a striking lack of correlation between the severity of the constitutional symptoms and impairment of renal function on the one hand, and histological appearances on the other. The main reason for this discrepancy is probably the focal nature of the disease.

The most important observation is that severe acute pyelonephritic lesions of the cortex, with inflammatory cell replacement of the tubules, can be obtained from patients who, clinically, have suffered only from a mild "pyelitis". In one series, such lesions were found in one quarter of a group of patients with clinical signs and symptoms of an acute upper urinary infection. As autopsy findings have shown that pyelonephritic lesions in general are focal, and more advanced in the medulla, these biopsy findings suggest that nearly all patients with an upper urinary infection have destructive lesions of the cortex and medulla.

It is interesting to note that it is unusual for these acute destructive lesions to be associated with any recognisable change in the intravenous pyelogram at the time of the infection. The abnormalities which may occur include a diminished density of the radio-opaque medium on the most affected side, localised renal swelling, and compression and elongation of one calyx. The difference in density is not a helpful finding, while the other two abnormalities are rare.

Sequelae of acute pyelonephritis

If the pyelogram is repeated a few months to a few years later, changes will be evident, the nature of which will depend on the patient's age. In children, serial pyelograms often reveal the development of gross cortical scarring with clubbing or distortion of one or more calyces. In adults, cortical scarring and clubbing and distortion of calyces rarely develop, but the kidneys often show a reduction in their lengths of 0·6 to 6·0 cm, which confirms the renal biopsy findings that clinical acute pyelonephritis in adults is usually associated with some destruction of the parenchyma. The radiological appearances of cortical scarring with distortion and clubbing of calyces are referred to as those of "chronic pyelonephritis". They may be found for the first time in children or adults who have never suffered from an overt attack of acute pyelonephritis. It must be stressed that as the radiological changes of "chronic pyelonephritis" rarely develop after childhood, they are nearly always evidence of childhood renal infection.

It is not clear why destruction of the renal parenchyma in children should be associated with such marked overall structural changes while in adults the overall effect is radiologically so much less pronounced. There is no doubt that ureteric reflux, which is nearly always present in those children who develop gross scarring, is somehow an important factor. Ureteric reflux is demonstrated by means of a technique known as a micturating cystogram. A radio-opaque liquid is placed into the bladder. Reflux is present if the liquid ascends either or both ureters during micturition. *It has been demonstrated that, in infants, gross reflux which distends the calcyces can produce focal scarring and progressive renal damage, in the absence of infection.* This may be due to the refluxed urine being pushed into the parenchyma of the kidney, a phenomenon which has been observed to occur particularly into the upper poles of children (intrarenal reflux). Gross reflux is rare in adults, but is present in 25 per cent of all infants with reflux. It is probable that another important adverse effect of reflux of any severity is that it prevents the child from emptying his bladder properly and that therefore heavily infected urine is repeatedly being flushed up the ureters towards the kidneys. In addition the presence of incomplete evacuation of the urine makes it very difficult to treat an infection. There is also some evidence that acute pyelonephritis is more destructive the younger the patient, regardless of ureteric reflux. And it is also probable that the distortion produced by those parts which have been destroyed may be accentuated by the continued growth of those parts which have escaped destruction.

Prognosis

An acute infection of the renal parenchyma may cause death, either if it is sufficiently extensive, or if it is superimposed upon pre-existing chronic renal disease.

Once the acute infection has been controlled, the risk of further attacks and the development of clubbing and scarring depends a great deal on whether there is permanent deformity of the renal tract such as bladder diverticulum, prostatic hypertrophy, or ureteric reflux. Usually such deformities precede infections, but the changes produced in the renal parenchyma and pelvis by sufficiently severe or recurrent infections may themselves perpetuate the tendency to infection. Even when the renal tract is radiologically normal the rate of recurrent bacteruria following an attack of acute pyelonephritis is 50 per cent at six months, and 80 per cent at 18 months.

It is essential to remember that a patient suffering from advanced renal failure secondary to an acute renal infection may rapidly recover once the infection is controlled; it is unwise, therefore, to give a prognosis during the acute phase of the infection.

Differential diagnosis

Fever, rigors, tenderness and pain in one or both loins suggest, and the finding of pus and organisms in the urine tend to confirm, the diagnosis. The higher the fever and the greater the loin tenderness the more likely is the urinary infection to be in the kidneys, but otherwise there is remarkably little correlation between the patient's symptoms and the site of the infection (see Table 23.1). A recent impairment in renal function and the presence of an abnormal IVP also increase the likelihood of the infection being in the kidney. Occasionally when local symptoms and signs are absent, the diagnosis only becomes apparent

TABLE 23.1. *Symptoms in Relation to the Site of the Infection*
(Fairley Test)

		Localisation of infection	
		Upper urinary tract	Lower urinary tract
Symptomatic patients	43	21 (49%)	22 (51%)
Frequency	32	18 (56%)	14 (44%)
Dysuria	35	18 (51%)	17 (49%)
Loin pain	31	15 (48%)	16 (52%)
Temp. < 38° C	19	13 (68%)	6 (32%)
Haematuria	6	3 (50%)	3 (50%)

after a routine examination and culture of the urine. The finding of a high serum antibody titre to the bacteria present in the urine is presumptive evidence that the organisms have invaded the parenchyma. *An acute urinary infection should always be kept in mind when the patient is known to suffer from some other chronic parenchymal renal disease.*

INVESTIGATION OF UNDERLYING URINARY TRACT ABNORMALITY. The structural integrity of the kidneys and of the urinary tract should be investigated following (1) any upper urinary infection occurring in a boy or a man, (2) a second infection in a woman, (3) a first infection in a woman when it is accompanied by renal colic, haematuria, impaired renal function, or followed by persistent proteinuria or large numbers of white cells in the urine. An intravenous pyelogram and a micturating cystogram are usually sufficient, though occasionally arteriograms and even laparotomy may be needed.

Treatment

PROPHYLACTIC. If organisms are introduced experimentally into a normal bladder which can empty completely, the bacteria are evacuated, persistent bacteruria does not develop and acute pyelonephritis is most unlikely to occur. On the other hand, if bacteria gain access to the bladder of any individual who suffers from some deformity of the renal tract including lesions which cause some residual urine to be present after voiding, the chances of developing persistent bacteruria and an overt symptomatic urinary infection thereafter are very great. Bacteria may gain access to the bladder during catheterisation and urological investigations. The incidence of bacteruria following these manoeuvres can be reduced by introduction into the bladder of an antiseptic or antibiotic at the end of the procedure. It is also wise to culture the urine of patients with known abnormalities of the renal tract from time to time. If the urine is infected it should be sterilised by a short course of antibiotic, routine cultures being continued thereafter. Another way in which organisms commonly enter a woman's bladder for the first time is at the beginning of active sexual life. At this time acute pyelonephritis occurs relatively frequently even in those who have a normal renal tract. There is much to be said for giving all virgins 50 mg of nitrofurantoin to take at night for the first two or three weeks after they cease to be virgins.

Acute pyelonephritis occurs predominantly in those individuals who have asymptomatic bacteruria. In schoolgirls the incidence of asymptomatic bacteruria is about 1 to 4 per cent. Immediately after puberty it rises to about 10 per cent: it then falls to about 5 per cent until the age of 60 to 70 when it rises again to 20–30 per cent in the elderly. The rise after puberty is due to sexual activity, for the incidence among nuns is the same as in schoolgirls before puberty. The incidence of acute pyelonephritis in women with asymptomatic bacteruria varies from group to group. For instance, it is highest in pregnant women in whom 25–30 per cent of those with asymptomatic bacteruria develop acute pyelonephritis. It is much less in women who are not pregnant (but the actual incidence is not known). There is no doubt that the detection of those pregnant women who have asymptomatic bacteruria and the sterilising of their urine with antibiotics can greatly reduce the incidence of acute pyelonephritis in pregnancy (p. 352). There is a growing feeling that a similar search for and treatment of asymptomatic bacteruria should be undertaken in infants and children. Unfortunately by the age of five most of the serious renal damage has already taken place. And to routinely monitor the urine of all children before the age of five is administratively impossible. Bacteruria in infants (using suprapubic technique) is so rare that, in the absence of compelling reasons, there seems little point in culturing the urine routinely. Routine screening of school children however does enable those with lesions to be identified and treated. They tend to be from poor homes and are of small stature.

CONTROL OF THE ACUTE INFECTION. Patients used to recover from acute upper urinary infections before antibiotics were available. It is probably true, therefore, that many infections would recover if treatment were limited to the administration of large quantities of water. In practice it is best to give an antibiotic in all upper urinary infections, for if the inflammatory process has penetrated into the renal parenchyma it is reasonable to suppose that quick control of the infection will lessen the residual damage.

Sulphonamides are usually administered without first identifying the organism responsible for the infection. The repeated success of this blind manoeuvre ensures its continuity, but there is no doubt that it is more satisfactory to culture the urine and determine the sensitivity of the organism. When there are recurrent infections it is imperative that this be done. Antibiotics are excreted in the urine at varying rates, but in all instances their urinary concentration is greater than their simultaneous concentration in body fluids. Contrary to original expectations it is only necessary to give sufficient antibiotics to obtain an effective urinary antibacterial level. In an acute upper urinary infection the administration of antibiotics should be continued for at least three weeks, and certainly *for some days after all trace of tenderness in the loins has disappeared.*

When there has been evidence of extensive parenchymal invasion, that is, if renal function has been depressed by the infection, it is advisable to continue treatment for two to three months.

The choice of antibiotic is determined by the sensitivity of the infecting organism, but if the diagnosis is clear cut it is unnecessary to wait 24 hours for the results of urine culture; treatment is started with either sulphadimidine (3 g followed by 1 g 6-hourly) or trimethoprim sulphamethoxazole (2 tablets twice a day), immediately after some urine has been obtained for culture. In this way no time will have been lost, whatever the result of culture. Other antibiotics are listed in the Table opposite. It is useful to remember that many antibiotics may themselves cause renal damage. A few, such as sulphamerazine, and bacitracin do this so frequently that they should be avoided.

During a course of treatment the urine should be cultured at least once to make certain that the antibiotic is effective. When the course of antibiotic is finished the urine should be cultured approximately 7, 14 and 30 days later and then at monthly intervals. The treatment and prevention of further attacks is discussed below.

PRECAUTIONS IN PATIENTS WITH RENAL FAILURE. Most drugs are excreted in large amounts in the urine so that their plasma and urine concentrations are closely related to the state of renal function. When renal function is impaired the plasma level of such drugs may rise to toxic levels (e.g. streptomycin and nitrofurantoin) while conversely their concentration in the urine may fall to such low levels that the concentration is insufficient to sterilise the urine, even if the organism is sensitive. Cephalexin, trimethoprim/sulphamethoxazole, penicillin and nalidixic acid are the safest drugs to use in the presence of severe renal impairment.

It is imperative that, with the exception of doxycycline, all other forms of tetracycline should be recognised to be highly poisonous for patients with renal failure. They cause a brisk rise in blood urea, with vomiting and a rapid deterioration of renal function.

PREVENTION OF FURTHER ATTACKS. The prevention of recurrence is sometimes a surgical procedure, with the repair or removal of a structural deformity or ureteric reflux. Otherwise the prevention of further attacks depends on keeping the urine sterile. This can be done in one of three ways. The first consists of giving a short course of an appropriate antibiotic in normal doses, each time the urine is found to be infected, *or* symptoms recur. In order that treatment should be prompt the patient keeps a supply of one of the wide spectrum oral antibiotics at home. Urine cultures are performed at regular intervals. Alternatively urinary sterility can be maintained by giving long courses of a simple urinary antibiotic in small doses. The antibiotic is given once in the 24 hours and is best taken at night on retiring. During the night the concentration of the urine is at its highest so that the concentration of the antibiotic is also at its highest, this urine remains in the bladder for some considerable time, and the bladder at this time is therefore in an advantageous position to repel any bacterial invasion introduced during sexual intercourse. Sulpha-

Antibiotic	Dose	Methods of administration	Comment
Trimethoprim/Sulpha-methoxazole (Septrin, Bactrim)	2 tab. b.d.	Oral.	Wide range. Few side effects. Do not use in first month of life.
Sulphadimidine (Sulphamezathine)	3 g loading dose 1 g 6-hourly	Oral administration—intramuscular and intravenous preparations available.	Particularly useful in acute infections. Emphasise need to drink much fluid.
Penicillin G	800,000 units 6-hourly.	Oral or intramuscular.	Wide range at this dosage. Toxicity minimal except for sensitivity. Useful in renal failure.
Nitrofurantoin (Furadantin)	100 mg 8-hourly. 50 mg daily for mainten-ance.	Oral—after meals preferably—intravenous preparations available.	Wide spectrum—particularly useful against *B. proteus* infections. Never use in chronic renal failure.
Ampicillin (Penbritin)	500 mg 8-hourly.	Oral and intramuscular.	Wide spectrum—frequent sensitivity in patients with renal failure.
Tetracycline	0·25 g 6-hourly.	Oral, intramuscular and intravenous.	Wide spectrum. Excellent for *Proteus morgani*. DO NOT USE IN RENAL FAILURE.
Doxycycline (Vibramycin)	100 mg o.d.	Oral.	Spectrum same as tetracycline. Can be used in renal failure.
Nalidixic acid (Negram)	1 g 6-hourly.	Oral.	Gram − ve, *B. proteus* particularly. Can be used in advanced renal failure.
Cephaloridine (Ceporin)	1 g b.d.	Intramuscular and intravenous.	Wide spectrum—can be used in advanced renal failure; nephrotoxic with very large plasma concentrations, particularly in association with frusemide administration.
Cephalexin (Ceporex)	500 mg t.d.s.	Oral.	Wide spectrum. Excellent in chronic renal failure. Not nephrotoxic.
Streptomycin	1 g. b.d. for 3 days or 1 g a day for 10 days.	Intramuscular. Best effect if urine is alkaline. Give sodium citrate 2 g 6-hourly.	Useful against organisms resistant to other anti-biotics, particularly recurrent infections. Best used as a short, heavy attack on the infection before beginning continuous therapy with some other drug. ADJUST DOSE TO G.F.R.
Kanamycin (Kantrex)	1 g per day.	Intramuscular and intravenous.	Same indications and complications as streptomycin.
Colistin methane sulphonate (Colomycin)	120 mg 8-hourly.	Intramuscular.	Particularly for *Pseudomonas pyocyaneus*. Ototoxic and nephrotoxic complications.
Gentamycin (Genticin)	1 mg/kg per day in 3 divided doses.	Intravenous or intramuscular.	Particularly useful against *Pseudomonas pyocyaneus* resistent to Colomycin. Ototoxicity marked.

dimidine 0·5 g, sulphamethizole 200 mg, nitrofurantoin 50 mg, cephalexin 125 mg and trimethoprim 20 mg/sulphamethoxazole 100 mg have each been found useful, particularly nitrofurantoin. Side effects on such small doses are most unusual.

Occasionally none of these methods prevents frequent reinfections of the urine but the patient does not develop overt clinical symptoms. This may happen if the patient has some residual urine which it is not possible to treat, or a renal stone. The administration of antibiotics presumably keeps the population of organisms below a critical number necessary to produce symptoms. In such a situation it is best to continue whichever treatment is being given and to watch and wait. If, on the other hand, frequent reinfections of the urine are associated with frequent attacks of overt and symptomatic attacks of urinary infection it may be necessary to give larger amounts of antibiotics and to use a different antibiotic each week to try and prevent the organisms becoming resistant. Nitrofurantoin 100–200 mg per day, 2 tablets trimethoprim sulphamethoxazole twice a day, cephalexin 500 mg three times a day, sulphamethizole 100 mg four times a day, doxycycline 250 mg once a day, nalidixic acid 2 g per day, benzyl-penicillin 500 mg four times daily and ampicillin 250 mg four times a day have been used in this way. Other drugs such as streptomycin, kanamycin and colistin, may be used in standard doses if infections occur in spite of this treatment.

CHRONIC PYELONEPHRITIS

Pathology

The diagnosis is based on the naked eye appearances. The microscopic appearances are relatively non-specific (see p. 299). The kidneys are small, coarsely and irregularly misshapen by scars and areas of hyperplasia of widely differing dimensions. The extent of the damage is often more pronounced on one side than on the other and is sometimes entirely unilateral. The cut surfaces show dilatation of some calyces with gross reduction of the thickness of the overlying parenchyma while other calyces are normal and surrounded by hypertrophied parenchyma. Fibrous scars extending from the pelvis to the capsule can also be seen.

The microscopic appearances consist of patches of intense infiltration with lymphocytes and plasma cells; these areas are distributed in a haphazard manner, but concentrated more in the medulla than in the cortex. The tubules in these sites are either small and atrophic, or dilated with flattened epithelium and contain collections of a homogeneous eosin staining material ("thyroid areas"). The glomeruli resist the inflammatory invasion better than the tubules; some may appear almost unchanged while others have normal tufts, though they are surrounded by a thick collar of fibrous tissue (Fig. 23.3); the remainder, however, show varying degrees of change in the tufts, including fibrosis and atrophy.

Sometimes the changes of acute pyelonephritis are found interspersed and superimposed upon those of chronic pyelonephritis.

The scarring is principally due to wedge-shaped areas of inflammation, but there may also be similar shaped areas of ischaemic infarction; often the two are histologically inseparable. The extent of the vascular changes is very variable, but in those patients who have suffered from severe hypertension, advanced

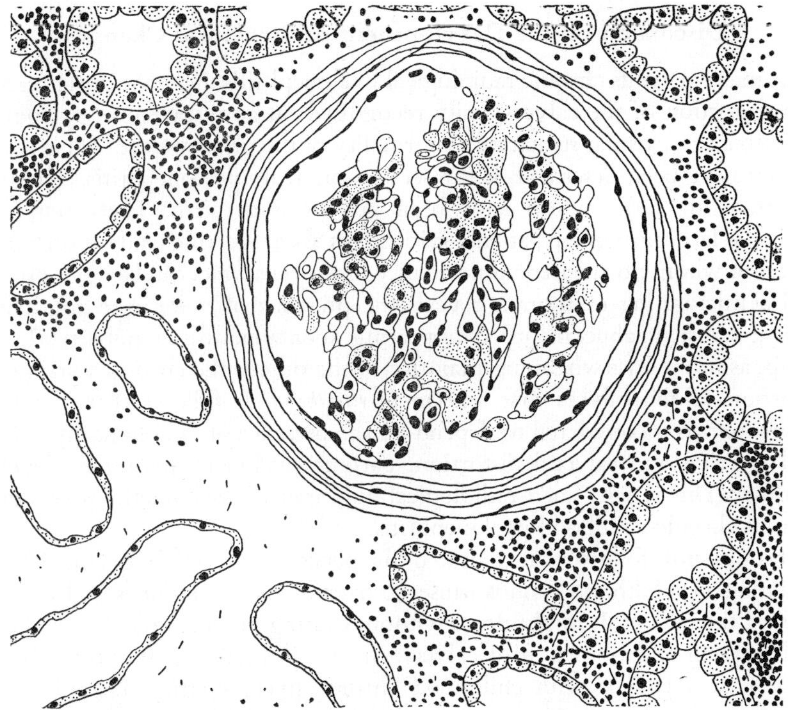

FIG. 23.3. Chronic pyelonephritis. Schema illustrating the following changes: a fibrous scar, atrophic tubules, chronic inflammatory cells, and one glomerulus which is surrounded by a thick halo of fibrous tissue but whose tuft is intact. The relatively normal tubules are separated by much intertubular material.

changes are always seen, both in the larger arteries and in the arterioles. The arcuate, interlobar and intralobular arteries show gross thickening of focal areas of the external elastic lamina with fibrous replacement of varying amounts of the arterial walls, including the elastic and muscle coats; they may also show extensive fibrocellular proliferation of the intima. These changes produce extreme narrowing of the lumen, though complete occlusion is rare. The arterioles show the changes associated with either malignant or non-malignant hypertension. Whenever there are malignant hypertensive changes there are also widespread and severe changes in the larger arteries.

Radiological Appearance

An intravenous pyelogram demonstrates the lesions which have been described above. Focal clubbing of calyces with thinning of the overlying parenchyma and asymmetry between the two kidneys. Usually some calyces are normal and they are covered by a particularly thick layer of hypertrophied parenchyma.

Discussion on the Development of Structural Changes

In many patients chronic radiological pyelonephritis, i.e. gross focal scarring with distortion of the calyces easily recognised on an intravenous pyelogram, is due to a pre-existing structural abnormality of the urinary tract. These abnormalities have been described in the section on acute pyelonephritis. The most important are those which have been present since birth. There remains a relatively large group of patients with gross focal scarring and distortion of calyces in whom no apparent abnormality of the renal tract can be demonstrated until a micturating cystogram reveals the presence of ureteric reflux. This is often a transient abnormality disappearing spontaneously at puberty. In this group, as in the overwhelming majority of the others, the cortical scarring and distortion of the calyces first *develop in childhood*. It follows that if chronic pyelonephritis is considered to depend on the presence of radiologically evident focal scarring and calyceal distortion, chronic pyelonephritis rarely develops in adults. This is why such radiological appearances are sometimes known as those of chronic childhood pyelonephritis.

It does not follow that repeated or persistent infection of the kidneys beginning in adulthood cannot cause destruction of the kidneys and eventual death of the patient. It might do so without causing gross radiologically evident focal scarring and distortion of calyces. Such a possibility is supported by the fact that if a patient with childhood chronic pyelonephritis, i.e. with gross scarring and calyceal distortion, survives into adulthood the radiological abnormalities will show little further change even though the patient may eventually die of chronic renal failure. Presumably continuing destruction of the kidneys by infection in adulthood does not cause further areas of focal scarring sufficiently extensive to be apparent radiologically. The suggestion that infection of the kidneys in an adult might cause destruction without gross scarring and calyceal distortion is also supported by the finding that acute pyelonephritis in adults is often followed by a reduction in the size of the kidneys, but as has been mentioned above cortical scarring and distortion of calyces rarely occurs.

If it is accepted that renal destruction by infection in adults can occur without the characteristic radiological appearances of "chronic pyelonephritis" it is clear that the diagnosis of chronic renal infection in adults is difficult. Renal biopsies are only of limited help while abnormalities in urine cultures and white cell excretion rates from bladder urine do not indicate the site responsible for the abnormality. The use of the Fairley bladder wash out technique (p. 304) to localise the site of infection is of immense help in differentiating such cases. The diagnosis is just as difficult at autopsy for it is well established that even in patients with the classical focal scarring and distortion of calyces who have died of chronic renal failure the kidneys may contain no organisms. In the *absence* of the characteristic macroscopic scarring and calyceal changes *and* organisms, the evidence on which a diagnosis of chronic renal infection can be made is limited to a subjective interpretation of the microscopical appearances.

The absence of organisms at *post-mortem* even in kidneys which have indubitably been the site of severe focal infection in the past, and in which the destruction has continued thereafter in a less focal way, is difficult to explain. In animal experiments there is some suggestion that bacterial antigens may remain in the kidneys after the death of the bacteria and cause a continuing inflammatory reaction in the absence of live organisms. It has been claimed that in some patients with sterile urines who have died of renal failure of unknown cause it has been possible to identify the presence of antigenic bacterial remnants in the renal parenchyma with an immunofluorescent technique. It is not clear however what significance to place on this finding for it is very possible that bacteria may become lodged in pre-existing scars. There is also some evidence that though conventional methods of bacterial culture may fail to reveal bacteria, other methods will reveal bacterial variants such as protoplasts. These are conventional organisms without their capsules. In this state they can only exist in hypertonic media. As the renal medulla is the only persistently hypertonic area in the body and as it is also particularly susceptible to infection it is possible that some of the continuing destruction of the kidneys in patients with "sterile" urine is due to infection with protoplasts.

Antikidney antibodies cannot be found in chronic pyelonephritis either circulating or deposited in the kidney. It does not appear therefore that the process of destruction is related to that involved in the immunological diseases of the kidney.

Clinical Features

Loin pain with or without febrile episodes is easily the commonest symptom with either unilateral or bilateral chronic pyelonephritis. Usually these attacks have been present for many years, often unaccompanied by any lower urinary symptoms. It is customary for the loin pain to have been ignored first by the patient and then by her doctor. A few patients first present with either hypertension, or with lower urinary symptoms such as frequency and dysuria with no upper urinary symptoms. Some patients are asymptomatic. Very rarely the presentation is one of asymptomatic proteinuria. Occasionally there is a history of acute pyelonephritis. It is very rare to obtain, from an adult, a history of urinary infection in childhood. Many patients, however, will admit to intermittent spells of tiredness, headache and loss of appetite in recent years.

Characteristically, the urine is infected (i.e. there are more than 100,000 organisms/ml of urine), and contains an excess number of white cells (i.e. more than 10 mm³ or more than 400,000/hr). In addition proteinuria is usually present though it is seldom greater than 5 g/24 hours. Some patients with active upper urinary tract infection have high antibody titres to the infecting organism. The absence of this abnormality does not exclude a diagnosis of chronic renal infection. When a diagnosis of chronic pyelonephritis has been made on radiological evidence, the absence of urinary abnormalities does not necessarily mean that the inflammatory process is quiescent. An injection of prednisolone phosphate intravenously may provoke a sudden rise in white cell excretion (p. 305) and demonstrate that a site active of inflammation does exist.

It must be stressed that the radiological appearances of chronic childhood pyelonephritis are no indication that the patient is suffering from an active renal infection even if the urine is infected and there is pyuria. The only way a diagnosis of renal infection can be made is to establish that organisms are descending the ureters from one or both kidneys. There are many patients with infections localised to the upper urinary tract who have normal intravenous pyelograms. Conversely there are others with the appearances of radiological pyelonephritis whose urinary infection is confined to the bladder.

It has been claimed that there is another group with normal radiological appearances and "renal" symptoms, who have progressive damage to the kidneys with deterioration of renal function but whose main abnormality is a sterile pyuria. It is alleged that if such patients are carefully followed up they will sometimes be found to have a small number of organisms in a suprapubic aspiration of urine, and that treatment with antibiotics brings the white cell content of the urine to normal.

In keeping with the focal nature of the chronic childhood pyelonephritis it is characteristic that there is often a marked difference in renal function between the two kidneys. This information can often be inferred from the inequality in renal size but is most accurately obtained with ureteric catheters. These are used mainly when a unilateral nephrectomy is being contemplated, particularly if there is hypertension. The investigation allows an assessment to be made of the likelihood of the remaining kidney being able to sustain life and may also give some indication whether the hypertension is due to a superimposed renal ischaemia and therefore whether unilateral nephrectomy for unilateral chronic pyelonephritis will reduce the blood pressure. In both pyelonephritis and ischaemia the ability to concentrate and the creatinine clearance will be reduced. In the predominently ischaemic kidney, however, the urinary sodium concentration will be lower and the creatinine concentration higher than on the opposite side whereas in the predominently pyelonephritic kidney the urinary sodium concentration will be the same or higher and the creatinine concentration lower than on the other side.

In general, renal functional impairment follows the same pattern as that described in the section on chronic renal failure. The presence of an active urinary infection, however, significantly reduces the ability to concentrate more than the glomerular filtration rate. But with antibiotic treatment this discrepancy disappears and it becomes apparent that persistent impairment in renal function is associated with parallel changes in glomerular filtration and in the ability to concentrate. The ability to acidify usually remains normal though occasionally a patient will present with a low plasma pH and plasma bicarbonate and a raised plasma chloride due to an inability to acidify.

In some patients with prolonged severe active chronic pyelonephritis there may be a considerable increase in the plasma concentration of gamma globulins together with a high erythrocyte sedimentation rate. A finding such as this in a patient in whom the presence of chronic pyelonephritis is not known may cause some confusion. The renal impairment and abnormal electrophoretic pattern may suggest a diagnosis of myelomatosis. After treatment with antibiotics the erythrocyte sedimentation rate and the plasma protein pattern gradually return to normal.

Relationship between clinical and structural features

There is little correlation between the amount of renal parenchyma involved, as gauged by radiology, and renal function. It is possible to find patients with chronic childhood pyelonephritis, who have had a nephrectomy on one side and a hemiphrectomy on the other with a normal blood urea, and a plasma creatinine below 1·2 mg/100 ml. In contrast renal function may deteriorate without any further measurable change in the radiological appearances.

Differential Diagnosis

The main point of differentiation between chronic childhood pyelonephritis and nearly all other renal diseases is its focal nature and that it so often affects one kidney more than the other. It is also useful to remember that chronic childhood pyelonephritis is the most common cause of predominantly unilateral renal disease.

When there are radiological changes suggestive of chronic childhood pyelonephritis the main problems of differentiation are phenacetin nephropathy, back pressure atrophy and ischaemic scars. The radiological appearances of phenacetin nephropathy (p. 322) are often sufficiently characteristic to suggest the correct diagnosis. The diagnosis can be confirmed by asking the relevant questions. Back pressure atrophy often follows a short period of ureteric obstruction, the radiological appearances remaining abnormal thereafter. Back pressure atrophy is characterised by a generalised and uniform loss of renal substance which is equal throughout the kidney, this change is nearly always associated with a uniform loss of papillae, and often with a dilatation of the renal pelvis and calyces. Radiologically focal ischaemic scarring is differentiated from pyelonephritic scarring by the fact that ischaemia does not distort the calyces.

Course and Prognosis

It is characteristic of the progress of chronic childhood pyelonephritis that renal function may either remain unchanged for 10–20 years, or suddenly become so impaired (due to an acute fulminating, untreated infection) that the patient dies within a few days. It is equally characteristic that, although an almost terminal state of renal failure may be provoked by an acute infection, an unexpected recovery may take place. For these reasons it is impossible to gauge the prognosis in an individual case until there is persistent and advanced renal failure, or malignant hypertension has developed.

The main cause of a gradual deterioration in renal function in chronic childhood pyelonephritis is either a surreptitious ingestion of phenacetin or bilateral severe reflux. Recurrent asymptomatic bacteruria rarely seems to affect renal function. And it is even difficult to detect a persistent impairment of renal function in adults with chronic pyelonephritis who have had several recent symptomatic upper urinary infections. It has been claimed that a very small number of patients gradually deteriorate without organisms appearing in their urine, or in whom organisms are found only intermittently and usually in small numbers, though there may be persistent sterile pyuria. Such patients may or may not have the characteristic radiological appearances of chronic childhood pyelonephritis. About half the patients with chronic pyelonephritis have a normal blood pressure, but it is nevertheless the renal disease which most frequently gives rise to malignant hypertension. Established hypertension is often aggravated by a clinically obvious flare-up of infection.

Chronic pyelonephritis is an uncommon cause of death in adults. This is best gauged by the proportion of patients with chronic pyelonephritis who are placed onto maintenance haemodialysis. It appears to be less than 5 per cent of adult females, and less than 2 per cent of all patients coming to dialysis.

Unilateral Chronic Pyelonephritis and Hypertension

It is difficult to predict which patients will have a fall in blood pressure following a unilateral nephrectomy. The combination of pyelonephritis and ischaemia makes the interpretation of individual renal functional studies difficult, for each produces opposing functional changes. A few patients have had their blood pressure successfully lowered in spite of ureteric studies which suggested that the kidney which was removed was not ischaemic. Many of the successful operations have been in patients who had an acute and accelerated form of hypertension of short duration, including malignant hypertension. Operations on patients with unilateral renal disease and hypertension should not be performed until the functional integrity of the other kidney has been investigated.

If one kidney is small the other should be large. If the supposedly normal side is not bigger than normal then it is itself diseased.

Some authorities consider that before deciding to do a nephrectomy a renal biopsy should be obtained from both kidneys (with an interval between the two biopsies), and that the likelihood of lowering the blood pressure will be greater in those in whom the kidney to be removed shows no arteriolar changes, whereas they are present on the other side. This demonstrates that there is some arterial occlusion between the main renal artery and the arterioles.

Chronic Pyelonephritis and Vesico–ureteric Reflux

The severity of ureteric reflux can be graded into four categories. The reflux extends up to the brim of the pelvis (grade 1), above the brim of the pelvis (grade 2), to the renal pelvis without causing calyceal distension (grade 3), to the renal pelvis causing distension of the calyceal system (grade 4). Grade 4 may be associated with pain in the loins immediately before and during the initial act of micturition. Among adult patients with the radiological appearance of chronic pyelonephritis reflux occurs in approximately 35 per cent of those with unilateral pyelonephritis, and in about 50 per cent of those with bilateral pyelonephritis. The reflux is less severe than in infants with ureteric reflux. For instance, whereas grade 4 gross reflux occurs in 25 per cent of infants with reflux, it is seen in less than 5 per cent of adult patients with reflux. Grade 4 reflux is the only type of reflux than can cause focal and generalised parenchymal destruction without an associated infection. This gross form should therefore be treated surgically as soon as it is detected. Other forms of reflux influence urinary infections because they prevent the patient totally evacuating his urine during micturition. This may need treatment surgically, if antibiotics are unable to control the infection. On the other hand there are now several reports that reflux, particularly in children, has disappeared following the prolonged administration of antibiotics.

Chronic Urinary Infection and Renal Stones

There is no doubt that the presence of renal stones often causes urinary infections, but there is also some evidence that infection itself may cause stone formation. The main factor which is probably responsible is the urea splitting properties of some organisms such as *B. proteus*; ammonia is formed and the urine becomes, and remains, highly alkaline, which leads to the precipitation of calcium phosphate. This mechanism is exacerbated if there is increased calcium excretion due either to excessive calcium intake (milk) or prolonged rest in bed (e.g. poliomyelitis).

Treatment

If the disease has extensively involved one kidney and the other is sound it is usually wise to remove the diseased kidney, for, if the blood pressure is not

L§

raised preoperatively, the operation will prevent its rising; and, if it is already raised, the operation may cause it to return towards normal. Nevertheless, if the kidney is not causing any symptoms, the urine is uninfected and the blood pressure is normal, it may occasionally be justifiable to do nothing except keep the patient under observation.

In bilateral disease any surgically treatable cause of urinary tract deformity, such as renal stone and ureteric strictures, should be attended to. Postoperatively these patients should be treated in the same way as those in whom no primary deformity of the urinary tract is discoverable, or in whom such a deformity is inoperable. The treatment of ureteric reflux has been discussed earlier.

Once a diagnosis of chronic pyelonephritis has been made, the aim of treatment is to try and prevent the infection from smouldering or suddenly flaring up. The ways in which further infections may be prevented are outlined on p. 312. Continuous and prolonged attention should be maintained by the patient and her doctor to detect any minor change in general condition, and the urine should be examined frequently. If the patient experiences similar symptoms to those she has had with previous attacks or if there is fever, pains in the loins, dysuria or a sudden increase in white cell excretion, antibiotics should be started at once, whether or not the urine contains organisms. If the patient is intelligent she can be given some antibiotic to keep at home and to take at the first sign of a recurrence. If there are frequent recurrences they can sometimes be controlled by the administration of one small dose of a single antibiotic each night, e.g. 50 mg of furadantin or 125 mg cephalexin. If this fails it is best to give intermittent courses of antibiotics all the year round, either every few days, or for a week once a month. Very occasionally when there is residual urine it may be necessary to give large doses of antibiotics every day throughout the year. The urine must be cultured at regular intervals during treatment to check on the sensitivity of the organism. During pregnancy, a woman known to suffer from chronic pyelonephritis should be given prophylactic antibiotics throughout.

The choice of antibiotic depends on the sensitivity of the organism and the patient's reaction to its administration.

Phenacetin Nephropathy

In 1967 the consumption of phenacetin in Great Britain was about 540,000 kg. Unfortunately, though the use of phenacetin in proprietary preparations is diminishing, it is still present in BP or BPC preparations such as Tab. Codeine co, and Tab. APC. More than four-fifths of the total phenacetin ingested is in the form of such preparations. Each of these tablets contains 250 mg of phenacetin. The prolonged ingestion of phenacetin causes papillary necrosis and death from chronic renal failure. The amount needed to produce radiological changes varies from 2 to 25 kg taken over two to more than 20 years (2 kg of phenacetin = Tab. Codeine co × 6 per day for four years).

There is no evidence that in man either aspirin or paracetomol cause papillary necrosis. Approximately 3,000,000 kg of aspirin were ingested in 1967 in Great Britain; 2,000,000 kg was in preparations that did not contain phenacetin. Nevertheless, there have been only two cases of papillary necrosis alleged to have been due to aspirin ingestion alone. Furthermore the arrest of further renal functional impairment which occurs upon ceasing to take phenacetin, still takes place if the patient switches to taking aspirin alone. These observations apply to man. Rats and rabbits are different. They appear particularly susceptible to the administration of aspirin and can be made to develop papillary necrosis with aspirin as well as with phenacetin. This difference in species susceptibility has thoroughly confused some authorities who, on the basis of the animal studies, claim that aspirin is as responsible as phenacetin in causing papillary necrosis in man. In the absence of these observations on animals, phenacetin would have been banned from all tablets which can casually be bought over the counter without a prescription. This restriction has been imposed in Sweden and Norway where the incidence of analgesic papillary necrosis is now declining. As phenacetin is a poor analgesic which proprietary firms have now removed from their products without loss of revenue it is incomprehensible why this potentially poisonous substance should continue to be available in BP and BPC preparations.

Pathology

The macroscopic appearances are the most characteristic and are due to the multiple loss of papillae. The macroscopic appearances are characteristic. Some papillae are green others are black and leathery with the tip slightly twisted away from its normal position. Other papillae are absent. The calyces are then clubbed but tend to be narrowed as they travel towards the pelvis. The overlying parenchyma is reduced in size but the gross asymmetrical distortions found in chronic childhood pyelonephritis do not occur. Microscopically the lesion consists of a chronic inflammation of the interstitial spaces which is particularly marked in the medulla and papillae. Tubules are eventually destroyed while the glomeruli tend to remain intact.

Clinical findings

Several groups of individuals are liable to take phenacetin in large amounts. The majority are women in whom the diagnosis is first made around the age of 50. The most understandable group is that which consists of persons who suffer from some chronic painful disease, such as rheumatoid arthritis, for which analgesics offer some relief. Another group consists of workers such as watch-makers who are liable to headaches. In some Swiss factories it used to be customary for the firm to distribute phenacetin free of charge to its workers. A third group are compulsive analgesic consumers. They have no pain or headache and they obtain no overwhelming pleasure from the ingestion of phenacetin. Their habit has usually started for some trivial reason and they can be induced to stop without much effort. Others are chronically neurotic, have an inadequate personality or suffer from reactive depression, often they are alcoholic. They tend to claim that the tablets are for their headache. The last group is a remarkable one and was first described from Sweden; it provided the first conclusive evidence of the toxicity of phenacetin. A whole village became addicted to phenacetin. The drug became a symbol of friendliness and sociability. When a few people gathered together they would offer each other a phenacetin tablet as a preliminary to conversation, while those who were invited out to dinner would take their hosts a packet of phenacetin.

The patient may first present for some other complaint when it is found that he has proteinuria, or he may appear with renal colic with haematuria, or chronic renal failure and hypertension. The renal colic is caused by the passage of necrosed papillae which can sometimes be recognised in the urine.

The diagnosis is made by asking the right questions. Apart from this the most characteristic findings are a sterile pyuria and pyelographic evidence of loss of papillae.

Radiological appearances

The main distinctions from chronic childhood pyelonephritis are (1) the disease is always bilateral, (2) and though it is focally distributed in that some papillae are more affected than others, there are no gross focal areas of renal destruction with accompanying hypertrophy of the remaining areas such as is seen in chronic childhood pyelonephritis. The characteristic appearance is one of bilaterally small kidneys with several abnormal calyces on both sides. These calyces are long and narrow and seem to stretch out towards the outer border of the kidney, in a slightly sigmoid fashion, known in France as "langue de chat". Patchy calcification often occurs, sometimes it lies on the surface of a devitalised papilla and thus appears as ring shadow. Occasionally another type of ring shadow is seen when contrast medium lies around a separated papilla. Sometimes a papilla may be only partially separated so that the contrast around it gives it an "egg in cup" appearance.

Functional and urinary changes

Phenacetin nephropathy causes severe impairment of the ability to concentrate long before there is any impairment in glomerular filtration rate, e.g. a maximum osmolality of 400 m.Osm/kg with a plasma creatinine of 1·0 mg/100 ml. Almost as often there is an impairment in the ability to acidify. There is also a tendency for there to be a sodium leak in that most patients with phenacetin nephropathy do not have hypertension; or may have had hypertension earlier which no longer needs treating as the disease progresses. They are therefore very susceptible to dehydration, vomiting and diarrhoea (see below). The urine often contains an increased number of white cells in the absence of infection though infection does occur from time to time.

Prognosis

The continued consumption of large amounts of phenacetin in a patient who has developed papillary necrosis leads to death. On the other hand, if the patient stops taking phenacetin, renal function nearly always stops deteriorating and often improves slightly. This makes the search for the disease particularly imperative. Surgical operations are dangerous for they may precipitate widespread necrosis of surviving papillae and a sudden deterioration in renal function. This is probably due to the routine dehydration, and the other multiple anaesthetic and surgical causes of renal ischaemia superimposed upon pre-existing damaged papillae. If surgery cannot be avoided it is best to use a local or spinal anaesthetic and to make certain that there is no dehydration by giving large amounts of intravenous saline before, during and after the operation.

Treatment

All cases are due to self-administration. Many patients will readily stop taking tablets containing phenacetin if they are told of the damage it causes. Patients who are in pain, however, must be advised that other analgesics are available; the censure implied by the term "analgesic abuse" to such patients is inappropriate and indefensible. If instead of taking phenacetin-containing tablets the patients are allowed to consume up to six tablets of aspirin or paracetomol per day for several years there is no further deterioration in renal function and sometimes there is some recovery.

BIBLIOGRAPHY

Pyelonephritis

ACQUATELLA, H., LITTLE, P. J., DE WARDENER, H. E., and COLEMAN, J. C. (1967). "The effect of urine osmolality and pH on the bactericidal activity of plasma." *Clin. Sci.*, **33**, 471.

ANDRIOLE, V. T. (1966). "Acceleration of the inflammatory response of the renal medulla by water diuresis." *J. clin. Invest.*, **45**, 847.

ANDRIOLE, V. T., and EPSTEIN, F. H. (1965). "Prevention of pyelonephritis by water diuresis: Evidence for the role of medullary hypertonicity in promoting renal infection." *J. clin. Invest.*, **44**, 73.

ANGELL, M. E., RELMAN, A. S., and ROBBINS, S. L. (1968). "Active chronic pyelonephritis without evidence of bacterial infection." *New Eng. J. Med.*, **278**, 1303.

AOKI, S., IMAMURA, S., AOKI, M., and MCCABE, W. R. (1969). " 'Abacterial' and bacterial pyelonephritis. Immunofluorescent localization of bacterial antigen." *New Eng. J. Med.*, **281**, 1375.

BAILEY, R. R., GOWER, P. E., ROBERTS, A. P., and DE WARDENER, H. E. (1971). "Prevention of urinary tract infection with low dose nitrofurantoin." *Lancet*, **2**, 1112.

BENGSTON, V., HOGDAHLIA, M., and HOOD, B. (1968). "Chronic non-obstructive pyelonephritis and hypertension. A long term study." *Quart. J. Med.*, **37**, 361.

BRAUDE, A. I., and SIEMIENSKI, J. S. (1965). "The influence of bacteriocins on resistance to infection by gram negative bacteria. I. The effect of colicin on bactericidal activity of blood." *J. clin. Invest.*, **5**, 849.

BRAUDE, A. I., SIEMIENSKI, J. S., and JACOBS, I. (1961). "Protoplast formation in human urine." *Trans. Ass. Amer. Phys.*, **74**, 234.

FAIRLEY, K. F., CARSON, N. E., GUTCH, R. C., LEIGHTON, P., GROUNDS, A. D., LAIRD, E. C., McCALLUM, P. H. G., SLEEMAN, R. L., and O'KEEFE, C. M. (1971). "Site of infection in acute urinary tract infection in general practice." *Lancet*, **2**, 615.

FAIRLEY, K. F., and BUTLER, H. M. (1970). Sterile pyuria as a manifestation of occult bacterial pyelonephritis with special reference to intermittent bacteriuria. "Renal Infection and Renal Scarring." Edited by P. Kincaid-Smith and K. F. Fairley. Mercedes Publishing Services, Melbourne, Australia.

HEPTINSTALL, R. H. (1966). "Pathology of the Kidney." Little, Brown & Co., Boston, Mass.

HODSON, C. J. (1967). "The radiological contribution toward the diagnosis of chronic pyelonephritis." *Radiology*, **88**, 857.

HODSON, C. J., and CRAVEN, J. D. (1966). "The radiology of obstructive atrophy of the kidney." *Clin. Radiol.*, **17**, 305.

HODSON, C. J., and WILSON, S. (1965). "Natural history of chronic pyelonephritis scarring." *Brit. med., J.*, **11**, 191.

HUTT, M. S. R., CHAMBERS, J. A., MacDONALD, J. S., and DE WARDENER, H. E. (1961). "Pyelonephritis: observations on the relationship between various diagnostic procedures." *Lancet*, **1**, 351.

KASS, E. H. (1957). "Bacteriuria and the diagnosis of infections of the urinary tract." *Arch. intern. Med.*, **100**, 709.

KIMMELSTIEL, P., KIM, O. J., BERES, J. A., and WELLMAN, K. (1961). "Chronic pyelonephritis." *Amer. J. Med.*, **30**, 589.

LITTLE, P. J., McPHERSON, D. R., and DE WARDENER, H. E. (1965). "The appearance of the intravenous pyelogram during and after acute pyelonephritis." *Lancet*, **1**, 1186.

LITTLE, P. J., and DE WARDENER, H. E. (1966). "Acute pyelonephritis. The incidence of re-infection of 100 patients." *Lancet*, **2**, 1277.

O'GRADY, F., and CATTELL, W. R. (1966). "Kinetics of urinary tract infection. 1. Upper urinary tract infection. 2. The bladder." *Brit. J. Urol.*, **38**, 149 and 156.

PARLOWSKI, J. M., BLOXDORF, J. W., and KIMMELSTEIL, P. (1963). "Chronic pyelonephritis. A morphologic and bacteriologic study." *New Eng. J. Med.*, **268**, 965.

ROLLESTON, G. L., SHANNON, F. T., and UTLEY, W. L. F. (1970). "Relationship of infantile vesicoureteric reflux to renal damage." *Brit. med. J.*, **1**, 460.

SHAND, D. G., NIMMON, U. C., O'GRADY, F., and CATTELL, W. R. (1970). "Relation between residual urine volume and response to treatment of urinary tract infection." *Lancet*, **1**, 1305.

SMELLIE, J. M. (1970). "Acute urinary tract infection in children." *Brit. med. J.*, **2**, 97.

STAMEY, T. A., GOVAN, D. E., and PALMER, J. M. (1965). "The localisation and treatment of urinary tract infections: The role of bactericidal urine levels as opposed to serum levels." *Medicine*, **44**, 1.

STEPHENS, F. D., and LENEGHAN, D. (1962). "The anatomical basis and dynamics of vesico-ureteral reflux." *J. Urol.*, **87**, 669.

VINNICOMBE, J., EYKYN, S., and SHUTTLEWORTH, K. E. D. (1971). "Localisation of urinary tract infection." *Brit. J. Urol.*, **43**, 39.

VIVALDI, E., CORTAN, R., ZANGWILL, D. P., and KASS, E. H. (1959). "Ascending infection as a mechanism in pathogenesis of experimental non-obstructive pyelonephritis." *Proc. Soc. exp. Biol. (N.Y.)*, **102**, 242.

WOODS, J. W. (1958). "Susceptibility of rats with hormonal hypertension to experimental pyelonephritis." *J. clin. Invest.*, **37**, 1686.

Phenacetin nephropathy

BELL, D., KERR, D. N. S., SWINNEY, J., and YEATES, W. K. (1969). "Analgesic nephropathy. Clinical course after withdrawal of phenacetin." *Brit. med. J.*, **3**, 378.

BURRY, A. F. (1970). The pathology and pathogenesis of renal papillary necrosis. "Renal Infection and Renal Scarring." Edited by P. Kincaid-Smith and K. F. Fairley. Mercedes Publishing Services, Melbourne, Australia.

BURRY, A. F. (1967). "The evolution of analgesic nephropathy." *Nephron*, **5**, 185.

CALDER, I. C., FUNDER, C. C., GREEN, C. R., HAM, K. H., and TANGE, J. D. (1971). "Comparative nephrotoxicity of aspirin and phenacetin derivatives." *Brit. med. J.*, **2**, 518.

EDWARDS, O. M., EDWARDS, P., HUSKISSON, E. C., and TAYLOR, R. T. (1971). "Paracetomol and renal damage." *Brit. med. J.*, **1**, 87.

GRIMLUND, K. (1963). "Phenacetin and renal damage at a Swedish factory." *Acta med. Scand.*, suppl. 105.

HODSON, C. J. (1970). Differential diagnosis between atrophic pyelonephritis and analgesic nephropathy. "Renal Infection and Renal Scarring." Edited by P. Kincaid-Smith and K. F. Fairley. Mercedes Publishing Services, Melbourne, Australia.

KOUTSAIMANIS, K. G., and DE WARDENER, H. E. (1970). "Phenacetin nephropathy with particular reference to the effect of surgery." *Brit. med. J.*, **2**, 131.

MURRAY, R. M., LAWSON, D. H., and LINTON, A. L. (1971). "Analgesic nephropathy: Clinical syndrome and prognosis." *Brit. med. J.*, **1**, 479.

MURRAY, R. M., TIMBURY, G. C., and LINTON, A. L. (1970). "Analgesic abuse in psychiatric patients." *Lancet*, **1**, 1303.

24

Polyuria

The functional disturbances which cause polyuria are (*a*) lack of circulating antidiuretic hormone (ADH), or (*b*) an inability of the kidneys to concentrate urine although ADH is present, because of (1) impaired ability of the tubule to respond to ADH, (2) a fault in the mechanism concerned with producing a hypertonic interstitial fluid in the medulla, and (3) an increased solute output (i.e. an osmotic diuresis). It may be difficult or impossible in an individual patient to disentangle which of these abnormalities is responsible for polyuria. The important point is that more than one abnormality may be present in any one form of polyuria. This is best demonstrated if the clinical causes of polyuria are listed under the various disturbances mentioned (see below). When the clinical condition is due to more than one functional abnormality, it is listed in italics under that abnormality which is considered to be the principal cause of the polyuria.

POLYURIA DUE TO DIMINISHED CIRCULATING ANTIDIURETIC HORMONE (ADH)

1. Because of an impaired ability to secrete ADH

(*a*) Persistent defect.
  (i) *Lesions of the supraoptico-hypothalamus, i.e. diabetes insipidus.*
(*b*) Transient defect.
  (i) Compulsive water drinking.
  (ii) ? Potassium deficiency.

2. Because of a diminished need to secrete ADH due to an increased intake of water due to increased thirst

(*a*) *Compulsive water drinking.*
(*b*) *Potassium deficiency.*
(*c*) *Lesion of thirst centre.*
(*d*) *Hypercalcaemia.*

3. Because of a circulating antibody to vasopressin

POLYURIA IN SPITE OF ADEQUATE CONCENTRATIONS OF CIRCULATING ADH

1. Because of an impaired ability of the tubule "wall" to respond to ADH

(a) Congenital.
  (i) A single tubular lesion, i.e. *nephrogenic diabetes insipidus.*
  (ii) One of several tubular lesions, i.e. *renal tubular acidosis, Fanconi's syndrome.*

(b) Acquired.
  (i) Compulsive water drinking.
  (ii) Diabetes insipidus.

2. Because of a fault in the mechanism concerned with producing a hypertonic interstitial fluid in the medulla

(a) Due to an impaired sodium transport in the loop of Henle.
  (i) Potassium deficiency.
  (ii) Hypercalcaemia and hypercalcuria.

(b) Due to a disturbed flow of blood in vasa recta, or structural damage to loop of Henle.
  (i) *Papillary necrosis.*
  (ii) Widespread gradual destruction of nephrons, i.e. most instances of chronic renal failure.
  (iii) *Hydronephrosis.*
  (iv) *Sickle cell disease.*

3. Because of an increased solute output per nephron (osmotic diuresis)

(a) Through a normal number of nephrons.
  (i) *Glycosuria.*
  (ii) *Salt diuresis following relief of urinary obstruction.*

(b) Through a greatly reduced number of nephrons.
  (i) *Chronic renal failure.*

Polyuria due to glycosuria is easily diagnosed by a routine test of the urine. Polyuria due to an antibody to vasopressin appears in pregnancy and recovers spontaneously after delivery.

The other causes of polyuria can be subdivided into those that are associated with a moderate rise in blood urea and in which the urine volume is usually only increased to about 3–4 litres per 24 hours, and those that have a normal or low blood urea, and in which the urine volume is usually above 5 litres per 24 hours (often up to 10–12 litres).

Those conditions in which there is a rise in blood urea and only a moderate rise in urine volume include chronic renal failure, potassium deficiency, some cases of hypercalcaemia, and renal tubular acidosis; while those with a normal blood urea and the excretion of large volumes of urine include diabetes insipidus, compulsive water drinking, some cases of hypercalcaemia, and familial nephrogenic diabetes insipidus:

A *Polyuria with urine volume usually less than 3–4 l/24 hr and blood urea raised*	B *Polyuria with urine volume often greater than 5 l/24 hr and blood urea normal*
1. Chronic renal failure (p. 180).	1. Diabetes insipidus.
2. Potassium deficiency (p. 219).	2. Compulsive water drinking.
3. Hypercalcaemia (p. 225).	3. Hypercalcaemia (p. 225).
4. Fanconi's syndrome (p. 236).	4. Familial nephrogenic diabetes insipidus.

The disturbances included in Group A have been discussed in earlier sections. Those in Group B are discussed below, except for hypercalcaemia, which has been discussed on p. 225.

CAUSES OF POLUYRIA IN WHICH THE URINE VOLUME USUALLY GREATER THAN 5 l/24 hr AND THE BLOOD UREA IS NORMAL

Familial Nephrogenic Diabetes Insipidus

This is a rare sex-linked condition which occurs in males and with such a marked familial incidence that sometimes there are several patients under the same roof with the same symptoms. The onset of symptoms is during infancy or childhood. Occasionally chronic dehydration with plasma hypertonicity in infancy may lead to severe and permanent mental retardation. Investigation of entire families has shown that they may contain symptomless heterozygous female carriers, in whom there is a mild impairment of maximum concentrating capacity.

The evidence that the primary defect is an inability of the tubules to utilise vasopressin is obtained by giving vasopressin intravenously. In nephrogenic diabetes insipidus the amount of vasopressin that then appears unchanged in the urine is much greater than in normal subjects. It must also be pointed out that microdissection of nephrons has revealed that in nephrogenic diabetes insipidus the proximal tubules are shorter than normal. The relevance of this finding to the inability of the tubule to utilise vasopressin is not clear. If, however, the shortening results in an increased amount of glomerular filtrate reaching the loop of Henle and the distal tubule it may be an additional cause for the hypotonicity of the urine.

The disease is characterised by an almost complete inability to raise the urine concentration above the concentration of plasma with either 5 units of vasopressin tannate in oil intramuscularly, or moderately severe fluid deprivation sufficient to cause a loss of up to 5 per cent of body weight; in both instances the urine usually remains around S.G. 1·004. If the vasopressin dosage is raised to toxic levels (i.e. 2 units of the aqueous solution intravenously), or the dehydration is so severe that it gives rise to distress and fever, the urine concentration may then rise to much higher levels; this is sometimes seen terminally in nephrogenic diabetes insipidus of infancy.

Treatment consists mainly in early recognition and the adequate administration of water. Infants also greatly benefit from a low electrolyte diet, for this produces a quicker return to normal plasma osmolality. Diuretics which cause much sodium loss such as frusemide or chlorothiazide can reduce the extent of the polyuria. They are useful for special occasions, but their prolonged administration may cause potassium deficiency. It is not known how they reduce the urine volume. It has been pointed out that this only occurs when the patient is in a negative sodium balance, and it has been suggested that this causes such an increased reabsorption of sodium from the proximal tubule that the quantity of tubular fluid which travels into the loop of Henle and emerges into the distal tubule as hypotonic fluid is greatly reduced.

Diabetes Insipidus

It has been mentioned above that diabetes insipidus is due to a diminished ability of the supraopticohypophyseal system to secrete ADH. This is usually an acquired defect associated with fracture of the base of the skull, tumours, infections and lipoid storage diseases. Not infrequently the cause is unknown. It is more common in men than in women. A few familial congenital cases have been described.

The onset of symptoms is usually gradual and, once polyuria and polydipsia have developed, the daily water exchange remains relatively constant. Sometimes 12–15 litres of fluid are ingested and excreted each day for many years; yet in spite of the great disturbance to sleep, there may be no other symptoms or signs. Loss of weight, exhaustion and constipation occur if the urine volumes become astronomical, i.e. 20–30 litres a day.

Differential diagnosis

The main difficulty in the differential diagnosis is to distinguish between diabetes insipidus and compulsive water drinking. Sometimes diabetes insipidus can be distinguished with relative certainty by finding other evidence of structural disease in the area of the neurohypophysis; or a diagnosis of compulsive water drinking can be inferred from the patient's disturbed mental state and previous history of psychiatric peculiarities. Often the distinction between these two conditions has to be made following the administration of vasopressin, a period of fluid deprivation, and on an estimate of the plasma osmolality (see below).

Treatment

The administration of vasopressin immediately relieves the thirst and polyuria. The duration of the relief depends on the vasopressin preparation and on the tubular capacity to concentrate the urine. The effect of vasopressin tannate in oil, 5 units intramuscularly, should continue for 2–3 days, whereas the effect of lysine vasopressin as a nasal spray wears off after 3–6 hours. The spray is best carried about in case of an emergency for sometimes the effect of the vasopressin tannate in oil wears off with an embarrassing rapidity. The disadvantages of vasopressin tannate in oil is that the sites of injection are apt to feel a little sore for 2–3 weeks. The disadvantage of the nasal preparation is the occasional development of rhinorrhoea or asthma. The incidence of such side effects with the synthetic lysine vasopressin spray, however, is much less than with the crude preparations of vasopressin snuff which used to be the only preparation available.

A newly synthesised analogue of vasopressin DDAVP (1 deamino-8-arginine) vasopressin has a higher antidiuretic potency, less pressor activity and a longer duration of action than lysine vasopressin. It may be administered intranasally or by injection. 2 μg intravenously has an effect for 10 hours. 10–15 μg intranasally twice a day induces a normal urine flow throughout the 24 hours. DDAV is particularly useful in pregnancy when lysine or arginine vasopressin may cause an abortion or miscarriage.

Chlorpropamide 250 mg b.d. is also useful in some cases. It acts by enhancing the effect of vasopressin in some manner which is not clear. It probably increases the sensitivity of the distal and collecting ducts to trace amount of vasopressin. The dangers of chlorpropamide are hypoglycaemia, and several toxic reactions such as rashes and nausea.

Compulsive Water Drinking

This is a much more common condition than diabetes insipidus. It is seen principally in middle-aged women. The onset of polydipsia and polyuria is often sudden and not infrequently it coincides with medical advice to drink more fluid (e.g. for constipation). The quantity of water which is consumed is apt to vary erratically from one day to the next, and frequently there is also a slow periodicity, with relapses and remissions varying from several weeks to months. Hysterical manifestations and depression are a part of the syndrome, and there is nearly always a long previous history of psychological disturbances; occasionally these patients are discovered to be magnifying the extent of their polyuria by pouring jugs of water into the bedpan.

A diagnosis of compulsive water drinking is usually suspected from the history and appearance of the patient, and often it is soon apparent that polydipsia and polyuria are the least of the patient's troubles. The differential diagnosis between diabetes insipidus and compulsive water drinking is discussed below.

Treatment

The only treatment which is likely to succeed is one that controls the particular psychological disturbance involved. Sometimes reassurance and encouragement are sufficient. Occasionally a rest in hospital will produce marked improvement and, if such a remission coincides with the administration of

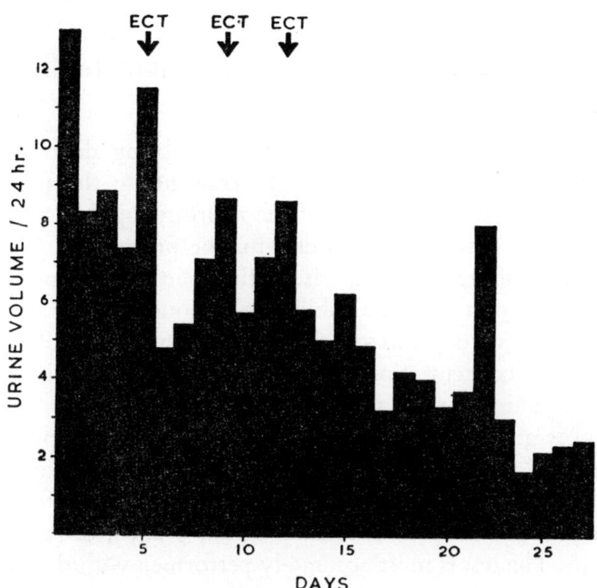

FIG. 24.1. The effect of electro-convulsive therapy (ECT) on a patient with compulsive water drinking and severe depression.

vasopressin, an erroneous diagnosis of diabetes insipidus may be made. Usually stronger measures have to be employed, such as electro-convulsive therapy for the depression (Fig. 24.1) and continuous narcosis for hysteria. Substantial remissions may be induced but the tendency to relapse is very great.

USE OF VASOPRESSIN AND FLUID DEPRIVATION TO DISTINGUISH BETWEEN DIABETES INSIPIDUS AND COMPULSIVE WATER DRINKING

As diabetes insipidus is due to a persistent defect in the ability to secrete ADH because of an abnormality of the neurohypophysis, and compulsive water drinking is simply an increased intake of fluid because of a mental abnormality, it should be possible to distinguish the two conditions by estimating the concentration of antidiuretic hormone in the blood during a period of fluid deprivation. It should be low in diabetes insipidus and high in compulsive water drinking. Unfortunately, there is as yet no reliable method of estimating the concentration of circulating ADH in the plasma directly. Its presence has to be deduced by observing changes in urine flow and urine concentration. For this reason, diabetes insipidus and compulsive water drinking have to be distinguished by (1) estimating and comparing the kidney's ability to concentrate the urine following the administration of vasopressin and after a period of fluid deprivation, (2) by observing the generalised effects of a long-lasting vasopressin preparation, and (3) estimating the osmolality of the plasma.

Urine Concentration after Vasopressin Administration, and Fluid Deprivation

Vasopressin is given when the patient is not being deprived of fluid to determine the efficiency of the kidney to concentrate the urine; and fluid deprivation is used to test the ability of the neurohypophysis to secrete ADH. It is logical to do these tests in this order, for the presence of ADH following fluid deprivation is inferred from the rise in the concentration of the urine; this, in turn, is dependent on the tubule's ability to respond to ADH. The interpretation of these two tests depends on the fact that when the ability to secrete ADH is normal the concentration of the urine after fluid deprivation is greater than after the administration of vasopressin.

Vasopressin is given at a time when the patient's consumption of water is perfectly free and uninhibited; it is administered either intravenously as 100 m.Units in 20 sec followed by 5 m.Units/min thereafter for one hour, or intramuscularly as (1) vasopressin tannate in oil, 5 units, or (2) aqueous vasopressin 2·5 units. The test is most accurately performed with the first technique, but it is more convenient to use vasopressin tannate in oil, for it is then unnecessary to catheterise the patient; nevertheless vasopressin tannate in oil may be dangerous for patients with compulsive water drinking.

A period of fluid deprivation stimulates ADH production because of the negative balance of water that results. The duration of such a period therefore is of secondary importance. For instance, a period of 12 hours' fluid deprivation is a stronger stimulus to ADH production in a polyuric patient unable to concentrate the urine, and who therefore excretes 3 to 5 litres of water, than is a 24-hour period of fluid deprivation in a normal person who only loses 1 litre. The most satisfactory method is to be guided by the weight that is lost during fluid deprivation, and to estimate the urine concentration after the loss of 3 to 5 per cent of the initial weight. If greater losses are allowed the urine may become concentrated by mechanisms other than the neurohypophyseal secretion, and the test becomes pointless.

Theoretically the result of these two tests in diabetes insipidus and compulsive water drinking should be as follows: patients with diabetes insipidus should concentrate their urine normally with vasopressin but not with fluid deprivation, whereas patients with compulsive water drinking should concentrate the urine normally with both vasopressin and fluid deprivation. Unfortunately, though this is frequently true, the situation is not always so straightforward.

Results of vasopressin and fluid deprivation tests in diabetes insipidus (Fig. 24.2). Patients with diabetes insipidus are, indeed, unable to concentrate their urine normally following fluid deprivation. And after vasopressin, the urine S.G. or osmolality rises to a concentration which is much greater than with dehydration alone. This phenomenon is best observed if vasopressin is given

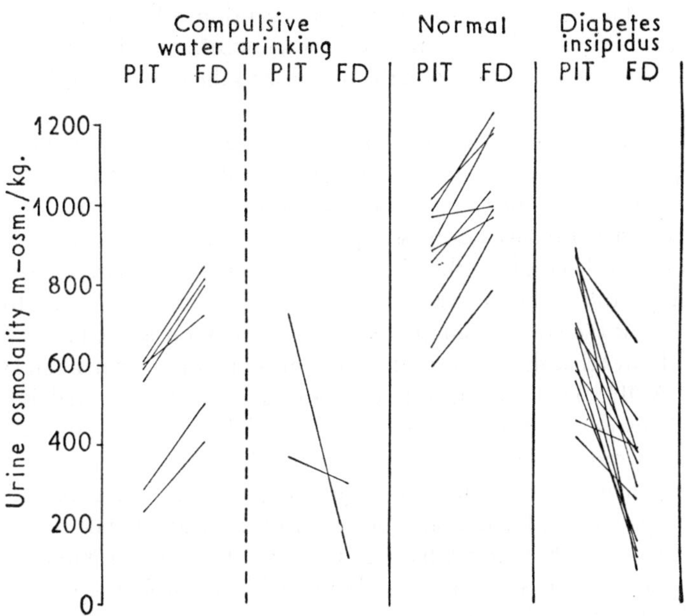

FIG. 24.2. Test of neurohypophyseal integrity by fluid deprivation and vasopressin. The urine osmolality after intravenous aqueous vasopressin (PIT) and after fluid deprivation (F.D.), in compulsive water drinking, normal individuals and in diabetes insipidus; each line represents one subject. (Barlow and de Wardener, 1959, *Quart. J. Med.*)

at the end of a period of dehydration when the urine osmolality suddenly increases by a substantial amount. A phenomenon which is totally abnormal. Occasionally, however, the response to vasopressin alone, though considerably greater than that following fluid deprivation, is still below normal.

Results of vasopressin and fluid deprivation tests in compulsive water drinking (Fig. 24.2). These patients may respond in a variety of ways and the multiplicity of their responses is very confusing. The following responses are seen:

1. The kidney's ability to concentrate the urine following vasopressin and fluid deprivation is normal, i.e. urine concentration rises to levels found in normal individuals and, what is more important, *the concentration after fluid deprivation is greater than after vasopressin.*

This indicates that both tubular function and the ability to secrete antidiuretic hormone are normal. Such a response is only found in patients whose daily urine volume is less than 5 litres.

2. The kidney's ability to concentrate the urine following both vasopressin and fluid deprivation is impaired, but the concentration after fluid deprivation is greater than after vasopressin.

This indicates that tubular function is impaired, but the ability to produce ADH is normal. In these patients the urine concentration after vasopressin may be around S.G. 1·010 and after fluid deprivation S.G. 1·014.

3. The kidney's ability to concentrate the urine following vasopressin is normal, but following fluid deprivation the concentration is considerably less than that following vasopressin (i.e. the response to the two tests is the same as in diabetes insipidus).

This indicates that tubular function is normal, but that there is an inhibition to ADH production which is not overcome by fluid deprivation. It may be difficult to differentiate such a patient from one suffering from diabetes insipidus, particularly if the aqueous vasopressin preparation has been used. If vasopressin tannate in oil has been given the distinction is usually easier (see below).

4. Finally, the kidneys are unable to concentrate the urine following vasopressin, but the concentration after fluid deprivation is even less.

This indicates that there is a combination of tubular impairment and inability to secrete ADH. These are identical responses to those obtained in diabetes insipidus. They demonstrate an ability to inhibit ADH secretion in spite of fluid deprivation, presumably due to the emotional stress of the test. This conclusion is confirmed by obtaining a normal response to fluid deprivation after treating the patient with some suitable psychotherapeutic manoeuvre.

DISCUSSION. It is not clear why the kidney's ability to concentrate the urine following vasopressin is impaired in both diabetes insipidus and compulsive water drinking. A similar impairment can be demonstrated in normal subjects drinking 8–12 litres of water a day (Fig. 24.3). It would appear to be unrelated to the expansion of the extracellular fluid or blood volume. It is more likely to be due to some change in the renal medulla consequent upon the increased rate of flow of hypotonic urine. In a patient with diabetes insipidus the ability to concentrate the urine takes several days or weeks to return to normal after starting treatment with vasopressin.

It is interesting to note that patients with long-standing polyuria and polydipsia excreting hypotonic urine may also have a reversible impairment in their ability to acidify the urine. To the unwary this combination of polyuria and polydipsia with an impaired ability to concentrate and acidify may suggest a diagnosis of renal tubular acidosis secondary to renal disease. This is a diagnostic trap into which only the sophisticated who measure these various tubular functions may fall. On the other hand, they are the ones best qualified to interpret these findings correctly.

The patient's ability to secrete ADH is sometimes tested by other means than fluid deprivation. For instance, the supraopticohypophyseal system can be stimulated by intravenous nicotine, or by suddenly raising the plasma osmolality with an infusion of hypertonic saline. Nicotine acid tartrate (3 to

6 mg) is given intravenously; it is only effective if it induces severe nausea and vomiting, but even if these unpleasant symptoms are produced some normal subjects may fail to respond. The hypertonic saline test is performed by infusing 2·5 g NaCl per 100 ml H_2O at a rate of 0·25 ml/kg of body weight per minute, an hour after the oral ingestion of 20 ml/kg of water. The urine flow should fall, but occasionally the water diuresis is replaced by a saline diuresis and the

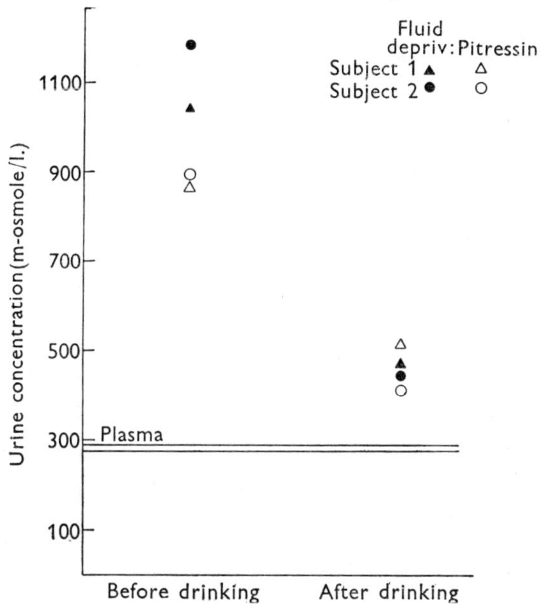

FIG. 24.3. Urine concentrations following the intravenous administration of vasopressin, and after a 26-hour period of fluid deprivation, before and at the end of drinking about 10 litres of water a day for 11 days. The plasma osmolarity varied between the limits indicated by the two parallel horizontal lines. (de Wardener and Herxheimer, 1957, *J. Physiol.*)

urine flow does not change materially (particularly in hypertensive women). Another disadvantage is that in elderly patients the large infusion of saline may precipitate heart failure. Neither of these two manoeuvres gives as much information as a properly controlled period of fluid deprivation, which is in any case a more physiological stimulus to ADH secretion.

General effects following the administration of a long-acting vasopressin preparation

If a patient suffering from compulsive water drinking is given a long-acting vasopressin preparation, i.e. vasopressin tannate in oil, there is a considerable decrease in urine flow even if the tubule's capacity to concentrate is seriously impaired* (see above). But usually thirst continues unabated, the intake of water

* Vasopressin can lower the urine flow from 10 to 3 ml/min without the concentration of the urine rising above S.G. 1·012; higher concentrations only occur at lower urine flows.

exceeds the output, and overhydration develops. There is abdominal distension, headache, drowsiness, and sometimes nausea and vomiting. In striking contrast, therefore, to patients suffering from diabetes insipidus, patients with compulsive water drinking complain of the vasopressin injections, often with much vehemence and bitterness. Occasionally, both the patient and his attendants are unaware that the onset of nausea, headache and drowsiness is related to the administration of vasopressin. Instead, these symptoms are considered to be additional evidence in favour of an intracranial lesion in the vicinity of the neurohypophysis, and therefore of a diagnosis of diabetes insipidus.

Plasma osmolality

The plasma osmolality of patients suffering from diabetes insipidus and compulsive water drinking is compared in Fig. 24.4 with that of normal

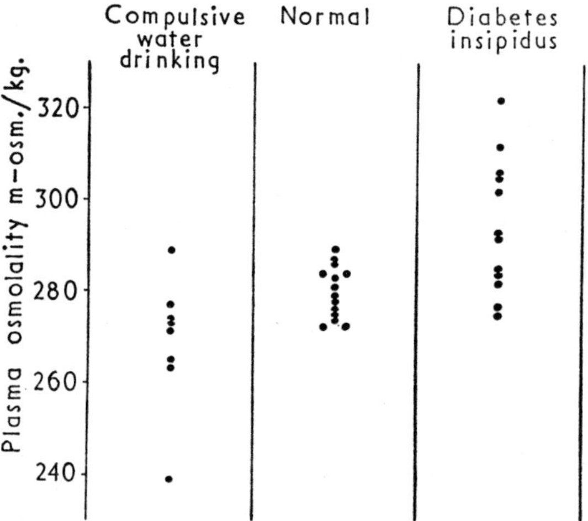

FIG. 24.4. Plasma osmolality in compulsive water drinking in normal subjects and in diabetes insipidus. (Barlow and de Wardener, 1959, *Quart. J. Med.*)

subjects. The mean osmolality in diabetes insipidus (295 ± 15 m.Osm/kg) is significantly higher than in the normal subjects (280 ± 6 m.Osm/kg), whereas in compulsive water drinking (269 ± 14 m.Osm/kg) it is significantly lower. These findings are in keeping with the aetiology of the two conditions. In patients with diabetes insipidus the initial disturbance is polyuria and the excessive drinking is a normal response to the contraction and concentration of body fluids, whereas in compulsive water drinking the initial disturbance is excessive drinking and the polyuria is the normal response to expansion and dilution of body fluids. There is a considerably overlap between the groups, but it appears that if the plasma osmolality of a patient with polyuria is greater than 290 m.Osm/kg the diagnosis is likely to be diabetes insipidus, and if it is less than 275 m.Osm/kg it is more likely to be compulsive water drinking.

BIBLIOGRAPHY

AVIOLI, L. V., LAKERSOLM, J. T., and LOPESTI, J. M. (1963). "Histiocytosis X (Schiller–Christian disease): a clinical pathological survey, review of 10 patients and the results of prednisone therapy." *Medicine*, **42**, 119.

BARLOW, E. D., and DE WARDENER, H. E. (1959). "Compulsive water drinking." *Quart. J. Med.*, N.S. **28**, 235.

BERDE, B., and CERLETTI, A. (1961). "Uber die antidiuretische Wirkung von synthetischen Lysin-vasopressin." *Helv. physiol. pharmacol. Acta*, **19**, 135.

BISSETT, G. W., and LEE, J. (1958). "Antidiuretic activity in the blood after stimulation of the neurohypophysis in man." *Lancet*, **2**, 715.

CAROME, F. A., and EPSTEIN, F. H. (1960). "Nephrogenic diabetes insipidus caused by amyloid disease." *Amer. J. Med.*, **29**, 539.

CARTER, C., and SIMPKISS, M. (1956). "The 'carrier' state in nephrogenic diabetes insipidus." *Lancet*, **2**, 1069.

DANIEL, P. M., and TREIP, C. S. (1961). The pathology of the pituitary gland in head injury. In H. Gardiner Hill, "Modern Trends in Endocrinology", 2nd series, p. 58. Butterworths, London.

DARMADY, E. M., OFFER, J., PRINCE, J., and STRANAK, F. (1964). "The proximal convoluted tubule in the renal handling of water." *Lancet*, **2**, 1254.

DICKER, S. E., and EGGLETON, M. G. (1960). "Hyaluronidase and antidiuretic activity in urine of man." *J. Physiol.*, **154**, 378.

DICKER, S. E., and EGGLETON, M. G. (1963). "Nephrogenic diabetes insipidus." *Clin. Sci.*, **24**, 81.

EPSTEIN, F. H., RIVERA, M. J., and CARONE, F. A. (1958). "The effect of hypercalcemia induced by calciferol upon renal concentrating ability." *J. clin. Invest.*, **37**, 1702.

HICKEY, R. C., and HARE, K. (1944). "The renal excretion of chloride and water in diabetes insipidus." *J. clin. Invest.*, **23**, 168.

MANITIUS, A., LEVITIN, H., BECK, D., and EPSTEIN, F. H. (1960). "On the mechanism of impairment of renal concentrating ability in potassium deficiency." *J. clin. Invest.*, **39**, 684.

MARTIN, F. I. R. (1959). "Familial diabetes insipidus." *Quart. J. Med.*, N.S. **28**, 573.

MILLER, M., DALAKOS, T., MOSES, A. M., FELLERMAN, H., and STREETEN, D. H. P. (1970). "Recognition of partial defects in antidiuretic hormone secretion." *Ann. Intern. Med.*, **73**, 721.

PANITZ, F., and SHINABERGER, J. H. (1965). "Nephrogenic diabetes insipidus due to sarcoidosis without hypercalcaemia." *Ann. Intern. Med.*, **62**, 113.

PERILLIE, P. E., and EPSTEIN, F. H. (1963). "Sickling phenomenon produced by hypertonic solutions. A possible explanation for the hyposthenuria of sicklemia." *J. clin. Invest.*, **42**, 570.

ROUSSAK, N. J., and OLEESKY, S. (1954). "Water-losing nephritis. A syndrome simulating diabetes insipidus." *Quart. J. Med.*, N.S. **23**, 147.

SHANNON, J. A. (1942). "The control of the renal excretion of water. (i) The effect of variations in the state of hydration on water excretion in dogs with diabetes insipidus." *J. exp. Med.*, **76**, 371.

STATIUS VAN EPS, L. W., PINEDO-VEELS, C., DE VRIES, G. H., and DE KRONING, J. (1970). "Nature of concentrating defect in sickle cell nephropathy." *Lancet*, **1**, 450.

VERNEY, E. B. (1946). "Absorption and excretion of water: the antidiuretic hormone." *Lancet*, **2**, 739 and 781.

WARDENER, DE H. E. (1960). "Polyuria." *J. chron. Dis.*, **11**, 199.

WARDENER, DE H. E., and HERXHEIMER, A. W. (1957). "The effect of a high water intake on the kidney's ability to concentrate the urine." *J. Physiol. (Lond.)*, **139**, 42.

WEBSTER, B., and BRAIN, J. (1970). "Antidiuretic effect and complications of chlorpropamide therapy in diabetes insipidus." *J. clin. Endocr. Metab.*, **30**, 215.

25

The Kidney, Glycosuria and Diabetes Mellitus

Glycosuria

IT has been pointed out in Section 5 that the quantity of glucose which passes through a glomerulus in one minute is the product of the filtration rate and the plasma glucose, and that normally the urine is free from glucose because this filtered glucose is reabsorbed in the proximal tubule. The rate at which glucose can be reabsorbed, however, is limited, and at normal glomerular filtration rates many of the tubules cannot reabsorb a greater amount than that which is delivered to them when the plasma glucose is about 170 mg per 100 ml. The appearance of glucose in the urine therefore denotes that either: (1) a normal tubular reabsorbing capacity for glucose has been exceeded by an increased rate of delivery through the glomerulus; or (2) a reduced reabsorbing capacity of some, or most, of the tubules has been exceeded, though the rate of delivery is normal.

Glycosuria is never due to an increased glomerular filtration rate, so that when the tubular capacity to reabsorb glucose is normal the appearance of glucose in the urine is due to hyperglycaemia, as in diabetes, thyrotoxicosis and Cushing's disease, or following a gastroenterostomy when there is an excessively rapid intestinal absorption of glucose.

Glycosuria associated with a diminished tubular reabsorptive capacity and a normal blood glucose is often a benign familial condition which is known as *renal glycosuria* (the condition is also known as "renal diabetes" and "pseudorenal diabetes", names which only confuse). If the reabsorbing capacity of only a few of the tubules is abnormal an estimation of the total capacity of the kidneys to reabsorb glucose (Tmg) may be within normal limits; but when more tubules are involved the total capacity to reabsorb glucose is reduced; familial renal glycosuria may be associated with either of these findings.

It is clear that when there is glycosuria the simplest way to differentiate between hyperglycaemic glycosuria, and renal glycosuria is to estimate the concentration of blood glucose. The blood should be taken at the midpoint of a short urine collection period, preferably during a fast. If this test is not decisive a glucose tolerance test should be done.

There are three other variations on this theme of glomerular supply and tubular reabsorption of glucose which are clinically important.

340

1. If, in a patient suffering from diabetes *and* renal glycosuria, insulin dosage is being adjusted according to the output of glucose in the urine, hypoglycaemia may be induced. This often occurs in pregnant diabetics.

2. Very occasionally, contraction of the extracellular fluid space in diabetic acidosis may cause such severe renal vasoconstriction and fall in glomerular filtration rate that, though there is hyperglycaemia, the amount of glucose being delivered to the tubule may still be within its reabsorbing capacity, and no glucose appears in the urine.

3. Finally, there are those rare cases of glycosuria associated with a normal blood sugar in which diminished tubular capacity to reabsorb glucose is not an isolated, benign functional lesion, but is only one of many similar but more serious abnormalities of tubular function, i.e. Fanconi's syndrome.

Diabetes Mellitus

The following renal disturbances occur:

1. Disturbances of renal function in the absence of ketosis.
2. Disturbances of renal function during ketosis.
3. Diabetic nephropathy.
4. Renal infections.

Disturbances of renal function in the absence of ketosis

The glycosuria of diabetes is secondary to hyperglycaemia. But its extent may give a misleading impression of the height of the blood glucose, for patients with diabetes often have renal glycosuria, and glycosuria may therefore be present when the blood glucose is normal. Paradoxically the glucose Tm is *raised* in diabetes; the cause of this teleologically reasonable phenomenon is not known; it tends to subside after the administration of insulin. The simultaneous presence of renal glycosuria and a raised glucose Tm is presumably due to a splaying out of the individual nephrons capacity to reabsorb glucose.

The osmotic diuresis provoked by the glycosuria causes many of the characteristic features of diabetes mellitus, for it is responsible for a high urinary excretion of water, sodium and potassium, which gives rise to polyuria, thirst and lassitude.

As glucose is a dense molecule, urine that contains glucose will tend to have a higher specific gravity than its colour would suggest, i.e. a pale urine may be found to have a specific gravity of 1·026.

Disturbances of renal function during ketosis

The urine in diabetic ketosis is acid and is characterised by an increased excretion of glucose, water, sodium, potassium and ketones, including β-hydroxybutyric acid. In severe cases there is metabolic acidosis, severe dehydra-

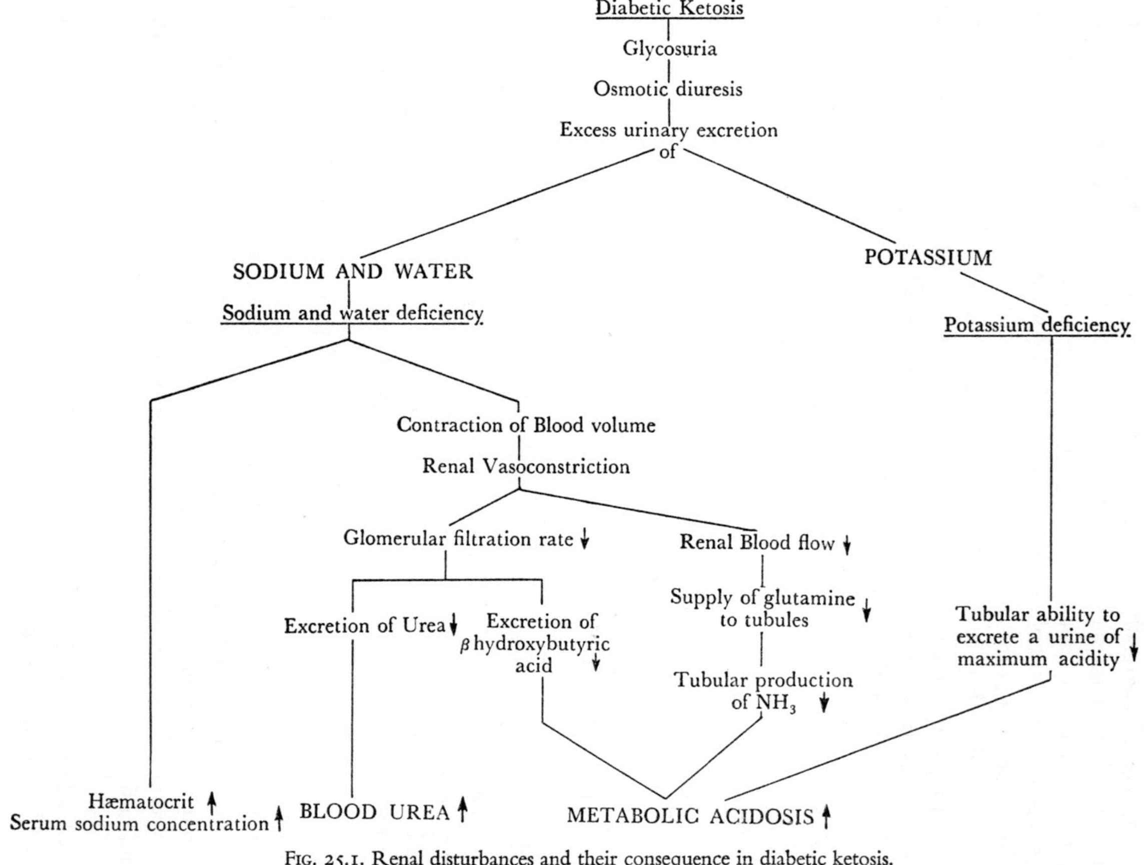

FIG. 25.1. Renal disturbances and their consequence in diabetic ketosis.

tion with a raised plasma sodium concentration, and a contraction of the extracellular fluid volume and the blood volume. The metabolic acidosis is caused principally by an accumulation of ketones due to an increased rate of ketone production, and ultimately there may also be some impairment in the kidney's ability to excrete hydrogen ions and ammonia. This impairment is due to both the sodium and potassium deficiencies which follow a prolonged osmotic glucose diuresis. Potassium deficiency diminishes the tubule's ability to form a urine of maximum acidity which reduces the transfer of ammonia from the tubule cell to the tubule lumen. And severe sodium deficiency decreases the tubule's capacity to form ammonia (Fig 25.1). In consequence the acidosis is increased and the ketones in the urine are excreted with sodium and potassium ions, thus aggravating their deficiencies. Although there is an overall potassium deficiency there is often a shift of potassium out of the cells so that the concentration of plasma potassium tends to be raised, a phenomenon which is reversed by the administration of insulin.

The loss of salt and water causes contraction of the extracellular fluid space and the blood volume; renal vasoconstriction follows and there is a reduction in renal blood flow and glomerular filtration rate, with a rise in blood urea. The fall in glomerular filtration rate also reduces the urinary excretion of ketones, and this further aggravates the metabolic acidosis. Occasionally, in very severe cases, filtration may fall to such a low rate that all the glucose *and ketones* which are filtered are reabsorbed by the tubules and none appear in the urine; this may cause considerable diagnostic confusion. The fall in glomerular filtration is also due in part to potassium deficiency, and this probably accounts for the slow recovery of renal function that sometimes follows the treatment of diabetic ketosis with only saline and insulin.

Acute renal failure with acute tubular necrosis may occur in the most severe cases.

Treatment

Insulin and antibiotics are given first, but to improve renal function it is essential to correct rapidly the negative sodium, water and potassium balances. Large quantities of isotonic sodium chloride and sodium bicarbonate are administered intravenously, and when the blood glucose has begun to settle, 5 per cent glucose is also given. It is unwise to give potassium solutions intravenously until, or unless, the urine flow is brisk, and the acute phase of the ketosis has passed, for the concentration of plasma potassium is often very high (see above).

These measures (except for potassium administration) are undertaken even in the presence of acute oliguria, for though they may be too late to prevent the development of acute tubular necrosis, their administration may limit the extent of the damage. Sometimes the blood pressure is very low, when it must be raised with plasma expanders, for a combination of renal vasoconstriction and hypotension is particularly likely to cause complete renal ischaemia and necrosis. In most instances the blood pressure rises and the urine flow returns within a few hours of giving saline, and it becomes clear that acute tubular necrosis has not occurred.

Diabetic Nephropathy

Widespread vascular abnormalities occur frequently in long-standing diabetes. They are known as diabetic microangiopathy. They differ from the common forms of hypertensive or atheromatous vascular changes and are situated in the retinal veins and arteries, the arteries to the peripheral nerves, the renal arteries and capillaries and the arteries of many other organs.

Pathology

The kidney may be of normal size or even a little larger than normal. The vascular lesions involve the glomerular capillaries and both the afferent and efferent arterioles. Their distribution may be widespread or focal, and the capillary lesions tend at first to involve only one part of a glomerulus.

In the gomeruli there are two principal lesions. One consists of globular, eosin staining, amorphous masses of basement membrane material focally distributed within the glomeruli. The other consists of mesangial stalk, and basement membrane thickening. The first lesion is known as the Kimmelstiel–Wilson lesion but it is probable that both are different stages of the same process for the globular lesions occur mainly after the diffuse lesions are well established. The globular masses tend to occur at the periphery of one of the capillary loops, and eventually, as they enlarge and multiply, they obliterate the tuft (Fig. 25.2). The capillaries which give rise to these excrescences are dilated and appear to be obstructed. The changes associated with mesangial stalk thickening may also obliterate the glomerulus, and may do so without the typical Kimmelstiel-Wilson lesion being present. Occasionally there are also some exudative lesions of protein-like substance containing high quantities of fat usually originating and attached to Bowman's capsule. Very rarely the appearances are identical to those of extra-membranous glomerular nephritis, with a diffuse even thickening of the glomerular capillary walls.

The electron microscope shows that the basement membrane is enormously thickened and that the globular masses at first lie in the endothelial cells. The epithelial cells often have disorganised foot processes; sometimes these are no longer distinct and instead are converted into large islets of cytoplasm covering the outer surface of the capillary.

The glomerular lesions are usually found in association with gross thickening of the afferent and efferent arterioles (mainly the afferent) of the glomeruli involved. The arteriolar walls keep their sharp outline (unlike the appearances in fibrinoid necrosis), but are widened by some material which stains a deep and vivid pink with haematoxylin and eosin; the composition of this substance is not known; it is not collagen or basement membrane-like material.

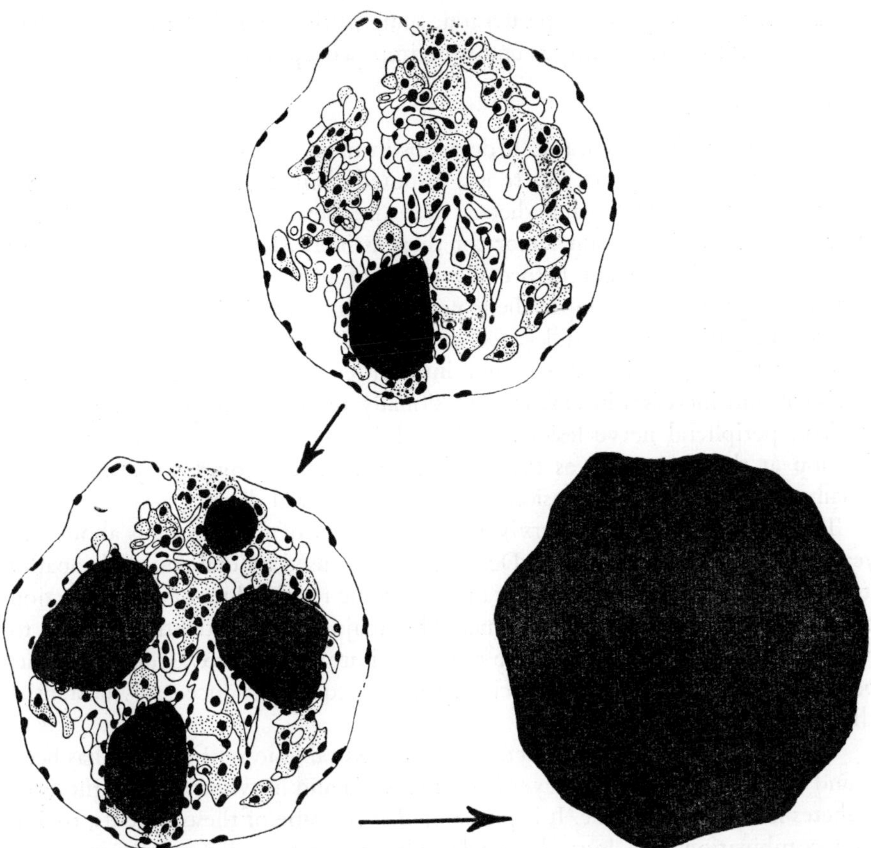

Fɪɢ. 25.2. Diabetes (Kimmelstiel–Wilson lesions). Schema illustrating the peripheral distribution in the glomerulus of the characteristic deposits of eosin staining material, and
how eventually they may entirely fill the glomerulus. The non-specific lesions which
also occur in diabetic nephropathy (see text) are not shown.

It is probable that diabetic microangiopathy including diabetic nephropathy is due to some immunological mechanism. Immunofluorescent techniques
demonstrate that the renal lesions contain insulin and globulin anti-insulin
antibodies which suggests that the lesions may be due to the deposition of
insulin anti-insulin antibody complexes. And circulating antibodies to endogenous insulin have been demonstrated in patients who have never received
exogenous insulin.

The tubules show similar changes to those found in persistent glomerular
nephritis, and very occasionally the proximal tubules contain large quantities
of glycogen. The interstitial tissues contain varying collections of chronic
inflammatory cells in proportion to the number of glomeruli which are
disintegrating.

M

Finally, the changes of hypertension, acute pyelonephritis, or chronic interstitial nephritis are frequently found superimposed upon those just described.

Clinical features

The first sign is proteinuria. It develops in most patients who have had the disease more than 10 years. There is a disputed claim that good control of the blood sugar with insulin and dietary measures lessens the incidence. This is unlikely to be an important factor for there is increasing biopsy evidence that the lesions can be present before the onset of glycosuria. Young males are particularly prone to develop diabetic nephropathy, though in absolute numbers most of the patients are middle-aged and elderly women.

At first the proteinuria is often intermittent, but gradually it becomes persistent and increases in extent. Occasionally there is a nephrotic syndrome. Retinal, peripheral nerve lesions and, in the older patients, severe atheroma, develop at the same time as the renal lesions. Patients over 50 years of age usually present with hypertension or peripheral arterial disease.

The average duration of survival after the onset of proteinuria is about five years; it is longest in the young. Death is rarely caused by diabetic nephropathy itself except in the young who may die of chronic renal failure or of an infection complicating a nephrotic syndrome. The majority of patients succumb to coronary thrombosis, hypertensive cardiac failure or cerebrovascular accidents before the renal lesions are sufficiently advanced to produce any substantial change in renal function.

Chronic renal failure associated with the classical lesions of diabetes has been found in patients who have never had glycosuria and in whom the diagnosis of diabetes has not been made. It is probable that in some of these patients, owing to a combination of a low glomerular filtration rate and a greatly increased ability to reabsorb glucose, there was no glycosuria, though there may have been hyperglycaemia. In a few patients the blood glucose has been measured and found to be normal, though at post-mortem there was, in addition to the characteristic diabetic renal lesions, widespread hyalinisation of the islets of Langerhans.

RELATIONSHIP BETWEEN CLINICAL AND STRUCTURAL FEATURES. Electron microscopy studies on renal biopsies from diabetic patients are beginning to show that the changes in the glomerular basement membrane probably precede the onset of proteinuria by several years. It has also been established that electron microscopy abnormalities appear about five years after the clinical onset of diabetes, whereas light microscopy changes begin to be obvious after 10 years. The histological changes are the same when the diabetes follows pancreatitis or haemochromatosis.

The extent of the proteinuria is greatest with severe structural changes, otherwise there does not appear to be any close relation between the histological appearances and renal function. Occasionally there may be well-marked histological changes without proteinuria or impairment of renal function. When light microscopy lesions are evident it is usual to be able to discern diabetic retinal lesions with an ophthalmoscope. This relationship is so close that the finding of retinal changes is a good indication that renal changes are present whether or not there is proteinuria.

It is important, though confusing, to point out that clinically it is impossible to predict the presence or absence of Kimmelstiel–Wilson lesions. Not infrequently these specific lesions will be found in patients who have never had proteinuria or other evidence of renal disease. Many diabetic patients dying from renal failure subsequent to a nephrotic syndrome may not show the characteristic focal lesion though all will have the diffuse lesions.

PLASMA GLUCOSE LEVELS AND CHRONIC RENAL FAILURE. A few diabetic patients require less insulin as they develop chronic renal failure. This may be due to the gradual obliteration of the kidney's ability to catabolise insulin. On the other hand some diabetic patients may need more insulin, and it is well known that non-diabetic persons who develop chronic renal failure have a diabetic type glucose tolerance curve. Both these observations are possibly due to the uraemia impairing hepatic function. Normally as plasma glucose rises, there is a rise in plasma insulin which inhibits further release of glucose from the liver into the blood. If normal liver slices are incubated in uraemic plasma however this response to insulin is less pronounced. It is inferred that the diabetic glucose tolerance curve of patients with chronic renal failure may be due to the liver continuing to supply glucose into the blood as glucose is being absorbed from the gut.

TREATMENT. Recently it has been demonstrated that the vascular lesions in the eyes either improve or do not progress following hypophysectomy. It is less certain whether diabetic nephropathy does as well. Perhaps in the future it may be possible to inhibit anterior pituitary function by some less irrevocable and dangerous method. Young patients dying of chronic renal failure due to diabetic nephropathy do well on maintenance haemodialysis. Theoretically, they are unsuitable to withstand the high doses of prednisone which are given after renal transplantation. But one centre has had good results transplanting young patients. Older diabetic patients do not do well with either maintenance haemodialysis or transplantation because of the widespread arterial disease.

Renal Infections

Diabetics are liable to infections in any site, and the kidneys are no exception. Acute and chronic pyelonephritis often accompany the renal vascular changes described above. Acute pyelonephritis is always accompanied by diabetic acidosis. Acute necrotising papillitis occurs from time to time in patients with an uncontrolled urinary infection. It usually gives rise to acute renal failure.

TREATMENT. Whereas the vascular lesions are untreatable, the infections can be controlled. It is of the greatest importance in diabetics to be always on the look out for urinary infections, for if they are overlooked the combination of infection and vascular damage is rapidly lethal. Renal infections should be treated in the way outlined earlier (p. 310).

BIBLIOGRAPHY

Glycosuria

BRADLEY, S. E., BRADLEY, G. P., TYSON, C. J., CURRY, J. J., and BLAKE, W. D. (1950). "Renal function in renal diseases." *Amer. J. Med.*, **9**, 766.

GOVAERTS, P. (1952). "The physiopathology of glucose excretion by the human kidney." *Brit. med. J.*, **2**, 175.

REUBI, F. C. (1954). "Glucose Titration in Renal Glycosuria." Ciba Foundation Symposium on the Kidney. J. & A. Churchill, London.

SMITH, H. W. (1951). "The Kidney. Structure and Function in Health and Disease." Oxford University Press, New York.

STARLING, E. H., and VERNEY, E. B. (1925). "The secretion of urine as studied on the isolated kidney." *Proc. Roy. Soc. B*, **97**, 321.

STEINITZ, K. (1940). "Studies on the condition of glucose excretion in man." *J. clin. Invest.*, **19**, 299.

Diabetes mellitus

BERGSTRAND, A., and BUCHT, H. (1959). "The glomerular lesions of diabetes mellitus and their electron-microscope appearances." *J. Path. Bact.*, **77**, 231.

BERNS, A. W., OWENS, C. T., HIRATA, Y., and BLUMENTHAL, H. T. (1962). "The pathogenesis of diabetic glomerulosclerosis. A demonstration of insulin-binding capacity of the various histopathological components of the disease with fluorescent microscopy." *Diabetes*, **11**, 308.

BERNSTEIN, L. M., FOLEY, E. F., and HOFFMAN, W. S. (1952). "Renal function during and after diabetic coma." *J. clin. Invest.*, **31**, 711.

BRODSKY, W. A., RAPOPORT, S., and WEST, C. D. (1950). "The mechanism of glycosuric diuresis in diabetic man." *J. clin. Invest.*, **29**, 1021.

CHURG, J., and DOLGER, H. (1971). Diabetic renal disease. In "Diseases of the Kidney". Edited by M. B. Strauss and L. G. Welt. Little, Brown and Company, Boston, U.S.A.

CORVILAIN, J., BRAUMAN, H., DELCROIX, C., TOUSSAINT, C., VEREERSTRAETEN, P., and FRANKSON, J. R. M. (1971). "Labelled insulin catabolism in chronic renal failure and in the anephric state." *Diabetes*, **20**, 467.

FARBER, S. J., BERGER, E. Y., and EARLE, D. P. (1951). "Effect of diabetes and insulin on maximum capacity of renal tubules to reabsorb glucose." *J. clin. Invest.*, **30**, 125.

FARRANT, P. C., and SHEDDEN, W. I. H. (1965). "Observations on the uptake of insulin conjugated with fluoresien isothinocyanate by diabetic kidney tissue." *Diabetes*, **14**, 274.

FRANKS, M., BERRIS, R. F., CAPLAN, N. O., and MYERS, G. B. (1948). "Metabolic studies in diabetic acidosis." *Arch. intern. Med.*, **81**, 42.

FREEDMAN, L. R. (1957). "Inapparent diabetes mellitus as a cause of renal insufficiency due to Kimmelstiel–Wilson lesions." *Johns Hopk. Hosp. Bull.*, **100**, 132.

HALL, G. F. M. (1952). "Factors in the aetiology of diabetic glomerulosclerosis." *Quart. J. Med.*, N.S. **21**, 385.

HEPTINSTALL, R. H. (1966). "Pathology of the Kidney." Boston, Little, Brown and Co., p. 465.

HOGEMAN, O. (1948). "Renal function in diabetic nephropathy." *Acta med. scand.*, suppl. 216b, **132**.

HORSFIELD, G. I., and LANNIGAN, R. (1965). "Exudative lesions in diabetes mellitus." *J. clin. Path.*, **18**, 47.

JOSLIN'S DIABETES MELLITUS (1971). Edited by A. Marble, P. White, R. F. Bradley and L. P. Krall. Lea and Febiger, Philadelphia.

McCANCE, R. A., and LAWRENCE, R. D. (1935). "The secretion of urine in diabetic coma." *Quart. J. Med.*, **28**, 53.

Monasterio, G., Oliver, J., Minesan, G., Pardelli, G., Marinozzi, V., and MacDowell, M. (1964). "Renal diabetes as a congenital tubular dysplasia." *Amer. J. Med.*, **37**, 44.

Rogers, J., Robbins, S. L., and Jeghers, H. (1952). "Intercapillary glomerulosclerosis. A clinical and pathological study." *Amer. J. Med.*, **12**, 688, 692 and 700.

Taft, H. P., Finckh, E. S., and Joske, R. A. (1954). "Biopsy study of kidney in diabetes mellitus." *Aust. Ann. Med.*, **3**, 189.

26

Renal Disturbances in Pregnancy

1. Physiological changes:
   Renal blood flow and glomerular filtration rate.
   Lactosuria and glycosuria.
   Orthostatic proteinuria.
   Ureteric and pelvic dilatation.
   Sodium and water retention.
2. Renal infections.
3. Renal changes associated with toxaemia of pregnancy and eclampsia.
4. Acute renal failure.
5. Pregnancy and pre-existing chronic renal disease.
6. The incidence of other renal diseases during pregnancy.

PHYSIOLOGICAL CHANGES

Renal blood flow and glomerular filtration rate

By the fourth month renal blood flow has increased by about 50 per cent and glomerular filtration rate by 30 per cent. This rise is related to increasing concentrations of circulating placental lactogen which has a growth hormone like effect.

The increase in glomerular filtration rate together with the diminished protein breakdown of pregnancy cause the blood urea to be considerably lower than normal, e.g. 15 mg per 100 ml. Unless this increase in glomerular filtration rate and fall in blood urea is appreciated, a false impression of renal functional efficiency during pregnancy may be held. Either an underlying renal disease is unsuspected because the filtration rate and blood urea are within normal (i.e. non-pregnant) limits, or a sudden deterioration in renal function after pregnancy is erroneously considered to be evidence that pregnancy has injured the kidneys. If during pregnancy the glomerular filtration rate is lower than the "non-pregnant" normal rate, or the blood urea is raised above the normal "non-pregnant" concentration, it is evidence of considerable impairment of renal function, and perhaps extensive structural damage.

Glycosuria and lactosuria

Most women during pregnancy excrete an increased quantity of both glucose and lactose. Glycosuria is due to a lowered renal threshold for glucose reabsorption. Lactosuria is simply related to the presence of lactose in the mother's blood; as it is not reabsorbed by the tubules all that is filtered through the glomerulus appears in the urine.

After delivery glycosuria rapidly disappears and there is an increase in both the incidence of lactosuria and the amount that is excreted.

At one time glycosuria after the oral ingestion of glucose was suggested as a test of pregnancy.

Orthostatic proteinuria

The incidence of orthostatic proteinuria varies considerably; some reports state that it is as high as 20 per cent. It is probably caused by (1) an exaggeration of the normal mechanism for orthostatic proteinuria, i.e. a lordosis which rotates the liver forwards, thus compressing the inferior vena cava and causing a rise in renal venous pressure; and (2) uterine compression of the left renal vein as it crosses the midline. The first mechanism causes protein to be excreted through both ureters, whereas with the second, protein is present only on the left side. In order, therefore, to distinguish orthostatic from other causes of proteinuria, the urine should be tested for protein, after the patient has been lying on her side.

Ureteric and pelvic dilatation

After the third month of pregnancy the ureters and renal pelves are usually dilated. Initially this is due to a ureteric and pelvic atony, possibly caused by hormonal changes accompanying pregnancy. Paradoxically the atony is associated with hyperplasia of the ureteric muscles and an increase in the connective tissue within the ureteric walls. Later, as the uterus enlarges, it compresses the ureters at the pelvic brim; this mechanical obstruction is superimposed upon ureteric atony and the combination results in considerable ureteric dilatation. The ureters and pelves may contain more than 100 ml of urine. It is interesting that during this period of ureteric dilatation there is no vesico ureteric reflux. Normally the uterus is tilted towards the right side and, in consequence, it is usual to find the ureteric dilatation on the right to be greater than on the left. After delivery ureteric dilatation gradually subsides in about three months. These changes are more marked in primigravidae than in multiparae. They are probably due to the increased concentrations of circulating oestrogens. Male rats given diethylstilboestrol develop similar changes in their ureters to those seen in pregnant female rats, and at the same time their susceptibility to renal infection also rises.

Sodium and water retention

Throughout a normal pregnancy there is a continued retention of sodium, potassium and water. The bulk of this is sequestered into the uterus and its contents. The mechanism responsible for this retention is not clear. Many pregnant women have a high aldosterone secretion rate and it has been established that both estriol and estradiol can increase aldosterone secretion in normal non-pregnant women. Nevertheless sodium and water retention occurs normally in those women who do not have a rise in aldosterone secretion rate. There is some evidence that estradiol itself has a direct effect on renal tubular sodium reabsorption.

RENAL INFECTIONS

Acute pyelonephritis* is the most common complication of pregnancy. It occurs in about 2 per cent of all pregnancies and is responsible for a great deal of discomfort and distress, and a few immediate deaths both of the mother and the foetus.

Aetiology

About three-quarters of all cases of acute pyelonephritis of pregnancy occur in the 5 to 8 per cent of women who have *persistent* bacteriuria throughout pregnancy. Unfortunately it is not possible to identify this group by any other means than performing a quantitative urine culture. Nearly all are asymptomatic, nor is the presence of bacteriuria related to previous catheterisation, past symptoms of urinary tract disease, or white cell excretion rate, and it occurs equally among women with or without anaemia. The incidence of acute pyelonephritis in women with previously sterile urine often follows catheterisation of the bladder during or shortly after delivery.

The remarkable severity and persistence of pyelonephritis in pregnancy is probably due to the dilatation, atony and compression of the ureters (see above).

Clinical features

The incidence of acute pyelonephritis begins at the fourth month and continues well into the puerperium. Much of the incidence in the puerperium is due to catheterisation. About 15 per cent of women have some difficulty in initiating micturation in the first few days of the puerperium because of episiotomies, prolonged labour, etc. They are liable to be catheterised in order to relieve overdistention of the bladder. Symptomatically the infection is either bilateral or, when unilateral, it is usually on the right side. The physical signs and symptoms have been described on p. 307. Mild cases only complain of backache; they may admit to occasional feverish symptoms or pain on passing water with some reluctance, considering that such symptoms are normal in pregnancy. Some attacks may be associated with such severe vomiting that the patient is thought to be suffering from hyperemesis gravidarum.

As in all forms of renal infection the most helpful diagnostic features are

---

* Obstetricians sometimes call the usual type of acute renal infection in pregnancy an acute pyelitis, and reserve the term acute pyelonephritis for those extremely severe infections with gross impairment of renal function which are usually due to a staphylococcal organism. This is a misleading use of the English language.

rigors, fever, tenderness in the costo-vertebral angles, an increased number of urinary white cells and a significant number of organisms in the urine.

An intravenous pyelogram should only be performed if there is reason to believe that there is a calculus, an ectopic kidney, or there are recurrent infections difficult to control. The number of films should be strictly limited, for recent statistical evidence suggests that acute leukaemia in children may follow foetal exposure to diagnostic X-rays. A unilateral *left-sided* infection is particularly likely to be due to some additional disturbance of the renal tract, such as a calculus.

Differential diagnosis

It is important to stress that often in acute pyelonephritis of pregnancy there are no lower urinary symptoms. If therefore a pregnant woman has an unexplained fever the urine should be cultured immediately. On the other hand it is now well established that over 70 per cent of pregnant women who do complain of lower urinary symptoms have a sterile urine.

Treatment

PROPHYLACTIC. It is possible by routinely culturing the urine of all patients at the beginning of pregnancy, to identify those among whom most of the attacks of acute pyelonephritis will occur. A week's course of a suitable antibiotic (e.g. sulphadimidine) will abolish the bacteruria for the rest of the pregnancy in the majority of bacteruric women. In about 15 per cent of such women, however, the urine will either remain infected or become reinfected. Recurrent reinfection can usually be treated with nitrofurantoin 50 mg in the evening until the end of pregnancy. Those in whom the urine cannot be made sterile with one antibiotic should be given another or a combination of antibiotics until the urine is sterile, and then placed on to nitrofurantoin 50 mg in the evening until delivery. With these measures the incidence of disabling attacks of acute pyelonephritis can be considerably reduced. The administration of antibiotics does not harm the foetus or give rise to an increased incidence of neonatal jaundice.

It has been proposed that urine culture should be undertaken as a routine antenatal service, for it has been claimed that it not only lowers the incidence of acute pyelonephritis but that it also substantially diminishes the incidence of toxaemia of pregnancy and the peri-natal mortality rate. There is no doubt that at one time this was true in certain underdeveloped parts of Boston, Mass., and the West Indies which contained an impoverished population in which the overall incidence of toxaemia of pregnancy and prematurity were extremely high; and in those women who had persistent bacteruria it was even higher. In other parts of the world, however, such as London and Aberdeen, the incidence of toxaemia and prematurity is much lower and is no greater in untreated bacteruric women than in women with sterile urine. Sterilising the urine of women with bacteruria in London and Aberdeen therefore cannot

M§

lower the incidence of toxaemia or the prematurity rate. In Melbourne the overall incidence of prematurity is low and yet it is considerably greater among the bacteruric women, nevertheless, sterilising the urine of bacteruric women does not lower the incidence of prematurity. It is probable that the high prematurity rate of bacteruric women in Australia is due to the high incidence of structural damage of the kidneys among such women (see below). And that this in turn is due to the high consumption of phenacetin prevalent in Australia. There is no evidence that bacteruria of pregnancy increases the incidence of abortion early in pregnancy. The incidence of bacteruria in women who do abort is no greater than in women who do not abort.

It now appears therefore that unless the overall incidence of toxaemia and prematurity is high, such as in Boston, Mass., or the West Indies, the only benefit to be obtained from treating asymptomatic bacteruria of pregnancy is to reduce the incidence of acute pyelonephritis. Some authorities consider that this is not a sufficient return for the expense and inconvenience involved in culturing the urine of all pregnant women. They point out that nowadays acute pyelonephritis is easily treated and rarely leads to protracted admission to hospital. Others point out that (1) the expense and inconvenience of culturing the urine can be reduced by certain simplifications; (2) that acute pyelonephritis is sometimes followed by recurrent ill health for some months after delivery; and (3) that if acute pyelonephritis is not prevented, it has to be treated, and to do this effectively it is necessary to have efficient bacteriological facilities for following up the patients. It is suggested that such facilities are better used to prevent the attacks of acute pyelonephritis. Whatever the result of these deliberations there is no doubt that pregnant women who are known to suffer from a pre-existing renal disease should always have their urine cultured. Many of the objections raised are no longer relevant if one of the commercially available dip slides or filter paper techniques for culturing the urine are used. The whole procedure can be carried out in the antenatal clinic and only samples which are suspicious need be looked at by a bacteriologist.

CURATIVE. The treatment of acute pyelonephritis has been discussed on p. 310. The liability for the urine to become reinfected is particularly great in pregnancy (80 per cent within six months), and treatment with antibiotics should be continued until delivery and for one month thereafter. Very occasionally antibiotic treatment is unavailing, the patient's condition deteriorates rapidly and pregnancy has to be terminated.

Prognosis

Intravenous pyelograms performed after delivery show that in England 35 per cent of bacteruric women who have developed acute pyelonephritis have some structural renal abnormality including scarring and clubbing of calyces. Similar lesions are found in 14 per cent of bacteruric women who have not developed acute pyelonephritis. There is now little doubt, that most if not all these abnormalities precede the acute attack of pyelonephritis. It is probable that most of the claims that acute pyelonephritis of pregnancy causes extensive renal damage, followed eventually by chronic renal failure, hypertension and death have been based on patients with childhood chronic pyelonephritis (p. 316) who happen to have had acute pyelonephritis during pregnancy.

Geographical differences

It is interesting to note that the incidence of radiological abnormalities of the kidneys in bacteruric women differs considerably from one place to another. In London it is 18 per cent whereas in Melbourne it is 57 per cent. It is becoming clear that the whole subject of renal infection in pregnancy presents striking regional differences and that these should be kept in mind when discussing any aspect of the subject.

RENAL CHANGES IN TOXAEMIA OF PREGNANCY AND ECLAMPSIA

The term toxaemia of pregnancy is a semantic curiosity attached to an ill-defined syndrome of unknown cause; its most severe form is associated with hypertensive encephalopathic convulsions, when it is called eclampsia. There is no convincing evidence that toxaemia of pregnancy is due primarily to a disturbance of renal function, though the kidneys are involved together with many other organs. Only the renal structural and functional disturbances are discussed here.

Pathology

The microscopical appearances have been studied by renal biopsy before and after delivery. There are two changes evident and they are both situated in the glomeruli. The one seen most frequently consists of minimal endothelial cell proliferation with widespread conspicuous swelling of the cytoplasm of both the endo- and epithelial cells of the glomerular tufts, more marked in the endothelial cells. These changes diminish the lumen of the capillaries and give the glomeruli a "solid" appearance. They disappear rapidly after delivery.

The other glomerular change is seldom found and is always in combination with the one just described. It consists of focal thickenings of the basement membrane; it appears to be less reversible than the first.

In autopsy material from multiparae or elderly primiparae who have died from eclampsia small crescents of proliferated capsular cells can be seen in the glomeruli.

Discussion on the cause of the renal structural changes

It is likely that the initial abnormality in toxaemia of pregnancy is ischaemia of the placenta. This may be due either to vascular disease of the uterine arteries such as that associated with pre-existing hypertension, or to some less obvious cause such as circulating placental antibodies formed by the mother. In some way that is not clear placental ischaemia then causes the release of clot-promoting agents into the circulation which produce intravascular clotting. Fibrin and its breakdown products then accumulate on the surface endothelium of the vascular system including the glomerular capillaries where it is absorbed into the endothelial cells and causes them to swell and proliferate.

This sequence is supported by the following evidence. (1) There is both anatomical and functional evidence that the irrigation of the uterus by blood is impaired in toxaemia of pregnancy. (2) The blood of pregnant women contains an increased concentration of cryofibrinogen, and this rises considerably in toxaemia of pregnancy (and when pregnancy is complicated by infection). (3) Immuno-fluorescent studies on renal biopsies have shown that there is a striking accumulation of fibrinogen derivatives within the endothelial cells, whereas gamma globulin and complement are not demonstrable which provides strong evidence against an immunological basis for the glomerular lesion. (4) In some especially severe cases occlusive masses of fibrin are found in the glomerular capillaries, sometimes leading to cortical necrosis. (5) Glomerular lesions similar to those observed in toxaemia of pregnancy can be produced in rabbits by inducing a slow prolonged state of intravascular coagulation.

Renal function

It is a remarkable fact that the renal blood flow in toxaemia of pregnancy is frequently within normal limits, though there is wide variation both above and below normal. The commonest abnormality is a fall in glomerular filtration rate; it may fall to 50 ml/min without a decrease in renal blood flow. It is possible that the depression in glomerular filtration rate is due to the cytoplasmic swelling of the cells lining the glomerular tufts. The fall in filtration rate often bears no relation to the clinical severity of the toxaemia. After delivery there is a sudden rise in filtration rate and for a short time it may reach 250 ml/min; there is an accompanying diuresis and urine volumes up to 550 ml an hour have been described.

In severe eclampsia there is a generalised peripheral vasoconstriction, and as in all clinical conditions associated with generalised vasoconstriction it is particularly marked in the kidney. Renal ischaemia may be sufficiently prolonged and extensive to cause acute tubular necrosis and acute renal failure.

The oedema and oliguria of toxaemia in pregnancy have not been explained satisfactorily. The urinary excretion of ketogenic steroids and aldosterone is either normal or decreased. Measurement of total exchangeable sodium has given conflicting results. There is no agreement whether the oedema is due to sodium retention or to a shift of sodium.

Hypertension is a constant accompaniment of toxaemia of pregnancy. It has repeatedly been shown that it can be present without any detectable change in renal blood flow. It would seem, therefore, that the hypertension of toxaemia of pregnancy is not caused by an overall change in renal circulation, but it may still be related to some intrarenal circulatory disturbance.

Proteinuria nearly always occurs and presumably results from the structural changes in the glomeruli.

Clinical features

Toxaemia of pregnancy occurs most frequently in primigravidae and in women who have a persistent rise in blood pressure before the start of pregnancy.

The disease is characterised by hypertension, oedema and proteinuria. It is not an acute nephritic syndrome, for the jugular venous and right auricular pressure are usually normal, i.e. pulmonary venous congestion does not occur, except very occasionally in the terminal phase of eclampsia. Nor does it fit within the definition of a nephrotic syndrome, for again, with the exception of very severe cases, the plasma protein concentrations are relatively normal or are altered to only a minor extent, and proteinuria is never greater than 5 g 24 hours.

The onset takes place after the first twenty weeks of pregnancy and is most common in the last six. It can be predicted to a certain extent, for it occurs in those women who have put on weight too rapidly, though 50 per cent of these will have a normal pregnancy. The first symptoms may be headache or dizziness due to the rise in blood pressure, or there may be oedema, or the patient may have symptomless proteinuria. The upper normal limit of the blood pressure in pregnancy is about 120/80 mmHg and a rise above this level may precede the onset of oedema, or proteinuria, by many weeks. As the blood pressure rises there may be visual disturbances from vascular changes in the retinae; hypertensive encephalopathy is nearly always preceded by intense, boring frontal headache. In some cases there may be epigastric pain, sometimes of great severity. From the initial symptom to the first convulsion the syndrome may be telescoped into a matter of hours; fortunately the development of symptoms is usually slower. There is always some degree of oliguria. With the convulsions there may be temporary anuria, and very occasionally acute renal failure develops. Unless there is acute renal failure the specific gravity of the urine during a period of oliguria is high.

After delivery the symptoms and signs usually subside rapidly, though in exceptional cases the most prominent features of the disease may occur in the first two or three days of the puerperium.

Relation between clinical and structural features

Excluding those exceptional cases of eclampsia who develop acute renal failure from tubular necrosis and widespread arterionecrotic lesions, there seems to be little relation between the severity of the pathological lesions and the clinical picture; the changes in mild toxaemia and in eclampsia may be identical. There is a good correlation, however, between the histological changes and the plasma concentration of uric acid. The rise in uric acid is due to a simultaneous rise in plasma lactic acid which accelerates tubular reabsorption of uric acid and thus diminishes uric acid excretion (p. 89). The cause of the rise in lactic acid is obscure: it is probably related to ischaemia of the placenta.

Differential diagnosis

It is essential to exclude contamination of the urine by protein from vaginal discharge.

If persistent proteinuria is found before the twentieth week it is most unlikely to be due to toxaemia of pregnancy. At this time the most common causes of proteinuria are orthostatic proteinuria and chronic renal disease. Excluding acute pyelonephritis, which is not difficult to diagnose, other acute renal diseases are very rare during pregnancy (p. 363). Other causes of proteinuria include cardiac failure, severe anaemia and renal tuberculosis.

If the urine is not examined before the twentieth week, and proteinuria is found subsequently, all these causes of proteinuria must be considered as well as the probability of toxaemia of pregnancy.

Not many patients with toxaemia of pregnancy have a urinary infection. But a large proportion of women with radiological evidence of childhood chronic pyelonephritis develop toxaemia when pregnant.

Prognosis

The immediate prognosis in toxaemia in pregnancy is excellent, unless there are fits; the mortality of eclampsia varies between 10–40 per cent, one of the causes of death being acute renal failure.

The ultimate prognosis is difficult to assess. Following toxaemia of pregnancy some women develop a persistent rise in blood pressure, and their prognosis is then that of hypertension, including its effects on the kidney. This would seem to indicate that toxaemia of pregnancy may cause persistent hypertension. Nevertheless statistical evidence shows that the incidence of hypertensive vascular disease in women is the same whether or not they have borne children. The conclusion, which is generally accepted, is that persistent hypertension following toxaemia of pregnancy only develops in women who were inevitably bound to have a rise in blood pressure later, and that the toxaemia of pregnancy has only accelerated its onset. The situation is complicated further by the fact that in a few patients it has been demonstrated that persistent hypertension following toxaemia has been due to renal artery stenosis. It is clear that persistent hypertension following toxaemia should always be thoroughly investigated.

The incidence of persistent hypertension following toxaemia of pregnancy varies considerably in different series. One report states that it is 20 per cent following eclampsia and 40 per cent following non-convulsive toxaemia. This paradox is attributed to (1) the fact that non-convulsive toxaemia usually lasts longer than eclampsia, for there is a positive correlation between the duration of toxaemia and residual hypertension, and (2) the diagnosis of non-convulsive toxaemia is often uncertain and may include some patients who had hypertension before pregnancy who may, therefore, have essential hypertension.

There is no published evidence that toxaemia of pregnancy gives rise to chronic renal disease other than that which may accompany the subsequent hypertension. Occasionally, however, a patient whose urine is known to have been protein-free before pregnancy develops persistent proteinuria without hypertension after pregnancy, having had toxaemia during pregnancy. Biopsy of such patients several years later shows persisting structural alterations in the glomeruli, particularly of the basement membrane. The prognosis in these patients is not known.

When a woman has had non-convulsive toxaemia of pregnancy in her first pregnancy the incidence of toxaemia in the second pregnancy is about 30 per cent. If a multiparous woman has had non-convulsive toxaemia the incidence of a recurrence of toxaemia with a subsequent pregnancy is about 60 per cent. These figures are slightly less following eclampsia, and greater in women with persistent hypertension between pregnancies.

Treatment

Toxaemia of pregnancy is unlikely to occur in women who avoid putting on more than 5 lb in any one month or more than 10 lb in the last three months. If these limits are exceeded a low-salt, high-protein, low-calorie diet is given until the position has been readjusted.

Once toxaemia of pregnancy has declared itself the best treatment is bed rest, sedatives and a similar diet to that described above, except that it should be as salt-free as possible. Infection should be looked for and treated vigorously. If the blood pressure continues to rise, with increasing proteinuria and the development of retinal changes, hypotensive drugs or spinal anaesthesia can be tried while the effect of the salt restriction and bed rest are given time to take effect; if there is a continued and uncontrollable deterioration, pregnancy must be terminated. The treatment of hypertensive encephalopathy consists in sedation, lowering the blood pressure, and termination of pregnancy.

It is important to keep in mind that acute renal failure may develop, in order that its treatment may not be delayed.

ACUTE RENAL FAILURE DURING PREGNANCY

Acute renal failure either occurs early in pregnancy when it is usually due to induced abortion, or it occurs at the end of pregnancy, when it is a complication of pre-eclamptic toxaemia, accidental haemorrhage or post-partum haemorrhage.

Acute renal failure complicating abortion

The main cause is loss of blood, reduction in blood volume and intense renal ischaemia (p. 103). The frequency with which this eventually causes renal failure in abortions is presumably related to the prolonged period of renal ischaemia which occurs before qualified medical help is sought. Many of these patients suffer from pelvic sepsis, often with *Cl. welchii* or *Staph. aureus*. Death occurs in approximately half the cases and is nearly always due to sepsis, not to renal failure. "Cortical necrosis" (see below) is nearly always associated with septicaemia.

Acute renal failure in late pregnancy

Again the cause of the renal lesion is renal ischaemia resulting from haemorrhage, and intravascular coagulation. It is possible that in addition there may be a direct nervous vasoconstricting stimulus from the uterus to the kidneys

Acute tubular necrosis is much more common with accidental haemorrhage (approximately 12 per cent of all cases) than following postpartum haemorrhage, and yet the blood pressure remains unchanged or rises in the former and tends to fall in the latter. Possibly the compensatory renal vasoconstriction which accompanies the reduction in circulating blood volume following postpartum haemorrhage is not so great or so prolonged as in accidental haemorrhage. It is more likely, however, that the main factor is the increased intravascular coagulation which takes place in accidental haemorrhage. It is sometimes associated with microangiopathic haemolytic anaemia.

Occasionally eclampsia may cause acute renal failure because of widespread arteriolonecrotic lesions, similar in all respects to those found in malignant hypertension.

Death occurs in an uncertain number and is usually due to irreversible renal failure associated with extensive cortical necrosis.

Acute renal failure developing a few weeks after delivery

In this peculiar syndrome a woman develops acute renal failure and a cardio-myopathy two to five weeks after a normal pregnancy and delivery. There may also be epileptic fits and haemolytic anaemia. The glomerular capillaries show evidence of thrombosis and endothelial proliferation while the inter-lobular arteries show marked intimal thickening with occasional thrombi. Death from cardiac failure may occur, in spite of maintenance haemodialysis. Or the patient finally survives with advanced and irreversible chronic renal failure. The cause is probably intravascular coagulation.

Pathology

Ischaemic tubular necrosis may be focal as described on p. 159, or may be so extensive that the entire cortex is involved, when the condition is known as "cortical necrosis". In the more severe and extensive lesions the arteries are also necrosed and contain thrombi.

Clinical features, course and treatment

Diagnosis is often delayed because the focus of concern is initially on the poor circulatory state of the patient. The clinical features and treatment of acute renal failure have been described on p. 165.

One of the aims of treatment is to prevent the development of acute renal failure. In eclampsia the use of hypotensive drugs or caudal anaesthesia to produce a widespread vasodilatation will not only lower the blood pressure and control the convulsions, but will diminish the renal vasoconstriction and prevent tubular necrosis. Often the quantity of blood that has been lost is underestimated for the clinical signs of blood loss may be trivial. Quick, repeated, bedside blood volume measurements with small computerised machines can be very helpful. If uterine stretch is considered to be an important factor in the acute renal failure of accidental haemorrhage it would seem reasonable to rupture the membranes as soon as the diagnosis of accidental haemorrhage is made.

The importance of infection in acute renal failure following abortion is such that all these patients should be given large doses of penicillin and ampicillin on admission (i.e. immediately after a high vaginal swab has been obtained for culture). Neither pelvic infection early in pregnancy nor an enlarged uterus late in pregnancy is a contraindication to peritoneal dialysis provided the catheter is inserted high in the abdomen.

PREGNANCY IN RELATION TO PRE-EXISTING CHRONIC RENAL DISEASE

Opinions vary. Addis, after a long experience, stated that "There is no instance in which we can be sure that the renal lesion interfered with pregnancy. There is no evidence that any of them have been harmed by pregnancy." Other authors are less sanguine.

Effect of Chronic Renal Disease on Pregnancy

In patients without renal failure

This group includes women with proteinuria of varying severity with or without hypertension, mainly suffering from glomerular nephritis. A third will develop "pre-eclampsia", and in a third of these the foetus will not survive. Because of the dangers of accidental haemorrhage it is usual to terminate pregnancy, if the foetus is sufficiently large, at about the thirty-third week. The use of the term "pre-eclampsia" in patients with pre-existing proteinuria or hypertension is confusing. Presumably the authors who use such a term do so when hypertension develops when originally only proteinuria was present, or hypertension becomes worse.

In patients with renal failure

Such women tend to be sterile. If the blood urea is raised above 60 mg/ 100 ml in the first few months of pregnancy it is unlikely that there will be a live birth. The patients either abort early or develop accidental haemorrhage later. Eclampsia is uncommon.

Effect of Pregnancy on Chronic Renal Disease

In patients without renal failure

In the absence of hypertension pregnancy rarely if ever causes a deterioration of renal function in patients with glomerular nephritis. In the presence of hypertension however about half the patients will develop persistent deterioration of renal function. It is not clear whether this is due to inadequate control of the blood pressure. The proteinuria of diabetic nephropathy often increases during pregnancy but improves after delivery.

In patients with renal failure

With glomerular nephritis the issue is relatively clear cut. Either there is a sudden deterioration in renal function, with increased proteinuria and a rise in blood pressure before the twentieth week, or pregnancy causes no harm. When there is an exacerbation of the renal disease some permanent additional impairment of function remains thereafter.

With other renal diseases, such as chronic pyelonephritis or polycystic disease, the prognosis depends more directly and less mysteriously on whether or not renal infections are allowed to develop.

Management

If a woman with chronic renal disease is anxious to have a child and is aware of the risks involved, it is reasonable that she should try and become pregnant only if her blood pressure is normal and renal function is not less than 50 per cent of normal. Once pregnancy has begun, renal infections should be prevented (p. 353), and renal function, the urine deposit, the extent of proteinuria and the height of the blood pressure carefully watched. Pregnancy is discontinued at once if there is evidence of an exacerbation of renal disease.

Some women with hypertension without renal failure, with or without renal disease may insist on becoming pregnant. The outcome is unpredictable. In some of these women the blood pressure during pregnancy may become normal without hypotensive therapy and they have an uneventful delivery with a live infant at term. The majority of women however continue to have hypertension which becomes more pronounced. Such women either abort or have a miscarriage and the foetus dies. Nevertheless with obsessional attention to treatment it is possible to obtain live births even in this group in whom the blood pressure is raised. The blood pressure has to be lowered and kept below a diastolic of 90 mmHg. One of the most useful drugs is propranolol together with a diuretic. The patient must be seen at least once a week in the first six months and twice a week thereafter. If the blood pressure starts to rise in spite of treatment the patients should be put to bed, monitored at least twice a day and hypotensive treatment rapidly adjusted accordingly. The patient may have to stay in bed during the last two months of pregnancy. Labour should be induced as soon as possible.

Women with chronic renal disease and moderately well advanced renal failure (blood urea 100 mg/100 ml or more) should not become pregnant, for any further deterioration in renal function may be crippling. Pregnancies should be terminated if they occur.

Occasionally a pregnant woman presents with advanced renal failure and refuses to have the pregnancy terminated. A few such patients have been successfully managed with conservative treatment. Others have been haemo-dialysed until the birth of a live infant.

Unilateral Kidney

When there is only one kidney pregnancy should not be attempted until the functional and structural state of the kidney has been examined; it should be remembered that a nephrectomy is often performed for a renal disease which may be bilateral.

Ectopic Kidney

If both kidneys are ectopic the foetus should be delivered by Caesarean section. If there is only one ectopic kidney it is worth attempting a normal birth, but if there are likely to be any complications such as a breech presentation, it is best to do a Caesarean section.

INCIDENCE OF OTHER RENAL DISEASES IN PREGNANCY

Excluding renal infections, the onset of a new renal disease during pregnancy is very rare. Acute glomerular nephritis is the most common. There is no difficulty in diagnosis if attention is paid to the jugular venous pressure and the urinary deposit. The sudden onset of pulmonary congestion and rise in blood pressure excludes other causes of proteinuria and oedema. If the acute phase of the disease is safely negotiated pregnancy may continue normally with no permanent deterioration of renal function evident.

Very occasionally nephrotic glomerular nephritis may develop for the first time during pregnancy. The massive proteinuria, the normal blood pressure and jugular venous pressure distinguish the diagnosis. Such patients have occasionally been successfully treated with cortisone or prednisone and had a normal pregnancy.

BIBLIOGRAPHY

ANDRIOLE, V. T., and COHN, G. L. (1964). "The effect of diethylstilboestrol on the susceptibility of rats to haematogenous pyelonephritis." *J. clin. Invest.*, **43**, 1136.

BAILEY, R. R. (1969). "Asymptomatic bacteriuria in 200 women undergoing uterine curettage following abortion." *New Zealand med. J.*, **70**, No. 446, 13.

BUCHT, H. (1951). "Studies on renal function in man with special reference to glomerular filtration and renal plasma flow in pregnancy." *Scand. J. clin. Lab. Invest.*, **3**, suppl. 3.

CHADD, M. A., HUMPHREYS, D. M., LEATHER, H. M., and WILLS, S. A. (1967). "Urinary leucocyte excretion in hypertension in pregnancy." *Brit. med. J.*, **2**, 655.

CHESLEY, L. C., and COSGROVE, R. A. (1955). "A continuation follow-up study of eclampsic women." *Obstet. Gynec. (N.Y.)*, **5**, 697.

FAIRLEY, K. F., BOND, A. G., ADEY, F. D., HABERSBERGER, P., and McCREDIE, N. (1966). "The site of infection in pregnancy bacteriuria." *Lancet*, **1**, 939.

FLYNN, F. V., HARPER, C., and DE MAYO, P. (1953). "Lactosuria and glycosuria in pregnancy and the puerperium." *Lancet*, **2**, 698.

GOLDSMITH, H. J., DE BOER, C. H., MENZIES, D. H., CAPLAN, W., and McCANDLESS, A. (1971). "Delivery of healthy infant after five weeks' dialysis treatment for fulminating toxaemia of pregnancy." *Lancet*, **2**, 738.

GOWER, P. E., HASWELL, H., SIDAWAY, M. E., and DE WARDENER, H. E. (1968). "Follow up of 164 patients with bacteriuria of pregnancy." *Lancet*, **1**, 990.

HANDLER, J. S. (1960). "The effect of lactic acid infusion in promoting reduced net excretion rate of urate." *J. clin. Invest.*, **39**, 1526.

HERWIG, K. R., MERIRLL, J. P., JACKSON, R. L., and OKEN, D. E. (1965). "Chronic renal disease in pregnancy." *Am. J. Obst. & Gynec.*, **92**, 1117.

HYTTEN, F. E., and THOMPSON, A. M. (1968). Maternal physiological adjustments. In Assali, N. S. (Ed.). "Biology of Gestation. The Maternal Organism". Academic Press, New York, Vol. 1, Chapter 8, p. 449.

KENNEY, R. A., LAWRENCE, R. F., and MILLER, D. H. (1950). "Haemodynamic changes in the kidney in 'toxaemia of late pregnancy'." *J. Obstet. Gynaec. Brit. Emp.*, **57**, 17.

THE KIDNEY IN PREGNANCY (1968). "Clinical Obstetrics and Gynaecology." Edited by J. B. Nettles. Hoeber, U.S.A., II, No. 2, p. 459.

LITTLE, P. J. (1966). "The incidence of urinary infection in 5,000 pregnant women." *Lancet*, **2**, 925.

NORDEN, C. W., and KASS, E. H. (1968). "Bacteriuria of pregnancy—a critical reappraisal." *Ann. Rev. Med.*, **19**, 431.

POLLAK, V. E., and NETTLES, J. B. (1960). "The kidney in toxemia of pregnancy: a clinical and pathologic study based on renal biopsies." *Medicine* **39**, 469.

ROBB, C. A., DAVIS, J. O., JOHNSON, A. J., BLAINE, E. H., SCHNEIDER, E. G., and BAUMBER, J. S. (1970). "Mechanisms regulating the renal excretion of sodium during pregnancy." *J. clin. Invest.*, **49**, 871.

ROBSON, J. S., MARTIN, A. M., RUCKLEY, V. A., and MACDONALD, M. K. (1968). "Irreversible post partum renal failure." *Quart. J. Med.*, **37**, 423.

RODBARD, S. (editor) (1964). "Supplement on hypertension, blood pressure and toxaemia of pregnancy." *Circulation*, **30**, suppl. 2.

SHEEHAN, H. L., and MOORE, H. C. (1953). "Renal Cortical Necrosis and the Kidney of Concealed Accidental Haemorrhage." Blackwell Scientific Pubs., Oxford.

SIMS, E. A. H. (1971). The kidney in pregnancy. In "Diseases of the Kidney". Edited by M. B. Strauss and L. G. Welt. Little, Brown and Company, Boston, Chapter 32, p. 1155.

SIMS, E. A. (1965). "Kidney disease in pregnancy." *Ann. Rev. Med.*, **16**, 221.

SMITH, K., McCLURE BROWN, J. C., SHACKMAN, R., and WRONG, O. M. (1968). "Renal failure of obstetric origin." *Brit. Med. Bull.*, **24**, 49.

SOLER, N. G., and MALINS, J. M. (1971). "Prevalence of glycosuria in normal pregnancy. A quantitative study." *Lancet*, **1**, 619.

STUDD, J. W. W., and BLANEY, J. D. (1969). "Pregnancy and the nephrotic syndrome." *Brit. med. J.*, **1**, 276.

VASSALLI, P., and McCLUSKEY, R. T. (1965). "The coagulation process and glomerular disease." (Editorial.) *Amer. J. Med.*, **39**, 179.

WARDLE, E. N., and MENON, I. S. (1969). "Fibrinogen in pre-eclamptic toxaemia of pregnancy." *Brit. med. J.*, **1**, 625.

27

Thrombosis of the Renal Artery and Vein

Renal Artery Thrombosis

An uncommon condition which occurs particularly either in elderly patients with advanced atheromatous vascular disease who have previously suffered from cerebral or coronary thrombosis, or peripheral arterial disease or in patients with long standing auricular fibrillation who have not been placed on anticoagulants.

Pathology

The thrombus is either in the main renal artery or it may be confined to one or two of its branches. With occlusion of the main vessel the kidney becomes smaller, pale and bloodless. If, however, some of the renal veins become thrombosed at the same time there will be localised areas of congestive and interstitial oedema.

Clinical features

In contrast to renal vein thrombosis the outstanding presenting symptom is severe pain. The patient usually presents as an acute emergency, either abdominal, if the pain is in the flank or hypochrondrium, or cardiac or respiratory if it radiates to the lower chest. Nausea and vomiting are common.

There is acute tenderness in the renal angle and flank, but there may be no rigidity. Haematuria sometimes occurs, presumably if there is a concomitant thrombosis of the renal veins; usually there is only a modest proteinuria.

A straight X-ray of the abdomen often shows a calcified abdominal aorta and an I.V.P. confirms that the condition is renal, for no dye is secreted on the side of the pain and tenderness. At cystoscopy no urine is seen emerging from the ureteric orifice, but a retrograde pyelogram shows a normal pelvis and calcyces. Subsequently the affected kidney becomes smaller while the normal kidney becomes larger. An aortogram confirms that there is a reduced blood flow into the renal artery of the affected kidney.

Prognosis

The immediate prognosis is more concerned with the functional integrity of the other organs, e.g. whether cardiac failure was present before the renal arterial thrombosis occurred.

Usually when the patient survives, the artery recanalises and renal function returns to normal. Very occasionally there is only a partial recanalisation, this produces a renal artery stenosis with the sudden onset of severe hypertension.

Treatment

The patient's general condition usually precludes any measures other than those of anticoagulant therapy, rest and symptomatic treatment.

If the thrombosis occurs in a young subject, because of a localised structural anomaly of the renal artery, the kidney should be removed, particularly if the blood pressure begins to rise.

Renal Vein Thrombosis

Thrombosis of the renal veins is an extremely rare condition. The thrombus may either originate in the inferior vena cava and spread laterally into the renal veins, or it may begin in the smaller veins within the parenchyma of a diseased kidney and spread medially.

Pathology

The usual biopsy specimen, obtained several weeks or months after the onset of the thrombosis, usually shows merely a few insignificant and unspecific changes, and is only of value in a negative sense. On occasions the appearances are the same as those of extra-membranous glomerular nephritis with deposits on the outer surface of the basement membrane. Renal biopsies performed a few days after the onset, show extensive interstitial oedema with tubular separation.

At autopsy the diagnostic feature is the finding of a thrombus in the renal vein with, in long-standing cases, the presence of large collateral venous channel between the capsule of the kidney and the surrounding tissues. Microscopically the glomeruli appear normal and the tubules are unchanged unless there has been much proteinuria, when the tubule cells will contain lipoid material and collections of an eosin staining substance, though in some long-standing cases there is considerable tubular atrophy and tubular separation.

Inferior vena caval thrombosis may be spontaneous, or may be due to invasion by neoplasm, or to external compression. The most common renal disease to give rise to intrarenal venous thrombosis in adults is renal amyloidosis. In infants renal vein thrombosis is often associated with acute pyelonephritis.

Clinical features

These depend on the rapidity of the thrombotic process, whether it is unilateral or bilateral, and if it is secondary to inferior vena caval thrombosis.

When the thrombosis is rapid, bilateral, and has spread from the inferior vena cava, there is sudden back pain extending into the flanks with oliguria, proteinuria and haematuria leading to renal failure with oedema of the lower limbs and the anterior abdominal wall. Death may occur rapidly from acute renal failure.

If the thrombosis is bilateral but the inferior vena cava is unobstructed there is no oedema of the lower limbs. In adults this is usually due to renal disease. In infants acute bilateral renal vein thrombosis often follows acute gastro-enteritis, when the thrombosis is presumably caused by intense renal ischaemia in otherwise normal kidneys; or it may be associated with acute pyelone-phritis; there is usually sepsis elsewhere, and the sudden onset of flank tender-ness and pyuria with a swinging fever may suggest the diagnosis. Acute renal failure and death are the usual outcome. An intravenous pyelogram usually shows a delayed and diminished density of contrast on the affected side. Very occasionally, however, there may be a dense nephrogram lasting up to 24–36 hours. This probably occurs if the renal vein thrombosis causes severe renal damage. Notching of the upper ureter by enlarged collateral veins is often seen. These may disappear as the thrombus dissolves.

Occasionally the onset of bilateral renal vein thrombosis in adults (whether or not it is associated with inferior vena caval thrombosis) is less acute and may pass unnoticed, or the initial disturbance is followed by a large measure of recovery. Some of these cases may subsequently develop a nephrotic syndrome and, unless it is accompanied by evidence of inferior vena caval thrombosis with large collateral channels on the anterior abdominal wall, the thrombosis of the renal veins is unsuspected. In a few patients all evidence of renal disturbance may disappear except for the continued presence of a mild proteinuria. It is questionable whether *unilateral* renal vein thrombosis can give rise to *bilateral* histological lesions of immunological renal disease, together with a nephrotic syndrome; or whether such histological changes always precede the renal vein thrombosis.

The clinical course probably depends on the ability to recanalise the thrombus and establish a collateral venous circulation.

Diagnosis

The sudden onset of oliguria, proteinuria, raised blood urea, and severe oedema confined to the lower limbs, without evidence of cardiac failure or hypoproteinaemia, should make one suspect the condition. Collateral venous channels on the anterior abdominal wall do not appear until several weeks or months after the onset, but once they are evident they greatly simplify the diagnosis in those cases of inferior vena caval and renal vein thrombosis who have survived the acute phase. Radiological verification of renal vein throm-bosis, particularly when it is unilateral, is difficult. Momentary occlusion of the inferior vena cava, however, by two rubber balloons, one above the renal veins and the other below, together with a simultaneous injection of radio-opaque material into this partitioned segment of vena cava may delineate the renal veins, and the intrarenal venous system, with remarkable clarity.

Treatment

If the onset is recognised in adults it is reasonable to give anticoagulants; otherwise treatment is usually symptomatic. There are, however, some reports of the successful surgical removal of the clot.

In infants with pyelonephritis a nephrectomy may prevent the spread of the septic thrombus into the inferior vena cava and across to the other kidney.

BIBLIOGRAPHY

Renal artery thrombosis

EHRLICH, A., BRODOFF, B. N., RUBIN, I. L., and BERKMAN, J. I. (1953). "Malignant hypertension in a patient with renal artery occlusions." *Arch. intern. Med.*, **92**, 591.

FERGUS, J. N., JONES, N. F., and LEATHOMAS, M. (1969). "Kidney function after renal arterial embolism." *Brit. med. J.*, **2**, 587.

GOLDSMITH, E. I., FULLER, F. W., LAMBREW, C. T., and MARSHALL, V. F. (1968). *J. Urol.*, **99**, 366.

GOODMAN, H. L. (1952). "Malignant hypertension with unilateral renal artery occlusion." *New Engl. J. Med.*, **246**, 8.

WOLFFE, J. B., and DONNELLY, D. J. (1942). "Thrombosis of renal artery simulating coronary thrombosis." *J. Amer. med. Ass.*, **119**, 27.

Renal vein thrombosis

BARENBERG, L. H., GREENSTEIN, N. M., LEVY, W., and ROSENBLUTH, S. B. (1941). "Renal thrombosis with infarction complicating diarrhoea of the new born." *Amer. J. Dis. Child.*, **62**, 362.

BLAINEY, J. D., HARDWICKE, J., and WHITFIELD, A. G. (1954). "The nephrotic syndrome associated with thrombosis of the renal veins." *Lancet*, **2**, 1208.

CORNOG, J. L., RAWSON, A. J., KARP, L. A., and ARVAN, D. A. (1970). "Immunofluorescent and ultrastructural study of the renal glomerulus in renal vein thrombosis." *Lab. Invest.*, **22**, 101.

DUNCAN, A. W., SCHORR, W., CLARK, F., and KERR, D. N. S. (1970). "Unilateral renal vein thrombosis and nephrotic syndrome." *J. Urol.*, **104**, 502.

McCLELLAND, C. Q., and HUGHES, J. P. (1950). "Thrombosis of the renal vein in infants." *J. Paediat.*, **36**, 214.

MILLER, G., HOYT, J. C., and POLLOCK, B. E. (1954). "Bilateral renal vein thrombosis and the nephrotic syndrome." *Amer. J. Med.*, **17**, 856.

MORRIS, J. F., GINN, H. G., and THOMPSON, D. D. (1963). "Unilateral renal vein thrombosis associated with the nephrotic syndrome." *Amer. J. Med.*, **34**, 867.

POLLAK, V. E., PIRANI, C. L., SESKIND, C., and GRIFFEL, B. (1966). "Bilateral renal vein and electron microscopic studies of a case with complete recovery after anticoagulant therapy." *Ann. Intern. Med.*, **65**, 1056.

RICHET, G., GILLOT, C., VAYSSE, J., and MEYEROVITCH, C. A. (1965). "La thrombose isolée de la veine rénale." *Presse Medicale*, **73**, 2035.

ROSENMANN, E., POLLAK, V. E., and PIRANI, C. L. (1968). "Renal vein thrombosis in the adult. A clinical and pathological study based on renal biopsies." *Medicine*, **47**, 229.

STEINER, R. E. (1957). "Venography in relation to the kidney." *Brit. med. Bull.*, **13**, 64.

28

Haemoglobinuria and Myoglobinuria

HAEMOGLOBINURIA is the term used for the appearance of free haemoglobin in the urine. It follows haemolysis of red cells, either in the blood stream or in the urine.

Free haemoglobin is about the biggest naturally occurring molecule that can pass freely through the normal glomerular membrane (mol wt 68,000). Haemoglobin in plasma is normally bound to protein and is present in a concentration of about 5 mg/100 ml. In a normal individual there is sufficient haemoglobin binding protein (haptoglobins) to bind concentrations of haemoglobin up to 100–125 mg/100 ml. The bound haemoglobin does not pass through the glomerulus. The unbound or free form of haemoglobin passes readily through the glomerulus, some is reabsorbed in the proximal tubule, and the rest promptly appears in the urine. Tubular reabsorption of haemoglobin is always associated with haemosiderinuria, for as the haemoglobin is processed through the tubule cell some of the molecule is converted into haemosiderin and excreted into the urine. Haemosiderinuria will therefore be present when there is free haemoglobin in the plasma whether or not there is haemoglobinuria.

Myohaemoglobin is a muscle protein with a molecular weight of 17,000; it is freely filtered through the glomerulus, and little seems to be reabsorbed by the tubule; it first appears in the urine when the plasma concentration is about 10 mg/100 ml, and its rate of excretion is extremely rapid. For this reason it is rarely detected in the blood.

Methods of Identification

Haemoglobin and myohaemoglobin

These can be identified in solution, either spectroscopically or by the colour that is produced when they react with tolidine. A few milligrammes of purified tolidine hydrochloride are dissolved in 5 ml of glacial acetic acid; 1 ml of this solution and 1 ml of freshly prepared hydrogen peroxide are added to 2 ml of urine. The presence of haemoglobin or myohaemoglobin in considerable amounts will turn the urine blue; a lesser amount will only produce a green colour. If, in the presence of such a positive test in the urine, a simultaneous sample of blood is obtained and centrifuged and the supernatant plasma is pink the material in the urine is haemoglobin whereas if the plasma is not pink the urine contains myoglobin.

Haemosiderin

In contrast to haemoglobin and myohaemoglobin which are in solution, haemosiderin in the urine is present in particulate form, either in disintegrating tubule cells or as amorphous debris. The test for haemosiderinuria consists, therefore, in using the Prussian blue reaction to stain the urine sediment. About 20 ml of urine is centrifuged and all but 1 ml of the supernatant fluid is discarded. 1 ml of 5 per cent hydrochloric acid and 0·5 ml of a 10 per cent aqueous solution of potassium ferrocyanide are then added to the 1 ml of urine in which the deposit has been resuspended. A drop is then examined under the microscope, when haemosiderin will appear as deep blue flecks lying free or within the tubule cells and casts.

Renal Changes Associated with Haemoglobinuria

Changes associated with acute haemoglobinuria

Large amounts of haemoglobin have been given experimentally both to normal man and animals. There are either no adverse effects on the kidneys or a transient reduction in glomerular filtration rate. Renal blood flow is unchanged through PAH clearance falls. There is also a transient fall in urine flow.

Under clinical conditions, however, haemoglobinuria is occasionally associated with acute renal failure. This is because the most common cause of acute renal failure associated with haemoglobinuria is the administration of incompatible blood. Though the associated haemoglobinuria facilitates the onset of the acute renal failure by blocking the collecting ducts (see below) the main determinant of the failure is the presence of the stroma of the destroyed incompatible red cells in the circulation. The patient's antibody fixes onto the blood group antigen on the membrane of the incompatible erythrocyte membrane to form a complex which causes intense renal ischaemia and acute renal failure. In addition to this immunological disturbance several other closely connected factors are responsible for the renal failure that follows clinical haemoglobinuria. Pre-existing oligaemia or dehydration are usually present, which causes renal vasoconstriction with an acute reduction in glomerular filtration rate. There is also a high concentration of circulating anti-diuretic hormone (ADH). This combination causes a maximal reabsorption of water from the glomerular filtrate so that the haemoglobin in the tubule lumen is highly concentrated; it then precipitates and causes obstruction of the nephron.

The pathological changes have been described in Section 12. There are focal areas of tubular necrosis, haemcasts and occasional collections of interstitial inflammatory cells. Large amounts of haemosiderin may be found in the tubule cells.

Changes associated with chronic haemoglobinuria

There are two functional changes; proteinuria and persistent haemosiderin-uria. Structurally the accumulation of haemosiderin in the tubule cell appears to be the only change which is specifically due to the haemoglobinuria. In addition, haemoglobin appears in the urine at lower plasma concentration of haemoglobin than in acute haemoglobinaemia. Following several haemo-globinuric crises haemoglobin may appear in the urine when the plasma concentration is only 25 mg/100 ml. This is because the normal rate of production of haemoglobin binding protein is insufficient to keep up with the large quanti-ties of haemoglobin that are liberated.

Aetiology

The following conditions may cause haemoglobinuria:

FOLLOWING INTRAVASCULAR HAEMOLYSIS:

1. Exercise: (*a*) Very strenuous exercise.
            (*b*) March haemoglobinuria.
2. Mismatched transfusion.
3. Paroxysmal nocturnal haemoglobinuria.
4. Blackwater fever.
5. Hypotonicity of the plasma (prostatic surgery).
6. Thermal and chemical injuries.
7. Paroxysmal cold haemoglobinuria.
8. Heat stress.

Other common causes of haemolysis, such as congenital spherocytosis or acquired haemolytic anaemia due to abnormal serum antibodies, rarely cause haemoglobinuria, for the rate of destruction is slower and the site of haemolysis is in the reticulo-endothelial system.

FOLLOWING HAEMOLYSIS IN THE URINE:

1. Any cause of haematuria when the specific gravity of the urine is below 1·007.
2. Renal infarction.

HAEMOGLOBINURIA FOLLOWING INTRAVASCULAR HAEMOLYSIS

Exercise

Any normal person who undergoes sufficiently severe and prolonged strenuous exercise will have haemoglobinuria and proteinuria. This has been shown particularly in marathon runners. It is a benign complication of strenuous exercise, with no late sequelae.

There are in addition certain individuals who develop considerable haemoglobinuria and proteinuria upon performing any moderate exercise, e.g. a brisk walk, or a short run. The cause of the phenomenon is unexplained. It is due to intravascular haemolysis which only occurs in the upright posture; vigorous exercise taken in the horizontal posture does not produce haemoglobinuria. It is a benign condition sometimes associated with increased aminoaciduria, and is known as March haemoglobinuria. There is no treatment. There are spontaneous fluctuations in the tendency to haemolyse; when relapses occur physical exercise should be curtailed. They can sometimes be prevented by putting sponge rubber insoles into the shoes, the implication being that haemolysis may result from damage to red cells in the soles of the feet.

Mismatched Transfusion

In temperate climates, this is the most common cause of haemoglobinuria to be followed by acute renal failure. Plasma concentrations of haemoglobin may rise to 1,000 mg/100 ml or more; there is fever, shivering, severe pains in the back, hypotension and discoloured urine.

Transfusions are most frequently given because of recent loss of blood. If, when blood is being administered, the patient develops symptoms which suggest that haemolysis is taking place, the transfusion should be stopped immediately. A sample of the *patient's blood* is then centrifuged and the supernatant plasma examined by naked eye for the presence of haemoglobin. If the plasma is not pink, then haemolysis is not the cause of the patient's symptoms and the administration of blood should be continued with a fresh bottle of blood. The previous bottle may have contained some other protein which caused the patient's reaction; it may, for example, have been infected. This is insufficient reason for abandoning the attempt to replace the lost blood.

If, however, the plasma clearly contains haemoglobin, then no further blood transfusions should be given. It is essential nevertheless to try and overcome the renal vasoconstriction of the oligaemia, and a plasma expander such as Dextran should be given in as large amounts as possible, e.g. about one to two litres. If this causes severe anaemia (as opposed to oligaemia) the patient should be given oxygen, for by increasing the plasma oxygen tension there may be sufficient improvement in his general condition to influence the extent of renal damage. It has been claimed that acute renal failure following mismatched transfusion can be avoided or cut short by immediate exchange transfusion. Cannulae are placed in the radial artery and cephalic vein, and the exchange begun with a litre of a plasma expander. It is continued with properly cross-matched blood. The duration of the exchange is determined by the concentration of the circulating haemoglobin in the plasma. An exchange of 5 to 8 litres can reduce the circulating concentration from about 800 mg to 100 mg/ml. In addition to eliminating the haemoglobin, exchange transfusion has added advantages in that it removes the circulating immune complexes and it supplies large quantities of fresh haemoglobin binding protein, so that a high proportion of the haemoglobin that remains is bound to protein and not filtrable.

Paroxysmal Nocturnal Haemoglobinuria

This is a rare disease characterised by an acquired abnormality of the red cells which greatly shortens their survival. Unlike most other causes of abnormal red cell destruction the cells in paroxysmal nocturnal haemoglobinuria are destroyed in the plasma, as opposed to the reticulo-endothelial system. This gives rise to high plasma concentrations of haemoglobin. The haemolytic process is particularly severe during sleep, so that the urine may be purple in the morning but a normal colour by evening. If the patient sleeps during the day the process is reversed. It has been demonstrated that the acceleration of haemolysis that occurs during sleep is not due to any accompanying change in plasma pH that may occur at that time.

The disease becomes manifest usually between the ages of 20 and 40, and occurs equally in both sexes. The tendency to haemolyse fluctuates, and during relapses haemoglobinaemia is continuous, though haemoglobinuria comes on in sudden sharp attacks. In addition to the discoloured urine these acute episodes are associated with headache, backache, muscular and abdominal pains. Acute haemolytic crises are sometimes brought on by mild infections. There may be severe anaemia and there is a continuous reticulocytosis; eventually the patient develops a pale brown pigmentation. Occasionally there may be remissions of a few weeks or months when the total blood haemoglobin concentration returns to normal, but haemosiderinuria continues uninterruptedly. Death usually occurs from thrombosis of visceral veins including the mesenteric, splenic and renal.

The anaemia cannot be treated with transfusions of ordinary blood, for these cause an intense haemolysis of the *patient's* red cells. This reaction is due to some substance present in the donated plasma, and can be avoided by giving red cells washed and suspended in saline.

Blackwater Fever

This complication of malignant tertian malaria usually occurs in those who have previously been treated with antimalarial drugs, particularly quinine, either prophylactically or for recurrent attacks of malaria. There is a sudden and severe haemolysis of unknown cause, sometimes followed by acute renal failure.

Hypotonicity of Plasma

Transurethral resections of the prostate are usually carried out with intermittent washouts of the bladder and urethra with water. If much water is absorbed during this procedure there may be haemolysis near the site of absorption, where the plasma osmolality is grossly reduced; there is haemoglobinaemia and, occasionally, haemoglobinuria; sometimes acute renal failure may develop.

Thermal and Chemical Injuries

Patients with severe burns may develop haemoglobinaemia and haemoglobinuria from destruction of the red cells contained in or near the affected areas. Acute renal failure occurs quite frequently and, though this is mainly due to renal ischaemia from the reduced blood volume, it is obvious that a superimposed haemoglobinaemia will only make its development more likely.

Arsine causes spherocytosis and acute haemolysis. Death from severe anaemia may occur a few hours later. The gas is produced when certain metals and acids containing arsenic come into contact.

Other chemicals which sometimes cause severe haemolysis and haemoglobinuria include naphthalene (moth balls), sulphonamides, and mephanesin.

Paroxysmal Cold Haemoglobinuria

This condition is characterised by sudden attacks of haemolysis which follow the cooling of a part or the whole of the body. It is due to an auto-haemolysin which only becomes attached to the red cells at body temperatures below normal. When such red cells circulate to parts of the body with a normal temperature they are haemolysed. Severe attacks are associated with rigors, fever and anaemia; acute renal failure can occur.

This disorder occurs in congenital and aquired syphilis, and sometimes follows certain acute infections such as "virus pneumonia".

Heat Stress

This condition is due to a combination of heat stress and physical exercise. It is most often seen in recruits training in the summer. There is diffuse destruction of muscle with raised serum aldolase, lactic dehydrogenase and serum glutamic oxaloacetic transaminase, with normal liver function tests. Acute renal failure develops together with persistent fever, in the absence of infection. Hypercatabolism and hyperkalaemia during the period of anuria are particularly striking. The kidneys are enlarged but show no lesions of the glomeruli or of tubular necrosis. The most consistent finding is the presence of pigmented casts in the lumina of the distal tubules, the collecting ducts and the thin limb of the loops of Henle.

HAEMOGLOBINURIA FOLLOWING HAEMOLYSIS IN THE URINE

If there is haematuria and the urine concentration falls below approximately S.G. 1·007 the red cells will haemolyse and there will be free haemoglobin in the urine. This is only important as a diagnostic trap. It will be recognised if the urine specific gravity is measured, and the deposit examined microscopically for red cells and casts.

It has been reported that acute renal infarction may be associated with unilateral haemoglobinuria.

MYOGLOBINURIA

Renal changes associated with myoglobinuria

There is no doubt that myoglobinuria may by itself cause acute renal failure. This has been clearly demonstrated in a patient who was being extensively investigated in hospital. Myoglobinuria could be induced by exercise. Following a particularly severe bout of exercise the patient developed acute renal failure and was oliguric for 14 days. Fortunately he recovered.

Usually when acute renal failure develops in combination with myoglobinuria the cause of the failure is as obscure and complicated as in haemoglobinuria. For instance, myoglobinaemia, myoglobinuria and acute renal failure can occur in crush injuries. But injuries are associated with acute renal failure in the absence of myoglobinuria. The importance of the myoglobinuria in the aetiology of acute renal failure following injury has always been, and is likely to remain, problematical.

The cause of the renal failure which follows myoglobinuria is not clear. Widespread tubular obstruction must be one of the factors, for casts of precipitated myoglobin can be seen in the tubular lumens.

Clinical features

Myoglobinuria results from rapid destruction of muscle. This may follow some obvious cause such as crush injuries, high voltage shock or localised muscle necrosis due to postural pressure during coma (e.g. gas poisoning, alcoholic intoxication, or hypothermia); it has also been described with sudden arterial occlusion and after severe convulsions. The other causes of acute muscle destruction are various biochemical disturbances which are not understood. One is said to be due to allergy to sea food, another is a variant of muscular dystrophy; and the most common is that known as idiopathic paroxysmal myoglobinuria.

Idiopathic paroxysmal myoglobinuria

The tendency to attacks fluctuates, but it is unusual to have more than one attack a year. It is usually precipitated by strenuous exercise. The patient wakes up complaining of severe pain and stiffness in those muscles which were involved in the exercise, and that his urine is dark brown. On examination, the affected muscles are firm, tender and exquisitely painful upon being stretched. Walking may not be possible. The urine is dark but clear. The diagnosis can be made in the ward by finding that the substance in the urine is tolidine positive, i.e. that the urine contains large quantities of either haemoglobin or myohaemoglobin. If the plasma has a normal colour it follows that the substance in the urine is myoglobin for if it were haemoglobin the plasma would be pink from haemoglobinaemia. Myoglobin is never present in the plasma in sufficient quantities to discolour it, for as it is not bound to protein and easily filtered at the glomerulus, it is rapidly excreted.

BIBLIOGRAPHY

Haemoglobinuria

BLACKBURN, C. R. B., HENSLEY, W. J., KERR GRANT, D., and WRIGHT, F. B. (1954). "Studies on intravascular haemolysis in man. The pathogenesis of the initial stages of acute renal failure." *J. clin. Invest.*, **33**, 825.

CROSBY, W. H. (1953). "Paroxysmal nocturnal haemoglobinuria. Relation of the clinical manifestations to underlying pathogenic mechanisms." *Blood*, **8**, 769.

GOLDBERG, M. (1962). "Acute haemoglobinuric renal failure without ischaemia." *J. clin. Invest.*, **41**, 2112.

HAM, T. H. (1955). "Haemoglobinuria." *Amer. J. Med.*, **18**, 990.

HUTT, M. P., REGER, J. F., and NEUSTEIN, H. B. (1961). "Renal pathology in paroxysmal nocturnal haemoglobinuria." *Amer. J. Med.*, **31**, 736.

LANDSTEINER, E. K., and FINCH, C. A. (1947). "Haemoglobinaemia accompanying transurethral resection of the prostate." *New Engl. J. Med.*, **237**, 310.

LATHEM, W. (1959). "The renal excretion of haemoglobin; regulatory mechanisms and the differential excretion of free and protein-bound haemoglobin." *J. clin. Invest.*, **38**, 652.

LIPPMAN, R. W. (1957). "Urine and the Urinary Sediment." 2nd ed. Charles C. Thomas, Springfield, Ill.

McDONALD, R. K., MILLER, J. H., and ROACH, E. B. (1951). "Human glomerular permeability and tubular recovery values for haemoglobin." *J. clin. Invest.*, **30**, 1041.

MACKENZIE, G. M. (1929). "Paroxysmal haemoglobinuria, a review." *Medicine*, **8**, 159.

MILLER, J. H., and McDONALD, R. K. (1951). "The effect of haemoglobin on renal function in the human." *J. clin. Invest.*, **30**, 1033.

SCHMIDT, P. J., and HOLLAND, P. V. (1967). "Pathogenesis of the acute renal failure associated with incompatible transfusion." *Lancet*, **2**, 1169.

SCHRIER, R. W., HENDERSON, H. S., TISHER, C. G., and TANNEN, R. L. (1967) "Nephropathy associated with heat stress and exercise." *Ann. Intern. Med.*, **67**, 356.

SPICER, A. J. (1970). "Studies on March haemoglobinuria." *Brit. med. J.*, **1**, 155.

SUSSMAN, R. M., and KAYDEN, H. J. (1948). "Renal insufficiency due to paroxysmal cold hemoglobinuria." *Arch. intern. Med.*, **82**, 598.

YUILE, C. L., VAN ZANDT, T. F., ERVIN, D. M., and YOUNG, L. E. (1949). "Haemolytic reactions produced in dogs by transfusion of incompatible dog blood and plasma." *Blood*, **4**, 1232.

Myoglobinuria

BLONDHEIM, S. H., MARGOLIASH, and SHAFIR, E. (1958). "Test of myoglobinuria." *J. Amer. med. Ass.*, **197**, 453.

HED, R. (1955). "Myoglobinuria in man with special reference to familial form." *Acta med. scand.*, suppl. 303.

SPAET, T. H., ROSENTHAL, M. C., and DAMESHEK, W. (1954). "Idiopathic myoglobinuria in man." *Blood*, **9**, 881.

WHEBY, M. S., and MILLER, H. S., Jr. (1960). "Idiopathic paroxysmal myoglobinuria." *Amer. J. Med.*, **29**, 599.

29

Porphyria

PORPHYRIA is a rare and often familial disorder of porphyrin metabolism which results in widespread abnormalities, particularly in the skin, gastro-intestinal tract and central nervous system. Frequently there are acute exacerbations which may be associated with renal disturbances.

Pathology

Porphyrins form part of the haemoglobin molecule. In porphyria their metabolism is disturbed, so that their concentration in the blood rises and they are excreted in increased quantities both in the urine and faeces. Several types of porphyrins are involved, but during an acute attack there is one, porphobilinogen, which is always present in large amounts.

Porphobilinogen is a colourless chromogen. Its presence, however, can sometimes be suspected on naked eye examination of the urine, for its break-down products on standing give the urine an orange or nectarine-like colour; this is usually overlooked for it is confused with the appearance of a concentrated urine. The presence of porphobilinogen is confirmed with Ehrlich's reagent (the same which is used for detecting the presence of urobilinogen). Both urobilinogen and porphobilinogen give a red colour within 20 sec; they are then differentiated by adding chloroform; if the red colour remains outside the chloroform the colour is due to porphobilinogen; if it goes into the chloroform the colour is due to urobilinogen.

Frequently, acute porphyria is associated with an increased excretion of other porphyrins which may turn the urine dark purple.

At autopsy large amounts of porphyrins can be identified in the tubule cells. These probably account for the disturbance of tubular function.

Clinical features of acute porphyria

Acute prophyria is often provoked by the administration of barbiturates. Its main clinical features are abdominal pain, constipation, tachycardia, hyper-tension and peripheral neuritis. Later, there may be coma, generalised flaccid paralysis and jaundice. In addition the most advanced cases develop an uncontrolled diuresis with extensive loss of sodium, potassium, chloride and water which may cause circulatory collapse and death. Acute intermittent porphyria is one cause of "inappropriate secretion of antidiuretic hormone".

N

Treatment

It is imperative that barbiturates, methyl dopa, sulphonamides and griseo-fulvin should not be given to patients who suffer from porphyria. To make sure of this the patient should be given a card on which it is clearly stated that she is suffering from porphyria and that these drugs, particularly barbiturates, must not be administered, however anxious and mentally disturbed the patient may appear.

Haemodialysis is a useful way to treat acute porphyria whether or not there is an associated acute renal failure, for it lowers the concentration of circulating porphyrins. Otherwise it is important to replace rapidly the water and electrolytes which may be aggravating the deterioration of renal function.

BIBLIOGRAPHY

EALES, L. *et al.* (1963). "The porphyrias." *South African J. clin. and lab. Med.,* **9,** 5, 81, 126, 143, 151, 162, 190, 347.

GOLDBERG, A., and RIMMINGTON, C. (1955). "Experimentally produced porphyria in animals." *Proc. Roy. Soc. B,* **143,** 257.

LINDER, G. C. (1947). "Salt metabolism in acute porphyria." *Lancet,* **2,** 649.

NIELSEN, B., and THORN, N. A. (1965). "Transient excess urinary excretion of antidiuretic material in acute intermittent porphyria with hyponatraemia and hypomagnesaemia." *Amer. J. Med.,* **38,** 345.

PRUNTY, F. T. G. (1949). "Sodium and chloride depletion in acute porphyria with reference to the status of adrenal corticol function." *J. clin. Invest.,* **28,** 690.

REES, H. A., GOLDBERG, A., COCHRANE, A. L., WILLIAMS, M. J., and DONALD, K. W. (1967). "Renal haemodialysis in porphyria." *Lancet,* **I,** 919.

WATSON, C. L., and SCHWARTZ, S. (1941). "Simple test for urinary porphobilinogen." *Proc. Soc. exp. Biol. (N.Y.),* **47,** 393.

WHITTAKER, S. R. F., and WHITEHEAD, T. P. (1956). "Acute and latent porphyria." *Lancet,* **I,** 547.

30

The Kidney, Gout, and Uric Acid

ABNORMALITIES of uric acid metabolism associated with a rise in plasma uric acid can cause chronic or acute renal failure. On the other hand abnormalities in renal function can cause a rise or fall in plasma uric acid.

Structural changes associated with hyperuricaemia

Chronic hyperuricaemia can cause chronic renal failure; the following changes are seen:

(*a*) Very occasionally there is an easily demonstrable deposition of urates within the renal parenchyma.
(*b*) Interstitial nephritis.
(*c*) Nephrosclerosis.
(*d*) Uric acid stones.

Urates are found in the interstitial spaces. They cause necrosis of the tubules in the immediate vicinity of the deposits, and are surrounded by focal concentrations of inflammatory cells. Very rarely the deposits can become sufficiently large to be macroscopically recognisable tophi. They are found particularly in the tip of the pyramids. The predominant histological abnormality is one of interstitial nephritis (usually called "chronic pyelonephritis" (p. 299). The vascular lesions are those sclerotic changes found in chronic hypertensive vascular disease, but hypertension is *not* essential for their presence. Uric acid stones contribute to the destruction of the kidneys by causing obstruction, and precipitating infection.

Acute hyperuricaemia can cause acute renal failure. This is due to precipitation of urates in the lumen of the tubules, the calyces and ureters. It only occurs when the plasma concentration of uric acid is extremely high.

Effect of hyperuricaemia on renal function

In man, a brief intravenous infusion of urates sufficient to cause a transient rise of plasma uric acid can cause a reversible depression of glomerular filtration.

A persistent rise in plasma uric acid is associated with a gradual retention of uric acid, and the deposition of uric acid in the tissues. This causes a gradual deterioration of renal function which may take 10 to 20 years to become important. The number of patients with "gout" who die of renal failure is uncertain. It is probably around 10 to 20 per cent.

A less prolonged persistent rise in plasma uric acid occurs in leukaemia, polycythaemia, congenital haemolytic anaemia, myelomatosis, and lymphosarcoma when it is due to the high turnover of cells containing large nuclei. The patient usually succumbs before the rise in plasma uric acid causes any detectable impairment in renal function. Occasionally, however, acute renal failure may be precipitated by treatment. This follows either the administration of cytotoxic drugs, or the beginning of radiotherapy. There is then an enormous rise in plasma uric acid (e.g. up to 50 mg/100 ml) because of the widespread destruction of cells; the large quantities of filtered uric acid precipitate in the tubules causing acute obstruction. Very rarely a previously healthy person, not on any treatment, may present with a rapid onset of renal failure due to a spontaneous high plasma uric acid occurring at the onset of leukaemia.

Effect of renal function on plasma uric acid

In some patients with persistent hyperuricaemia the rise in plasma uric acid is due to a selective impairment of the kidney to excrete uric acid. Initially the glomerular filtration rate is normal. Many of these patients also have an increased production of uric acid and have therefore considerable rises in their

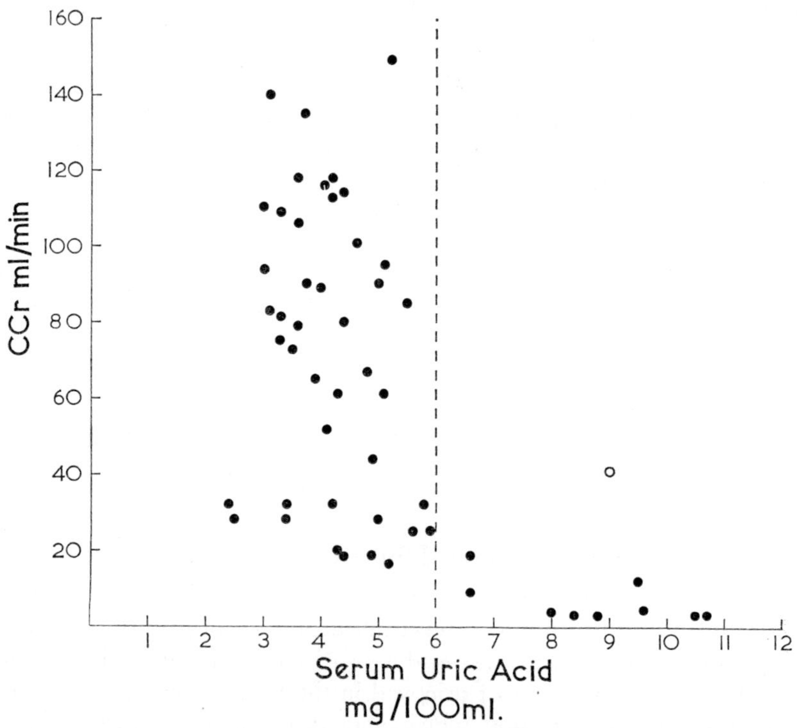

FIG. 30.1. Creatinine clearance plotted against plasma uric acid in women admitted to hospital; ○ = patients with a history of gouty arthritis; ● = patients with no history of gouty arthritis. (Pollard, A. C., personal communication.)

plasma concentration of uric acid. This group includes those with acute arthritis (gout) and those with familial hyperuricaemia without arthritis.

A similar selective impairment in the ability to excrete uric acid, but without overproduction of uric acid, occurs in a number of other conditions where it may cause a mild rise in plasma uric acid. It is probable that in all these conditions the kidney's inability to excrete uric acid is due to a raised plasma lactic acid which is a known inhibitor of uric acid excretion. This phenomenon occurs in a proportion of patients with "essential hypertension", myxoedema, toxaemia of pregnancy, glycogen disease, ketotic conditions such as starvation and following the ingestion of alcohol.

The ingestion of pyrazinamide, pempidine, mecamylamine and many diuretics, including particularly chlorothiazide and frusemide also directly inhibit tubular secretion of uric acid and may cause quite brisk rises in plasma uric acid.

The advent of renal functional deterioration in a person who already has an impaired ability to excrete uric acid will aggravate the uric acid retention and cause the rise in plasma uric acid to be more pronounced. But the development of renal failure in persons with no previous impairment in the ability to excrete uric acid does not cause a rise in plasma uric acid until the creatinine clearance is below 20 ml/min (Fig. 30.1).

On rare occasions acute poisoning with some exogenous substance may so damage the proximal tubule's ability to reabsorb uric acid that there is a uric acid leak and a *fall* in plasma uric acid.

Clinical features of hyperuricaemia

If a patient is known to have a persistent rise in plasma uric acid, renal disturbances should be anticipated. The main difficulty is the variety of ways in which a patient with hyperuricaemia may present for the first time. There may be the typical arthritis of gout, or multiple aches and pains which are shrugged off as "rheumatism". The young with familial hyperuricaemia may have hypertension which is first discovered either at a routine medical examination or as a sequel to toxaemia of pregnancy. Sometimes asymptomatic proteinuria is the first abnormality to be noticed, or the patient first presents with acute pyelonephritis. A few patients will present with uric acid stones.

It is an excellent rule to measure the concentration of uric acid in the plasma of all patients suffering from proteinuria or any other renal disturbance, hypertension, arthritis or vague aches and pains. The finding that the prognosis in essential hypertension is much worse in patients with a raised plasma uric acid makes this increasingly important.

URIC ACID STONES may occur in any patient with hyperuricaemia due to overproduction of uric acid. The stones are formed because of the increased quantity of uric acid being excreted in the urine. The majority of uric acid stones, however, occur in patients with a normal plasma uric acid who are not excreting an excess amount of uric acid in the urine. In these patients the stones are formed because the urine is persistently acid. Whereas in a normal individual the urinary pH rises to 6 or higher during the day, the urinary pH of these patients remains below 6, or more usually below 5·5 throughout the 24 hours. The cause of this functional disturbance is not clear. It is associated with a moderate impairment in the ability to excrete ammonia which must contribute to the persistent acidity.

The formation of stones is associated with renal colic, haematuria, proteinuria, pyelonephritis and urinary obstruction.

Treatment

Persistent hyperuricaemia can be corrected either by blocking uric acid reabsorption by the tubules, or by inhibiting the production of uric acid by the liver. If renal function is only moderately impaired the daily administration of probenecid will increase uric acid excretion by about a third and lower plasma uric acid. As renal failure develops probenecid will become less effective. It then becomes necessary to use allopurinol to inhibit xanthine oxidase activity and thus the production of uric acid from xanthine.

A sudden brisk rise in plasma uric acid with uric acid precipitation in the tubules such as that which may complicate the treatment of leukaemia can be avoided by the administration of allopurinol, and by preventing the patient from becoming dehydrated from vomiting.

It is very important to remember that most diuretics, and severe weight reducing diets, may cause a rise in plasma uric acid. In some patients this may precipitate gout or some deterioration of renal function. In a patient with some pre-existing impairment of renal function this risk should be prevented by the administration of allopurinol as soon as the plasma uric acid begins to rise. In a patient with normal renal function the plasma uric acid can be controlled if necessary with probenecid.

Uric acid stones associated with a persistently acid urine are best treated with an increased intake of fluid, and 50–100 mEq of sodium bicarbonate per day. In elderly subjects it is important to avoid precipitating pulmonary congestion. They can be given acetazolamide in the evening; this will increase sodium excretion and keep the urine alkaline during the night.

BIBLIOGRAPHY

BERKOWITZ, D., and GLASSMAN, S. (1965). "Effects of hypertriglyceridemia on urinary uric acid outputs." *Circulation*, **32**, suppl. ii, 2.
BERLINER, R. W., HILTON, J. G., YÜ, T. F., and KENNEDY, T. J. Jr. (1950). "The renal mechanism for urate excretion in man." *J. clin. Invest.*, **29**, 396.
BLUESTONE, R., KIPPEN, I., and KILINENBERG, J. R. (1969). "Effect of drugs on urate binding to plasma proteins." *Brit. med. J.*, **2**, 590.
BRECKENRIDGE, A. (1966). "Hypertension and hyperuricaemia." *Lancet*, **1**, 15.
COOMBES, F. S., PECORA, L. J., THOROGOOD, E., CONSOLAZIO, W. V., and TALBOTT, J. H. (1940). "Renal function in patients with gout." *J. clin. Invest.*, **19**, 525.
DUNCAN, H., and DIXON, A. St. J. (1960). "Gout, familial hyperuricaemia, and renal disease." *Quart. J. Med.*, N.S. **29**, 127.

EPSTEIN, F. H., and PIGEON, G. (1964). "Experimental urate nephropathy. Studies of the distribution of urate in renal tissue." *Nephron*, **1**, 144.

FINEBERG, S. K., and ALTSCHUL, A. (1956). "The nephropathy of gout." *Ann. intern. Med.*, **44**, 1182.

GONICK, H. C., RUBINI, M. E., GLEESON, I. O., and SOMMERS, S. C. (1965). "The renal lesion in gout." *Ann. intern. Med.*, **62**, 667.

GUTMAN, A. B., YÜ, T. F., and BERGER, L. (1959). "Tubular secretion of urate in man." *J. clin. Invest.*, **38**, 1778.

GUTMAN, A. B., and YÜ, T. F. (1957). "Renal function in gout." *Amer. J. Med.*, **23**, 600.

HANDLER, J. S. (1960). "The effect of lactic acid infusion in promoting reduced net excretion rate of urate." *J. clin. Invest.*, **39**, 1526.

HENNEMAN, P. H., WALLACH, S., and DEMPSEY, E. F. (1962). "The metabolic defect responsible for uric acid renal stone formation." *J. clin. Invest.*, **41**, 536.

KRITZLER, R. A., (1958). "Anuria complicating the treatment of leukemia." *Amer. J. Med.*, **25**, 532.

LATHEM, W., and RODMAN, G. (1962). "Impairment of uric acid excretion in gout." *J. clin. Invest.*, **41**, 1955.

LIEBER, C. S., JONES, D. P., LOSOWSKY, M. S., and DAVIDSON, C. S. (1962). "Inter-relation of uric acid and ethanol metabolism in man." *J. clin. Invest.*, **41**, 1863.

MAURICE, P. F., and HENNEMAN, P. H. (1961). "Medical aspects of renal stones." *Medicine*, **40**, 315.

MIKKELSEN, W. M., DODGE, H. J., and VALKENBURG, H. (1965). "The distribution of serum uric acid values in a population unselected as to gout and hyperuricaemia." *Amer. J. Med.*, **39**, 242.

NUGENT, C. A., MACDIARMID, W. D., and TYLER, F. H. (1964). "Renal excretion of urate in patients with gout." *Arch. Int. Med.*, **113**, 115.

NUGENT, C. A., and TYLER, F. H. (1959). "The renal excretion of uric acid in patients with gout and in nongouty subjects." *J. clin. Invest.*, **38**, 1890.

PAK POY, R. K. (1965). "Urinary pH in gout." *Australas. Ann. Med.*, **14**, 35.

PEARCE, J., and AZIZ, H. (1969). "Uric acid and plasma lipids in cerebrovascular disease. Part I. Prevalence of hyperuricaemia." *Brit. med. J.*, **2**, 78.

SCOTT, J. T., HALL, A. P., and GRAHAME, R. (1966). "Allopurinol in treatment of gout." *Brit. med. J.*, **2**, 321.

SEEGMILLER, J. E., GRAYZEL, A. I., HOWELL, R. R. and PLATO, C. (1962). "The renal excretion of uric acid in gout." *J. clin. Invest.*, **41**, 1094.

SNAITH, M. L., and SCOTT, J. T. (1971). "Uric acid clearance in patients with gout and normal subjects." *Annals of the Rheumatic Diseases*, **30**, 285.

STEELE, J. H., and RISELBACH (1963). "The contribution of residual nephrons within the chronically diseased kidney to urate homeostatis." *Am. J. Med.*, **43**, 876.

TALBOT, J. H., and TERPLAN, K. L. (1960). "The kidney in gout." *Medicine*, **39**, 405.

VIDEBACK, A. (1950). "Polycythaemia vera." *Acta med. Scand.*, **138**, 179.

YÜ, T. F., and GUTMAN, A. B. (1964). "Effect of allopurinol (4 hydroxypyrazolo (3,4d) pyrimidine on serum and urinary uric acid in primary and secondary gout." *Amer. J. Med.*, **37**, 885.

YÜ, T. F. (1950). "Uric acid metabolism and gout." *Amer. J. Med.*, **9**, 812.

31

Renal Disturbances in Monoclonal Gammopathies

MONOCLONAL gammopathies are characterised by an increase in the plasma concentration of one of the immunoglobulins (IgA, IgG, IgM). When the increase in IgA or IgG is associated with lymphoid cellular proliferation the condition is known as multiple myelomatosis; and when there is an increase in IgM and cellular proliferation it is known as Waldenström's macroglobinaemia. An increase in the plasma concentration of an immunoglobulin without an accompanying cellular proliferation is referred to as a benign gammopathy. Multiple myelomatosis is often associated with renal failure whereas it is unusual in Waldenström's macroglobinaemia. Renal failure does not seem to occur in benign gammopathies.

Pathology

There are a variety of renal lesions, including renal infection secondary to a neurological bladder from myelomatous tumours compressing the spinal cord, or small collections of neoplastic myeloma cells within the renal parenchyma; in addition renal amyloidosis occurs in 5–15 per cent of all cases.

Many patients show none of these changes; instead they develop the following structural disturbances. In multiple myelomatosis the characteristic lesion is the presence in the collecting tubules of wide and dense laminated casts. Often these are surrounded by a ring of disintegrated tubular cells, the whole complex lying within a collecting tubule whose cells appear normal. In addition there is extensive tubular atrophy, but the glomeruli remain relatively unchanged. There may also be multiple focal deposits of calcium in the casts, the tubule cells, and the interstitial spaces. The appearances suggest that much of the renal functional impairment is due to blocking of the collecting tubules.

With an IgM gammopathy there are, in contrast, no tubular lesions but instead there are occasional large round deposits, like thrombi, found on the endothelial aspect of the basement membrane of the glomerular capillaries. They can be so large that they obstruct the lumen. There is no associated cellular proliferation. The deposits consist of IgM, they do not contain fibrin or B_1C complement.

Clinical features

In the early stages, though proteinuria and mild renal functional impairment may be present, the main clinical features which usually predominate are unrelated to the kidney. The renal complications of myelomatosis are due to (*a*) abnormal protein metabolism, (*b*) hypercalcaemia, (*c*) hyperuricaemia and (*d*) amyloidosis. Another cause of renal failure is that the tubular reabsorption of paraprotein causes crystals to appear in the tubule cells.

DISTURBANCES OF PROTEIN METABOLISM. Each normal plasma cell produces only one type of antibody, that is, a single immunoglobulin. In myelomatosis the multiplying plasma cells are all producing the same antibody. It is therefore assumed that they have all originated from a single plasma cell precursor; the monoclonal concept of myelomatosis. Though there is a large concentration of circulating immunoglobulins the abnormal immunoglobulin appears as a narrow band on electrophoresis when it is called a paraprotein. Immuno-globulin molecules consist of long (heavy) chains and of short (light) chains combined together in a characteristic manner. Each plasma cell normally manufactures both long and short chains in the right proportions so that no excess residue of long or short chains remain after the immunoglobulin mole-cules are assembled. In 50 per cent of patients with myelomatosis, however, the proliferating clone of cells produces an excess of light chains which spill out into the circulation. These free light chains are best known as Bence-Jones' protein. Complete immunoglobulins are too large to pass through the glomerular filter so that in myelomatosis the concentration of the abnormal immuno-globulin is high in the plasma and low in the urine. Bence-Jones' protein however has a molecular weight of about 22,000. It therefore appears in high concentrations in the urine and low concentrations in the plasma, unless very large amounts are being manufactured.

The precipitation of this small molecular weight protein in the collecting ducts is one cause of renal failure in myelomatosis. This precipitation is some-times induced acutely by the preliminary period of dehydration which precedes an intravenous pyelogram. There is also "in vitro" evidence that free light chains are cytotoxic to tubular epithelial cells. The proteinuria of myelomatosis nearly always contains albumin whether or not Bence-Jones' protein is also present. Occasionally, however, Bence-Jones' protein is the only protein present; it is important to remember that Bence-Jones' protein cannot be detected with Albustix. The most accurate way to detect the presence of Bence-Jones' protein is to examine the urine electrophoretically. It can also be identi-fied by warming the urine; the protein at first comes out of solution and appears as a white precipitate, but as the urine becomes warmer the precip-itate redissolves and the urine becomes clear. If, however, other proteins are present, the persistent precipitate which they form on heating obscures the presence of Bence-Jones' protein. To establish the presence of Bence-Jones' protein when other proteins are present it is therefore necessary to filter the urine immediately after it has been brought to the boil. The precipitated albumin and globulins will then be separated from the Bence-Jones' protein which remains in the clear filtrate. This filtrate is observed as it cools and Bence-Jones' protein will appear when the temperatures falls to 70° C. It is important that the warmed urine should not be allowed to cool before it has passed through the filter, for otherwise the Bence-Jones' protein is precipitated on the wrong side of the filter and does not appear in the filtrate. To keep the urine warm it is best to filter small amounts at a time, to reheat the urine at frequent intervals, and to place the filter paper upon a warm funnel. It is characteristic of multiple myelomatosis that if Bence-Jones' protein is present, it appears in large quantities; Bence-Jones' proteinuria is sometimes found in other conditions but only in small amounts.

IgM is a large molecule, therefore, an IgM gammopathy causes a large increase in plasma viscosity. This may give rise to renal failure due presumably to the viscosity of blood in the post-glomerular circulation becoming so great that it impedes renal blood flow. It is characteristic of monoclonal gammopathies that the plasma concentration of those immunoglobulins which are not manufactured by the abnormal clone of cells is low. It is probable that the low plasma levels of IgG or IgM are responsible for the increased susceptibility of patients with gammopathies to infection, including renal infection.

HYPERCALCAEMIA, HYPERURICAEMIA AND AMYLOIDOSIS. Renal failure can be caused by the hypercalcaemia which sometimes accompanies the massive bone resorption induced by the lesions in the bone marrow. In these lesions there is also a high turnover of nucleoproteins and therefore an increased production of uric acid. This may cause a sufficient rise in plasma uric acid to be responsible for a rapid deterioration of renal function. Sometimes treatment which destroys the myeloma cells releases large amounts of nucleoprotein and causes a brisk rise in plasma uric acid. Amyloidosis occurs in 10 per cent of patients with myelomatosis and may also contribute to the renal functional impairment. It is most often seen in patients with Bence-Jones' proteinuria. If a patient with multiple myelomatosis develops a nephrotic syndrome it is nearly always an associated amyloidosis.

Treatment

Death is frequently due to renal failure. Often this is precipitated by dehydration and the consequent precipitation of protein in the tubules. The patient should therefore be encouraged to drink large volumes of fluids. When the daily excretion of Bence-Jones' protein is high the fluid intake should amount to about 4 litres a day. The rate of excretion of Bence-Jones' protein can sometimes be controlled by the administration of Melphalan or cyclophosphamide. Hypercalcaemia can sometimes be controlled in the same way, or with prednisone. This acts in part by inhibiting the multiplication of the myeloma cells. It is also helpful to avoid bed rest. Hyperuricaemia can be avoided or controlled by the administration of allopurinol. If the plasma viscosity rises to dangerous levels it can be lowered quickly by plasmapheresis. This often has to be done as an emergency because of a rapid deterioration of renal function.

In order to try to prevent renal failure in myelomatosis therefore, it is imperative to measure the rate of Bence-Jones' protein excretion, and the plasma concentrations of calcium and uric acid at frequent intervals.

Prognosis

Fifty per cent of all patients with myelomatosis who present with a blood urea greater than 80 mg/100 ml die within the next 10 weeks in spite of treatment. Other poor prognostic signs are a Bence-Jones' protein concentration in the blood greater than 200 mg/100 ml, a plasma albumin of less than 3·0 g/100 ml and a haemoglobin of less than 7·5 g/100 ml. IgA myelomatosis is sometimes associated with a rapid onset of renal failure of unknown cause; at *post mortem* the kidneys are histologically normal and do not bind immunofluorescent stains.

Renal Disturbances with IgG–IgM

Cryoglobulinaemia

IgG–IgM cryoglobulins can be found in systemic lupus erythematosus, diffuse proliferative glomerular nephritis, and in association with an IgM monoclonal gammopathy. They may also occur alone. The renal symptoms which they cause may vary from acute and chronic renal failure to no detectable abnormality. The characteristic histological lesions are in the glomeruli where there are deposits of IgG, IgM and B_1C complement together with moderate to severe endocapillary proliferation. They may cause an acute necrotising arteritis or on the other hand there are often no renal lesions. When they occur they resemble the passive deposition of immune complexes. It is possible that the IgG–IgM globulin is a form of immune complex, the IgG being the antigen and the IgM the antibody.

BIBLIOGRAPHY

ABRAHAMS, C., PIRANI, G. L., and POLLAK, V. E. (1966). "Ultrastructure of the kidney in a patient with multiple myeloma." *J. Path. Bact.*, **92**, 220.

ARGANI, I., and KIPKIE, G. F. (1964). "Macroglobulinaemic nephropathy: acute renal failure in macroglobulinaemia of Waldenström." *Am. J. Med.*, **36**, 151.

ARMSTRONG, J. B. (1950). "A study of renal function in patients with multiple myeloma." *Amer. J. med. Sci.*, **219**, 488.

BENTZEL, C. J., CARBONE, P. P., and ROSENBERG, L. (1964). "The effect of prednisone on calcium metabolism and ^{47}Ca kinetics in patients with multiple myeloma and hypercalcaemia." *J. clin. Invest.*, **43**, 2132.

FEIZI, T., and GITLIN, N. (1969). "Immune complex disease of the kidney associated with chronic hepatitis and cryoglobulinaemia." **2**, 873.

GOLDE, D., and EPSTEIN, W. (1968). "Mixed cryoglobulins and glomerulitis." *Ann. Intern. Med.*, **69**, 1221.

GREY, H. M., KOHLER, P. F., TERRY, W. D., and FRANKLIN, E. C. (1968). "Human monoclonal G-cryoglobulins with anti-globulin activity." *J. clin. Invest.*, **47**, 1875.

Hobbs, J. R. (1971). "Immunocytoma. O' mice an' men." *Brit. J. Med.*, **1**, 67.

Larcan, A., Rauber, G., and Strieiff, F. (1962). "Les manifestations rénales de la maladie de Waldenström." *J. Urol. Paris*, **68**, 57.

MacAlister, C. L. O., and Addison, N. V. (1961). "Renal aspects of myelomatosis." *Brit. J. Urol.*, **33**, 141.

Morel-Maroger, L., Basch, A., Danon, F., Verroust, P., and Richet, G. (1970). "Pathology of the kidney in Waldenström's macroglobulinaemia." *New Eng. J. Med.*, **283**, 123.

Myeloma Workshop (1971). *Brit. med. J.*, **1**, 319.

Putnam, F. (1962). "Structural relationships among normal human gamma globulin, myeloma globulin and Bence-Jones protein." *Biochem. biophys. Acta (Aust.)*, **63**, 539.

Verroust, P., Mery, J-P., Morel-Maroger, L., Clauvel, J. P., and Richet, G. (1971). Glomerular lesions in monoclonal gammopathies and mixed essential cryoglobulinaemia IgG–IgM. "Advances in Nephrology." Year Book Medical Publishers, **1**, 161.

32

Renal Amyloidosis

AMYLOID is an eosinophilic substance which appears structureless on light microscopy but which has a characteristic fibrillary pattern on electron microscopy; it may be distributed throughout all the organs of the body. Its deposition is possibly related to an immunological disturbance in that amyloid material contains a fragment which is part of the light chain of immunoglobulin molecules. In experimentally produced amyloidosis there is first a proliferation of reticulum cells which when they degenerate leave behind a deposit of amyloid. There is some connection between amyloidosis and myelomatosis, for (*a*) amyloid deposits contain immunoglobulins, (*b*) the bone marrow of patients with amyloidosis often contains an excess number of plasma cells, and (*c*) 10 per cent of patients with myelomatosis develop amyloidosis.

Pathology

The kidneys are usually smooth, resilient and enlarged. The cut surface shows that both the cortex and medulla are broader than normal and the demarcation between them is sharp; the glomeruli can be identified as small translucent deposits which stain dark brown upon the addition of iodine. Occasionally there is considerable disorganisation, the kidneys are small and scarred and the cortex and medulla difficult to recognise.

Under the microscope amyloid material is found in the walls of all vessels, including the glomerular capillaries and the peritubular venous capillaries. In a renal biopsy specimen it is characteristic that the glomeruli may appear to be almost entirely replaced by amyloid material at a time when the glomerular filtration rate may be only moderately impaired. The first changes consist of a lobular stalk thickening due to amyloid deposits in the mesangium. Apart from the characteristic staining reactions, the appearances are much the same as those found in post-streptococcal glomerular nephritis and diabetes. Electron microscopy reveals that the basement membrane is normal; the deposits of amyloid lying on either side. At autopsy the glomeruli mostly consist of solid, structureless, compact masses of amyloid of about the same size as a normal glomerulus. The amyloid material, which is laid in the peritubular venous capillaries, may be very thick but does not invade the tubule cells.

The tubule cells show the characteristic changes found in nephrotic glomerular nephritis, i.e. those changes found with heavy proteinuria, intracellular deposits of lipoid, and collections of an eosin-staining material of uncertain origin. Tubular atrophy is also present.

Without the use of special stains it is easy to confuse renal amyloidosis with diabetic nephropathy, and particularly persistent glomerular nephritis. But even the special stains may occasionally mislead. Amyloidosis can sometimes be demonstrated on electron microscopy when all special stains are negative.

Clinical features

Amyloidosis used to be seen most commonly in sanatoria in patients suffering from chronic tuberculosis of the bones or lungs. It can occur as a complication of chronic sepsis from any cause. Now, it is most often seen in rheumatoid arthritis and other diseases in which there is no sepsis, e.g. myelomatosis. Amyloid also occurs as a familial condition. In one type of familial amyloidosis which is characterised by polyneuropathy, cardiomyopathy and splenomegaly, renal involvement is unusual. In the other the amyloidosis is a complication of Familial Mediterranean Fever. In this type the amyloid deposits in the kidney are the usual cause of death.

Amyloidosis can also occur in patients with no accompanying disease and with no family history of the condition. This form is usually known as primary amyloidosis.

The first indication of renal amyloidosis is proteinuria, and the most common clinical manifestation is the development of a nephrotic syndrome. This may be particularly severe, for the hypoproteinaemia may not only be due to proteinuria but also to a decreased rate of protein synthesis as a consequence of hepatic amyloidosis, and also to an impaired absorption of amino- acids because of amyloid deposits in the mucous membrane of the small bowel.

It is very rare for the presenting symptoms to be those of chronic renal failure; and it is characteristic that the blood pressure may often remain normal for a considerable time after its onset. In some cases this is due to the deposition of amyloid in the sympathetic chains. This may cause hypotension. "In chronic failure, postural hypotension in spite of large administrations of salt, is amyloid" is a useful aphorism.

Occasionally there is a sudden onset of acute renal failure due to renal vein thrombosis. The thrombosis appears to begin in the intrarenal veins and extend medially. A few remarkable cases have been described which have suffered from severe polyuria and polydipsia over many years. In one of these the collecting ducts and vasa recta at *post-mortem* were found to be surrounded by a thick layer of amyloid material.

Diagnosis

The diagnosis of renal amyloidosis is confirmed by finding the characteristic deposits in a renal biopsy. If it is inappropriate to perform a renal biopsy, a rectal biopsy can be performed. A rectal biopsy will show amyloid deposits in

75 per cent of patients with renal amyloidosis, whereas a liver biopsy will only be positive in less than 50 per cent, and a gum biopsy in less than 20 per cent.

It is important that all renal biopsies which show any deposits of eosinophilic material should be stained for amyloid. Otherwise the diagnosis will be missed.

Treatment

If the disease with which amyloidosis is associated can be controlled, particularly if a septic lesion can be excised, renal function may improve, and the blood pressure will return to normal. Familial Mediterranean Fever has recently been treated with cyclophosphamide with some success. In a few children there has been definite renal biopsy evidence of a diminution in the amount of amyloid. Otherwise treatment is symptomatic and is that of the nephrotic syndrome and chronic renal failure. Serial renal biopsies from adult patients with rheumatoid arthritis suggest that once renal amyloidosis is sufficiently severe to cause some impairment in renal function, the renal lesions are irreversible. Treatment with adrenal steroids may produce a remission of symptoms, and proteinuria may cease, but the renal lesions remain.

BIBLIOGRAPHY

BARCLAY, G. P. T., CAMERON, H. MACD., and LOUGHRIDGE, L. W. (1960). "Amyloid disease of the kidney and renal vein thrombosis." *Quart. J. Med.*, N.S. **29**, 137.

BELL, E. T. (1933). "Amyloid disease of kidneys." *Amer. J. Path.*, **9**, 185.

COHEN, A. S. (1965). "The constitution and genesis of amyloid." *Int. Rev. exp. Path.*, **4**, 159.

HEPTINSTALL, R. H., and JOEKES, A. M. (1960). "Renal amyloid: a report on 11 cases proven by renal biopsy." *Ann. Rheumat. Dis.*, **19**, 126.

McGEKEE, H. A., GORDON WALKER, W., and YARDLEY, J. H. (1963). Renal involvement in myeloma, amyloidosis, systemic lupus erythematosus and other disorders of connective tissue. "Disorders of the Kidney." Ed. by Strauss, M. B., and Welt L., G. J. & A. Churchill, London, p. 575.

MOVAT, H. Z. (1960). "The fine structure of the glomerulus in amyloidosis." *Arch. Path.*, **69**, 323.

MUEHRCKE, R. C., PIRANI, C. L., POLLAK, V. E., and KARK, R. M. (1955). "Primary renal amyloidosis with the nephrotic syndrome studied by serial biopsies of the kidney." *Guy's Hosp. Rep.* **104**, 295.

PLATT, R., and DAVSON, J. (1950). "Clinical and pathological study of renal disease: Diseases other than nephritis." *Quart. J. Med.*, N.S. **19**, 33.

REIMANN, H. A. (1935). "Recovery from amyloidosis." *J. Amer. med. Ass.*, **104**, 1070.

33

Scleroderma

THE generalised form of scleroderma not only affects the skin but also the gastro-intestinal tract, the lungs, the heart and the kidney.

Pathology

Renal lesions are uncommon. They consist mainly of a striking thickening of the intralobular arteries and afferent arterioles. One type of thickening consists of intimal proliferation. This may be found in renal biopsies obtained many years before death.

The other lesions develop in the last few weeks of life and rapidly cause the death of the patient from renal failure. The kidneys are swollen and pale, while the cut surface shows a mottled congestion of the cortex which is due to a patchy necrosis. The necrotic lesions are due to occlusion of the proximal portions of many intralobular arteries by a mucoid substance which lies in concentric layers in the intima. The distal parts of some of the intralobular arteries and the afferent glomerular arterioles also show necrosis and fibrinoid changes. Many pathologists find these lesions indistinguishable from those found in malignant hypertension. Isolated polyarteritic lesions and "wireloop" lesions have also been described, but both changes are inconstant. There are no immunofluorescent deposits.

Clinical features

Proteinuria may be present for many years. This is usually associated with some reductions in renal blood flow but little impairment in renal function. Once renal function begins to deteriorate death usually follows within a few weeks. Some patients develop a catastrophic rise in blood pressure. They present with convulsions and rapidly go into coma. Occasionally, the acute deterioration of renal function appears to have been provoked by the use of adrenal steroids, when these have been used to alleviate some of the other symptoms of scleroderma.

Treatment

Treatment is symptomatic.

BIBLIOGRAPHY

CALVERT, R. J., and OWEN, T. K. (1956). "True scleroderma kidney." *Lancet*, **2**, 19.

GOLDSMITH, H. J., PETERS, J. H., and ZOMENO, M. (1963). "The evolution of renal disease in scleroderma. (A clinico-pathological study based on renal biopsies)." *II Int. Nephrology Congress, Excerpta Medica.* International Congress Series no. 67.

HANNIGAN, C. A., and HANNIGAN, M. H. (1956). "Scleroderma of the kidneys." *Amer. J. Med.,* **20,** 793.

MOORE, H. C., and SHEEHAN, H. L. (1962). "The kidney of scleroderma." *Lancet,* **1,** 68.

URAI, L., NAGY, Z., SZINAY, G., and WILTNER, W. (1958). "Renal function in scleroderma." *Brit. med. J.,* **2,** 1264.

34

Radiation Nephritis

RADIATION nephritis has been described in patients with malignant tumours of the testicle following irradiation of the periaortic abdominal glands, and after irradiating the stomach to treat peptic ulceration.

Pathology

There is little to see with the naked eye except some fibrous tissue between the kidney and the peritoneum. The capsule, however, is free and the kidney normal in size.

Microscopically the capsule shows considerable fibrous thickening. The glomeruli are smaller than normal and the glomerular loops show replacement with variable quantities of an eosin-staining material. Many of the tubules are atrophic and they are separated by large amounts of intertubular material which in some places includes fibrous tissue.

The larger vessels show no changes, the intralobular arteries and the arterioles may show sclerotic changes, and the glomerular capillaries occasionally show necrotic lesions similar to those found in malignant hypertension. These necrotic lesions may be present in the kidney even though they are absent from other organs, and the patient has not suffered from malignant hypertension clinically.

Following irradiation of the kidneys in animals the blood pressure rises before any abnormal microscopical changes are evident. It seems probable, therefore, that the vascular lesions that are seen later are due to the hypertension or irradiated vessels$_3$ the cause of the hypertension is unknown.

Acute Radiation Nephritis

Clinical features

The onset of symptoms attributable to changes in the kidney occurs after a latent period of six to twelve months from the start of radiotherapy. The reason for this interval is not known; it is one of the most interesting points about the disease.

Symptoms develop gradually; they include oedema, dyspnoea, hypertension, headache, nausea and vomiting, lassitude, and nocturia. In most instances the patient has to retire to bed within a month. There is no clear-cut acute nephritic syndrome or nephrotic syndrome. The condition usually

394

appears as chronic renal failure of rapid onset. In all cases there is proteinuria and hypertension, but widespread oedema and cardiac failure seem rather to follow a hypertension of increasing severity than to be an integral part of the initial disturbance. Proteinuria is rarely greater than 5 g/day and hypoproteinaemia has not been recorded. Some degree of renal failure occurs in all cases and is characteristically associated with severe anaemia.

Course

A third to a half of the cases reported in one series died within 4–12 months of the onset of symptoms. Death was due to hypertensive cardiac failure, hypertensive fits and renal failure. The remainder survived, but continued to have proteinuria, hypertension and some diminution in glomerular filtration rate.

Prognosis

A rise in blood urea above 200 mg per 100 ml at some time during the first three months or the development of pleural effusions without generalised oedema are stated to be signs indicative of a poor prognosis.

The duration of the latent period, the age of the patient, and the height of the blood pressure in the first five months, have no prognostic significance.

Treatment

Prophylactic. With the greatest care, the dose of X-rays needed for secondary seminomas is perilously close to that which can damage the kidney. The use of the cobalt bomb should enable the field of irradiation to be so narrowed that renal damage, if it occurs, is limited to one kidney and the damaged kidney can then be removed.

Curative. It is imperative to decide if the renal damage is unilateral or bilateral, for if it is unilateral the blood pressure can be lowered by nephrectomy.

Otherwise treatment is symptomatic and includes the control of hypertension, cardiac failure, oedema and renal failure. The necessity for blood transfusions appear to be greater than in other forms of renal failure; their administration is frequently accompanied by generalised reactions.

Chronic Radiation Nephritis

Some patients never develop a period of acute renal disorder, but 18 months to several years after irradiation they are found to be suffering from proteinuria, hypertension and some impairment of renal function. The cause of this form of radiation nephritis is obscure. Some cases have shown no tendency to further deterioration.

Malignant Hypertension

Occasionally there is a sudden onset of malignant hypertension. It may or may not be accompanied by renal failure. Death occurs within a few weeks.

BIBLIOGRAPHY

HARTMAN, F. W., BOLLIGER, A., and DOUB, H. P. (1927). "Functional studies throughout the course of roentgen-ray nephritis in dogs." *J. Amer. med. Ass.*, **88**, 139.

LUXTON, R. W. (1953). "Radiation nephritis." *Quart. J. Med.*, N..S **22**, 215.

PAGE, I. H. (1936). "Production of nephritis in dogs by roentgen rays." *Amer. J. med. Sci.*, **191**, 251.

THOMPSON, P. L., MACKAY, I. R., ROBSON, G. S. M., and WALL, A. L. (1971). "Late radiation nephritis after gastric x-irradiation for peptic ulcer." *Quart. J. Med.*, **40**, 145.

WILSON, C., LEDINGHAM, J. M., and COHEN, M. (1958). "Hypertension following X-irradiation of the kidneys." *Lancet*, **1**, 9.

35

Congenital, Macroscopic, Structural Lesions of the Kidney

THE term "macroscopic" is inserted in the title of this section in order to exclude the congenital microscopic structural lesions of the tubules which are associated with innate functional defects (p. 230).

The following malformations will be discussed:

Renal agenesis:
   (a) Bilateral.
   (b) Unilateral.
Renal hypoplasia:
   (a) Bilateral hypoplasia.
   (b) Unilateral dwarfed kidney.
Renal ectopia.
Anomalies due to fusion:
   (a) Horseshoe kidneys.
   (b) Unilateral fused kidney, crossed renal ectopia.
Duplication of pelvis and ureter.
Cystic disease of the kidneys:
   (a) Polycystic kidneys.
   (b) Solitary cysts.
   (c) Cystic disease of the medulla.
   (d) Sponge kidney.

RENAL AGENESIS

Bilateral Agenesis

Bilateral agenesis is not compatible with life, though occasionally the infant may live for two to three days. Not only are the kidneys absent but the ureters are often rudimentary. Other congenital abnormalities, such as spina bifida, are always present. Bilateral agenesis can sometimes be suspected during pregnancy for it is often associated with oligohydramnios.

Clinical Note Unilateral congenital renal structural abnormalities are often associated with a homolateral illshaped external ear. There may only be some prominence, shortening or absence of the lobe, or there may be severe distortion. This can sometimes be a useful clue in a child with a fever of unknown origin.

Unilateral Agenesis

Unilateral agenesis (Fig. 35.1) is more common than bilateral agenesis and may not be discovered until autopsy for some other disease. It occurs equally in both sexes and is more frequent on the left side. The remaining kidney hypertrophies and often weighs as much as a normal pair of kidneys.

Other congenital abnormalities may be found; in children gross abnormalities, such as meningocoele are not infrequent; in adults they are found less often and occur mainly in the genital tract, for instance, there may be a bicornuate or a double uterus.

RENAL HYPOPLASIA

Bilateral Hypoplasia

Bilateral hypoplasia usually causes death shortly after birth. Very rarely it may produce a state of chronic renal failure after two to three years of life.

Unilateral Hypoplasia

Unilateral hypoplasia has to be differentiated from acquired unilateral disease, for chronic urinary obstruction or infection may also result in a remarkably small kidney. As this differentiation is sometimes very difficult, the term *unilateral dwarfed kidney* is used to include those kidneys which are unequivocally hypoplastic, and those in which hypoplasia is the most likely diagnosis.

By combining the incidence of unilateral agenesis and hypoplasia, Bell has calculated from his autopsy records that in persons over one year of age the chance of there being only one kidney capable of sustaining life is about 1/200.

RENAL ECTOPIA

Ectopic kidneys are usually situated either in the iliac fossae, including the brim of the pelvis, or in the pelvic cavity (Fig. 35.1). They occur equally in the two sexes, and are rather more common on the left side. In the iliac fossae they show no major structural alteration, but when they are in the pelvis they may be seriously distorted. Frequently the kidney is hypoplastic; the renal pelvis is usually directed forward and the ureter is often dilated and tortuous. The renal artery arises from the nearest part of the aorta or the common iliac artery.

Ectopic kidneys may function normally, but they are liable to hydronephrosis and pyelonephritis.

Clinical features

Lower abdominal pain or discomfort, dysuria, frequency and haematuria are the presenting symptoms; or proteinuria may be found during a routine examination. Occasionally an ectopic kidney may first be diagnosed during

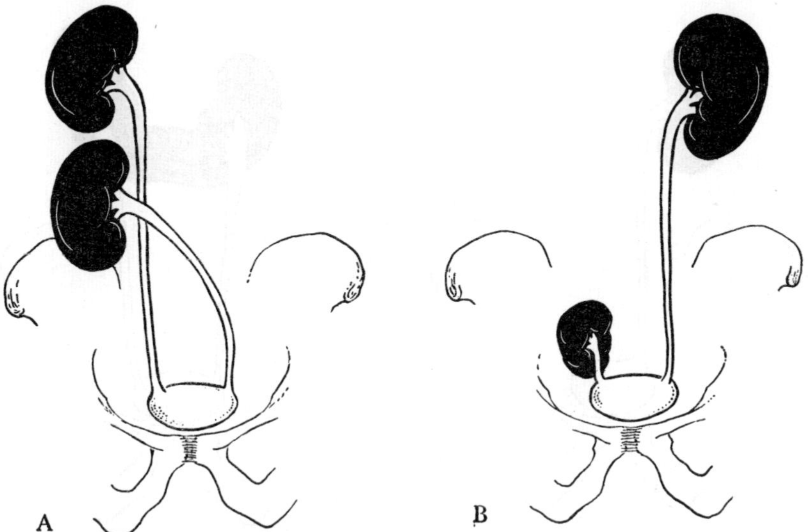

FIG. 35.1. Renal ectopia: (*a*) Both kidneys on the same side, and (*b*) Unilateral pelvic kidney.

pregnancy and may be confused with a tumour or pelvic abscess; an intravenous pyelogram allows the right diagnosis to be made only if the kidney can excrete the radio opaque material; at other times a retrograde pyelogram or laparotomy is necessary.

Often there are other congenital abnormalities.

Movable Kidney

The mobility of the kidney may be greater than normal but it is extremely doubtful if excess mobility is ever the cause of symptoms, or makes the kidney more liable to infection or other disorders. At one time, however, numerous operations were performed to secure errant kidneys into more conventional sites. Most of the operations were performed in that notorious group of middle-aged women who complain of vague abdominal pains.

ANOMALIES DUE TO FUSION

Horseshoe Kidney

This malformation consists in the fusion of two poles of the kidneys, usually the lower poles, across the midline. The two pelves are always separate and point in a forward direction, the two ureters travelling anteriorly over the surface of the lower poles (Fig. 35.2).

Horseshoe kidneys occur more frequently in males. In persons over one year of age Bell found the incidence to be 1 : 400. There is no conclusive evi-

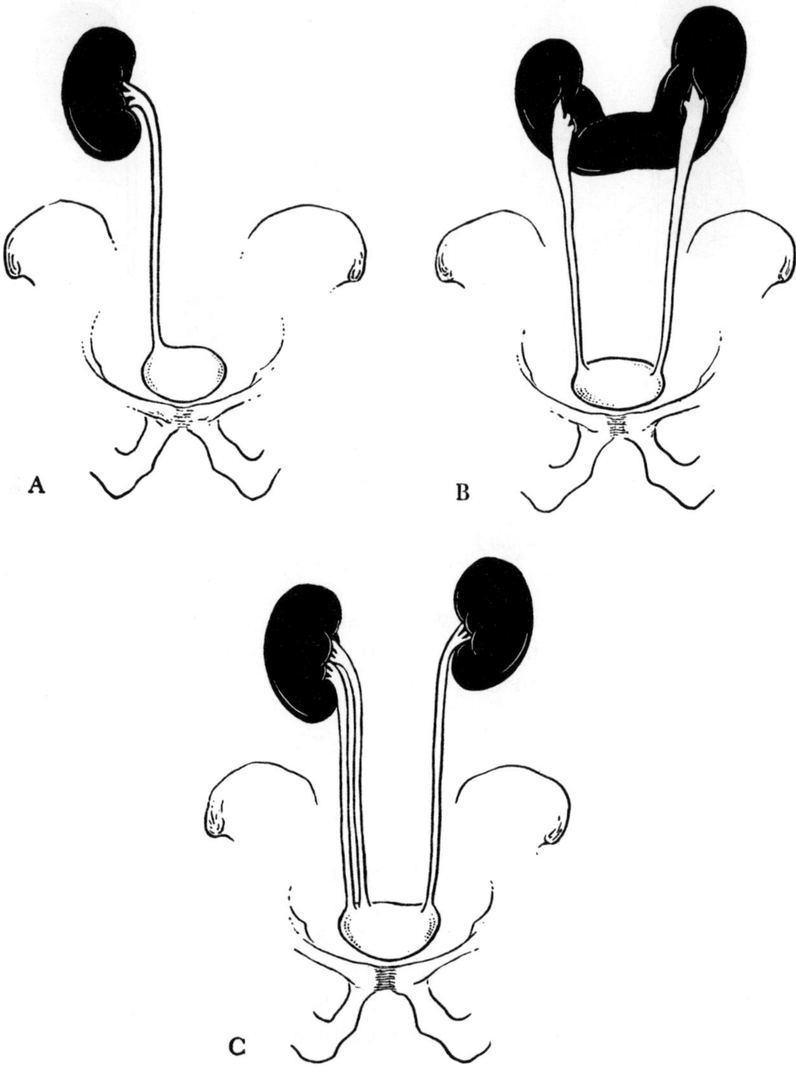

FIG. 35.2. (*a*) Unilateral agenesis, (*b*) Horsehoe kidney, (*c*) Double ureter.

dence that this abnormality is associated with a greater frequency of renal diseases than are normal kidneys.

Unilateral Fused Kidney

Very rarely both kidneys may be fused together on one side of the body. Both ureters enter the bladder in their normal sites, so that one ureter has to travel across the midline and is thus more liable to cause hydronephrosis and infection.

DUPLICATION OF PELVIS AND URETER

This anomaly is more common in women and is found most frequently on the left side; it is not unusual for it to be bilateral, when it is more extensive on one side than the other. The two ureters from one kidney may be completely separate in their course to the bladder, so that there are two ureteric orifices to one side of the midline (Fig. 35.2). At other times the two ureters fuse together either in the bladder wall or somewhere between the pelvis and the bladder. Occasionally one ureter may enter the vagina, the urethra, the seminal vesicles or the vas deferens. This is often the ureter from the upper part of the kidney while the ureter from the lower part enters the bladder in the normal place.

Duplication of the pelves and ureters is often associated with ureteric reflux, pain, hydronephrosis and recurrent urinary infection.

CYSTIC DISEASE OF THE KIDNEYS

A malformation which may be unilateral or bilateral. Bilateral cystic disease of the kidneys is far more frequent and important clinically.

Bilateral Polycystic Kidneys

This is a hereditary condition which declares itself clinically either in infancy (the neonatal form), or in middle age (the adult form); in childhood and up to the age of 20 the incidence falls off to negligible proportions. The reason for this remarkable division of incidence is not known. It is possible that the two forms of the disease, though they appear almost indistinguishable structurally, may stem from different aetiologies. In favour of this theory is the fact that the adult form appears to be inherited as an autosomal dominant in families in which there are a number of other cases, whereas the neonatal form appears to be due to an autosomal recessive. There are no records of adult and neonatal cases occurring in the same family.

Both forms occur equally between the two sexes.

Pathology

Both kidneys tend to be considerably enlarged, though the degree of enlargement may be unequal (Fig. 35.3). Each consists of a compact mass of cysts. On section the cysts are seen to be scattered equally in the cortex and medulla, and usually there does not seem to be any intact parenchyma. On rare occasions the cysts may be limited to one pole. In the neonatal disease all the cysts tend to be of a similar size, whereas in adults they vary considerably and some may be exceedingly large.

o

The cysts are filled with a watery fluid which may be clear, blood-stained from recent haemorrhage, or brown from an old haemorrhage; some may be filled with pus. They are lined by a single layer of epithelium and occasionally a normal glomerular tuft may be found invaginated into the cavity of a cyst, when the cyst is then considered to be the distended capsular space of that glomerulus. Cysts do not often communicate with the pelvis of the kidney.

It can be demonstrated that the contents of some cysts are in a continuous flux with the circulation, e.g. inulin placed in the cysts will appear in the blood

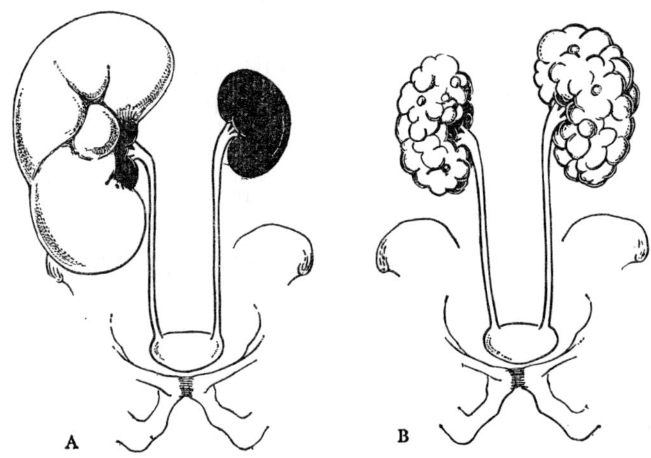

FIG. 35.3. (*a*) Solitary cyst, (*b*) Polycystic kidneys.

and vice versa. It has been suggested therefore that the cysts have some renal "functional" capacity, however trivial. Unless the cysts are joined to the pelvis, however, this is of no consequence whatever its extent.

Liver cysts are found in one-third of patients with polycystic kidneys and there is also a significant association with aneurysms of the cerebral arteries.

Pathogenesis

There are many theories but "nothing certain is known" (Dalgaard, 1971).

Clinical features

NEONATAL FORM. Usually neonatal bilateral cystic kidneys cause stillbirth, and sometimes their size may cause serious difficulties during delivery. The infant may live for a few months or one to two years, only to succumb to chronic renal failure.

ADULT FORM. The onset of the presenting symptoms usually occurs when the patient is about 40 years old, but the age of onset may range from 8 years to 77 years. These may be entirely renal with haematuria, clot colic, or acute pyelonephritis, or they may be more generalised, when they are due to renal failure or hypertension. Sometimes the patient complains of abdominal distension, or pain following some relatively minor trauma. Proteinuria is always present and may be the first abnormality to draw attention to the renal disease.

Hypertension develops in only about 50 per cent of cases, is rarely malignant and comes on late. As renal failure develops the usual fall in haemoglobin tends to be less pronounced than in other forms of renal disease. In some patients there is no significant fall in haemoglobin.

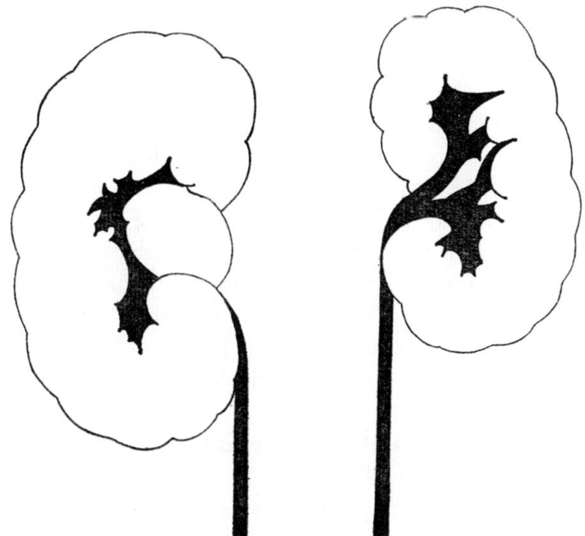

FIG. 35.4. Polycystic kidneys. An intravenous pyelogram, illustrating the distortion of the pelvis and calyces by the cysts.

By the time the patient begins to complain of symptoms the kidneys are usually easily palpable and have a characteristic "knobbly" feel. The diagnosis is confirmed by an intravenous pyelogram which shows the pelvis to be elongated with the calyces stretched out, and their peripheral ends shaped into crescents of varing sizes (Fig. 35.4). Early disease showing only unilateral abnormalities may be difficult to differentiate from solitary cysts or a tumour.

Prognosis

The rate of renal impairment and the pattern of events varies enormously from patient to patient, but certain families show a tendency towards a recurring pattern. Death is due either to chronic renal failure from compression of the renal parenchyma by the enlarging cysts, and chronic renal infection; or from hypertensive cardiac failure, and cerebrovascular accidents. Cerebral aneurysms are present in about 20 per cent of patients. Hypertensive cardiac failure is the most common immediate cause of death.

The average age of death is about 50 years, i.e. the average duration of the disease once it has become manifest is 5 to 10 years. There are wide variations around these means, however. If renal infections are promptly treated some patients live many years without appearing to deteriorate.

Treatment

If the disease is almost confined to one kidney which is subject to recurrent infections and is functionally useless it may be wise to remove it, after first establishing that the function of the other kidney is adequate.

When the disease is bilateral the only measure which may cause any improvement is the evacuation of some of the larger cysts in order to relieve the pressure upon the residual parenchyma. The functional results of such operations, however, have not often been investigated; attention has been paid rather to the improvement in appearance of the intravenous pyelogram, and the continued survival of the patient. Until now there has not been a convincing demonstration that the operation will in fact prolong life; some authorities categorically deny that renal function is improved. Nevertheless, there is general agreement that the operation is sometimes most useful in the relief of recurrent pain and haematuria and that occasionally there has been relief of hypertension. It is considered that the operation should only be performed on one side at a time, for there is often a relatively severe transient post-operative deterioration in renal function.

Otherwise, treatment is symptomatic and is that of renal failure, renal infection, hypertension and cardiac failure.

If the patient suffers from migraine or has a cerebrovascular accident special attention should be given to the possibility of cerebral aneurysm. If renal function is good, prompt treatment of the aneurysm may extend life.

Solitary Renal Cysts

Small cysts are frequently found during routine autopsies; their size usually precludes them from having caused any ill effects.

Large "solitary" cysts are rarely single, but occur in clusters of two or three (Fig. 35.3). They are more common on the right side, and more often seen in women. They may be situated in either pole, or in the middle of the kidney; nearly always they spring from the parenchyma, but occasionally they may be entirely sub- or extracapsular. The parenchyma near the cyst is always considerably compressed. They only rarely have a connection with the pelvis. The contents of the cysts contain 500–1,000 ml of yellow or blood-stained fluid and sometimes considerably more. The walls of the cysts are composed of thin fibrous tissue in which a few atrophic tubules may be seen.

Clinical features of large cysts

The main complaint is of intermittent attacks of abdominal pain interspersed by long remissions. The attacks tend to become more frequent as the years go by and the total duration of the history may be 20–30 years. The pain may be associated with fever, dysuria and occasionally with haematuria. Painless haematuria is sometimes the first symptom.

Cysts in the upper poles are particularly difficult to palpate and when on the right side may cause symptoms resembling cholecystitis. Lower-pole cysts cause gastric and intestinal symptoms, with nausea or diarrhoea; they are also liable to obstruct the ureter and cause renal infections.

The diagnosis should be evident from an intravenous pyelogram, which may show compression of the calyces and elongation of the pelvis. Often the appearances are difficult to differentiate from those of a tumour, and sometimes the radiological appearances are normal.

Treatment

This is surgical. If possible, a heminephrectomy is performed, otherwise a total nephrectomy is necessary.

Cystic Disease of the Renal Medulla

This condition destroys the patient either in adolescence or early adult life. The patient presents with severe thirst and polyuria and is found to have renal failure with a pronounced urinary sodium leak. The intravenous pyelographic changes have not been described. The kidneys at *post-mortem* show multiple cysts in the medulla and sometimes a few in the cortex together with cortical atrophy.

Sponge Kidney

This is a radiological diagnosis of a relatively benign condition which is not usually diagnosed until adulthood. The I.V.P. may be performed because of a urinary infection or haematuria. The preliminary picture may show areas of calcification in the medulla. After the dye has been injected the I.V.P. shows multiple discrete opacifications in the pyramidal areas before the pelvis and calyces become opacified. These medullary opacities are grouped at the tips of the calyces and appear to branch away from them like a bouquet of flowers. It is characteristic that a retrograde pyelogram shows a completely different picture, for most of the cysts have such small connections into the calyces that they are not filled from below. There are very few descriptions of the structural changes and these are mainly from surgical specimens. They show collections of small cysts in the pyramids and medulla but the cortex is normal.

BIBLIOGRAPHY

BAXTER, T. J. (1965). "Polycystic kidney of infants and children." *Nephron*, **2**, 15.
BELL, E. T. (1946). "Renal Diseases." Henry Kimpton, London.
BRICKER, N. S., and PATTON, J. F. (1955). "Cystic disease of the kidneys." *Amer. J. Med.*, **18**, 207.

CAIRNS, H. W. B. (1925). "Heredity in polycystic disease of the kidneys." *Quart. J. Med.*, **18**, 359.
DALGAARD, O. Z. (1971). Polycystic disease of the kidneys. In "Diseases of the Kidney", 2nd edition. Edited by M. B. Strauss and L. G. Welt. Little, Brown and Company, Boston, U.S.A., p. 1223.
DARMADY, E. M., OFFER, J., and WOODHOUSE, M. A. (1970). "Toxic metabolic defect in polycystic disease of kidney." *Lancet*, **1**, 547.
DAVIS, J. E. (1925). "Congenital polycystic kidneys." *Amer. J. Obstet. Gynec.*, **9**, 758.
FERGUSSON, J. D. (1949). "Observations on familial polycystic disease of the kidney." *Proc. roy. Soc. Med.*, **42**, 806.
LAMBERT, P. P. (1947). "Polycystic disease of the kidney. A review." *Arch. Path.*, **44**, 34.
OSATHANONDH, V., and POTTER, E. L. (1964). "Pathogenesis of polycystic kidneys." *Arch. Path.*, **77**, 510.
POTTER, E. L. (1946). "Bilateral renal agenesis." *J. Pediat.*, **29**, 68.
RUBIN, E. L., ROSS, J. C., and TURNER, D. P. (1959). "Cystic disease of the renal pyramids (sponge kidney)." *J. Fac. Radiol. (Lond.)*, **10**, 134.
SIMON, H. B., and THOMPSON, C. J. (1955). "Congenital renal polycystic disease. A clinical and therapeutic study of three hundred and sixty-six cases." *J. Amer. Med. Ass.*, **159**, 657.
STRAUSS, M. B. (1971). Microcystic disease of the renal medulla. "Diseases of the Kidney", 2nd edition. Ed. by Strauss, M. B., and Welt, L. G. J. & A. Churchill, London, p. 1259
YATES-BELL, J. G. (1957). "Rovsing's operation for polycystic kidney." *Lancet*, **1**, 126.

Appendix 1

Diets

HIGH PROTEIN, LOW SODIUM DIET

Protein Content 180–190 g. Sodium Content 30–40 mEq

Meal	oz	g	Food	Protein g	Sodiu mm Eq
Breakfast	5	142	Porridge	2	0·3
	2	57	Unsalted bread	4	0·2
	½	14	Unsalted butter or margarine	—	0·2
	4	114	2 eggs, cooked in any way	14	6·6
			Milk from daily allowance for porridge and tea or coffee	—	—
			Sugar as desired	—	—
	½	14	Marmalade, honey or jam	—	0·2
Dinner	5	142	Lean meat, cooked weight	35	4·1
	4	114	Potatoes, boiled, roasted or fried	2	0·2
			Vegetable or salad, average helping	0·5	0·5
			Stewed or tinned fruit, average helping	0·5	0·5
			Pudding using high protein Edosol milk from daily allowance		
Tea	2	57	Unsalted bread	4	0·2
	½	14	Unsalted butter or margarine	—	0·2
	2	57	Lean meat as sandwich filling	14	2·2
			Tea with milk from daily allowance		
			Sugar as desired		
	1	28	Cake made from low sodium ingredients (see general instructions)	2	0·4
Supper	6	170	Fried fish (cooked weight)	35	12·0
	4	114	Potatoes, boiled, roasted or fried	2	0·2
			Vegetable or salad, average helping	0·5	0·5
			Fruit, average helping	0·5%	0·5
			Pudding using high protein Edosol milk from daily allowance		
Daily	4	114	Ordinary milk for tea	4	2·5
	25	710	Edosol milk	25	1·1
	1½	43	Casilan for drinks and puddings	39	1·8
				184	34·4

All foods cooked without salt.

In this diet, if ordinary milk is substituted for Edosol the sodium will rise by 14·6 mEq, and if ordinary bread and butter are substituted for the low sodium varieties the sodium will rise by 22 mEq.

General instructions for high protein, low sodium diet

Edosol is a low sodium synthetic milk powder made by Trufood reconstituted according to the directions on the tin. Casilan is a calcium caseinate, a 90 per cent soluble protein made by Glaxo.

The mixture of Edosol and Casilan can be used in place of ordinary milk to make cereal milk puddings, custard, egg custard and milk jelly as well as in drinks flavoured with milk shake, syrups, and coffee. It is not suitable for use in tea.

To make a low sodium diet more interesting, use pepper, mustard, vinegar, lemon juice, home made unsalted chutney and unsalted pickles. Herbs such as bay leaves, thyme and sage, and spices such as curry, cayenne pepper, paprika, cloves and nutmeg can also be used. To improve the flavour further, fry potatoes and other vegetables, toast the bread and use garlic and onion liberally.

Foods low in sodium not mentioned previously

All frozen vegetables except spinach.
Lard, dripping, olive oil, double cream, unsalted butter.
Matzos, Rakusen's unsalted crackers, salt free Ryvita.
Shredded and Puffed Wheat, Oatmeal.
Low sodium canned peas and baked beans in tomato sauce (Dietade) and Banmene unsalted yeast extract are available through most branches of Boots and Health Food Stores.
Sugar, glucose, Hycal, Caloreen, jams, honey, marmalades (see overleaf)
Fruit juices, boiled sweets, peppermints.
Wheatstarch and plain flour, Cornflour.

Recipe for low sodium baking powder for use with plain flour:

Starch	28 g
Potassium bicarbonate	40 g
Tartaric acid	8 g
Potassium bitartrate	56 g

This recipe can be made up by any chemist. It should be used like ordinary baking powder.

Foods to be avoided

All bread if not specially made without salt.
Crispbreads such as Ryvita, cream crackers (unless salt free).
Ordinary cakes and biscuits.
Self raising flour.
Cornflakes and other cereals (except Puffed Wheat and Shredded Wheat).
Shop-prepared meats and pies, tinned meat and fish, sausages, bacon, ham, meat and fish pastes.
Cheese except home-made unsalted.
Salted butter and margarine.
Tinned vegetables, tinned tomato juice.
Tinned and packet soups, shop pickles, sauces, salad cream.
Meat and yeast extracts (except salt free Banmene). Gravy mixes.
Golden syrup. Black treacle. Rennet.
Potato crisps and salted nuts.
Chocolates. Toffees. Liquorice.
Beers and Lagers.
Health salts and indigestion tablets.
Milk beverages, e.g. Ovaltine, Horlicks, etc.
Evaporated or condensed milk.
Culinary salts (e.g. garlic salt) and foods containing mono-sodium glutamate (e.g. Alomat).

Low Protein, Low Sodium Diet

Protein Content 40 g, Sodium Content 28 mEq

Meal	oz	g	Food	Protein g	Sodium mEq
Breakfast	1	28	Milk	0·9	0·62
	2	56	Egg	6·8	3·3
	1	28	Bread, ordinary	2·4	6·8
	½	14	Butter	—	1·5
	4	112	Fruit and Sugar	0·4	0·1
	½	14	Marmalade, honey, syrup	—	—
Dinner	1½	12	Meat, cooked weight	10·5	1·2
	3½	98	Green vegetables	1·2	0·3
	3½	98	Root vegetables	0·7	1·0
	4	112	Potato	1·6	0·2
	4	112	Fruit and sugar	0·4	0·1
	1	28	Double cream	0·4	0·3
Tea	1	28	Milk	0·9	0·62
	1	28	Bread, ordinary	2·4	6·8
	½	14	Butter	0·05	1·5
	½	14	Jam, honey or syrup	—	—
	4	112	Fruit	0·4	0·1
Supper	1	28	Meat, poultry, offal or fish	7·0	1·2
	3½	98	Green vegetables or salad	1·2	0·4
	3	84	Potato	1·2	0·15
	½	14	Butter	—	1·5
	4	112	Fruit and sugar	0·4	0·1
	1	28	Double cream	0·4	0·3
Daily	3½	98	Sugar	—	—
				39·2	28·09

General instructions for low protein diets

To make certain that a positive nitrogen balance is obtained at least 3,000 calories should be taken per day. The calorie content of the 20 g and 40 g protein diets are 1,500 and 2,000 calories respectively. The additional calories are derived from the following foods:

Hycal, caloreen, glucose, fruit squash, fruit juice, lemonade, coca-cola, boiled sweets, peppermints, jam, honey, marmalade, butter (unsalted if necessary), lard, cooking oils, wheat starch, protein free pastas, and protein free bread and biscuits.

In the low protein diets with a sodium restriction all foods should be cooked without salt. In addition all salty foods listed on p. 408 should be avoided.

Hycal, produced by Beecham Laboratories, is a high calorie electrolyte free drink (one bottle contains 425 calories). Caloreen is a high calorie electrolyte free sugar substitute which is instantly soluble. It is manufactured by Scientific Hospital Supplies Limited, Liverpool. Protein free flour, bread and biscuits, either salted or unsalted, are available from Welfare Foods (Stockport) Ltd. Wheatstarch can be obtained from Energen Foods, Ashford, Kent, and low protein pasta is produced by Carlo-Erba, Milan. All these items may be prescribed on form E.C.10.

Very Low Protein Normal Sodium Diet

Protein Content 20 g

Meal	oz	g	Food	Protein g
Breakfast	4·0	112	Fruit average helping raw or stewed with sugar	0·5
	1	28	Bread, plain or toasted—1 slice from a cut loaf	2·2
			Butter or margarine	
			Marmalade, honey or jam	
			Tea with sugar and lemon or coffee with sugar	
Dinner	1	28	Meat or cheese or	
	1½	43	Fish or	
	2	56	Egg	7
	1	28	Bread or	
	5	140	Potato—2 medium sized, fried if desired	2
			Vegetables or salad, average helping, not including peas or butter beans	0·5
			Fruit, average helping, raw or cooked with sugar	0·5
Tea	1	28	Bread	2·2
			Bread or margarine	
			Jam or honey	
			Tea with sugar and lemon	
Supper or High Tea		56	As Dinner (omitting meat or alternative)	3·0
Daily	2		Milk—4-tablespoons	1·8
				19·7

Very Low Protein, Low Sodium Diet

Protein Content 20 g, Sodium Content 20 mEq

Meal	oz	g	Food	Protein g	Sodium mEq
Breakfast	4	112	Grapefruit segments	0·8	0·1
	1	28	Bread, plain or toasted, ordinary	2·4	6·8
	½	14	Butter	—	1·5
			Marmalade	—	—
			Tea or coffee	—	—
	1	28	Milk	0·9	0·62
Dinner	1	28	Meat or	7·0	0·82
	1½	43	Fish or	7·0	3·0
	1	56	Egg	7·0	3·3
	2	56	Potato	0·8	0·1
	3½	98	Root vegetable	0·7	1·0
	3½	98	Green vegetable	1·2	0·3
	4	112	Fruit	0·4	0·1
	1	28	Cream	0·4	0·3
Tea	½	14	Bread, ordinary	1·2	3·4
	½	14	Butter, ordinary	—	1·5
			Jam or salad		
			Tea or coffee with 1 oz milk	0·9	0·62

Supper	2	56	Potato		0·8	0·1
	3½	98	Root vegetable	} or salad	0·7	1·0
	3½	98	Green vegetable		1·2	0·4
	4	112	Fruit		0·4	0·1
	1	28	Cream		—	—
	3½	98	Daily Sugar		—	—
					20·2	19·06

PROTEIN, SODIUM AND POTASSIUM CONTENT OF CERTAIN FOODS

Food	Protein g/100 g	Sodium mEq/100 g	Potassium mEq/100 g
Cheese (Cheddar)	24·9	26·6	3·0
Chocolate	5·6	6·5	7·5
Cow's milk	3·3	2·2	4·1
Cream (double)	1·5	1·1	2·0
Edosol milk (reconstituted)	3·5	0·1	18·2
Complan	31·0	17·4	28·2
Casilan	90·0	4·3	0·1 (less than)
Ice cream	4·1	3·4	4·3
Horlicks	14·4	30·0	29·0
Egg	11·9	5·9	3·5
Beef (steak with fat, grilled)	25·2	2·9	9·4
Beef (stewed lean only)	30·8	1·7	3·9
Mutton (leg with fat, roasted)	25·0	3·1	8·9
Mutton (chop, fried, lean only)	22.8	5·0	9·0
Chicken (boiled)	26·2	4·3	9·8
Ham (boiled)	23·1	91·3	11·6
Liver (calf, fried)	29·0	5·3	10·5
Tongue (ox, pickled)	19·1	81·0	3·9
Veal (cutlet, fried)	30·4	4·6	10·8
Sausage (pork, fried)	11·5	43·0	5·3
Cod (steamed)	18·0	4·3	9·2
Cod (fried in batter)	20·7	7·0	8·8
Cod (grilled)	27·0	4·8	10·5
Herring (fried)	21·8	4·4	10·6
Oysters	10·2	22·0	6·6
Plaice (steamed)	18·1	5·2	7·1
Plaice (fried in batter)	18·0	5·4	5·6
Porridge (cooked)	1·4	0·2	1·8
Cornflakes	6·6	45·6	2·9
Energen flakes	36·8	0·3	3·9
Bread (white)	8·1	17·1	1·8
Ryvita	6·8	26·7	12·0
Cream crackers	8·5	19·0	3·3
Puffed wheat	13·9	0·25	11·5
Bread (unsalted, white)	8·1	0·3	1·8
Energen rolls (per roll)	2·0	0·1	0·1
Flour	8·6	0·01	4·5
Spaghetti	9·9	0·2	4·01
Rice (boiled)	2·1	0·1	1·0
Butter or margarine	—	9·8–14·0	0·1–1·0
Butter or margarine (unsalted)	—	0·1	0·1–1·0

Foods High in Potassium and Low in Protein

	Food	Potassium mEq/100 g
Cereals	All Bran	24·5
	Malt bread	9·5
	Ryvita	12·0
Fruit and nuts	Apricots—dried, stewed	20.0
	Apricots—tinned in syrup	6·6
	Bananas	8·9
	Dates	19.3
	Figs—dried, stewed	14.8
	Grapes—black	8·1
	Prunes—dried, stewed	8·5
	Chestnuts—shelled	12·7
Vegetables	Beetroot, boiled	9·0
	Mushrooms, fried	14·5
	Potatoes, old and new boiled	8·4
	Potatoes, baked in skin	17·4
	Potatoes, roasted	19·1
	Potatoes, chips	26·2
	Spinach, boiled	12·6
	Tomatoes, fried	8·6

	Food	mEq per teaspoon of concentrate
Drinks	Bovril	5·5
	Marmite	4·4
	Instant coffee	10
	Instant tea	7

	Food	mEq/100 g
Others	Black treacle	10·5
	Salt substitutes, e.g. Selora	12·68

Food values have been obtained from McCance and Widdowson's tables*; in some instances average figures have been used.

The author would like to thank Miss M. M. Ramsey and Miss E. P. Skinner of St. Thomas's Hospital and Miss F. Toy and Miss P. Grant of Charing Cross Hospital for their work in writing Appendix I.

* McCance, R. A. and Widdowson, E. M. (1960 amended 1969). "The chemical composition of food." *Med. Res. Coun. Spec. Rep. Ser.*, No. 235.

Appendix 2

Some Normal Values

RENAL FUNCTIONAL CAPACITY

Some Normal Values for Young Subjects, 1·73 m_2 Surface Area

Renal plasma flow	612±68 ml/min
Renal blood flow	Approximately 1,200 ml/min
Glomerular filtration rate: .	
1. Inulin clearance	112±15 ml/min
	Adult males by age groups*:
	20–29 yr 123±16 ml/min
	50–59 yr 99±15 ml/min
	80–89 yr 65±20 ml/min
2. Creatinine clearance	Approximately the same as inulin.
Urea clearance (at urine flows greater than 2 ml/min) . .	75 ml/min
Maximal Tubular Capacity (Tm):	
1. To reabsorb glucose	323±64 mg/min
2. To secrete PAH	68±11 mg/min
Ability to concentrate (Fluid deprivation)	800 to 1,200 m.Osmol/l
	(i.e. S.G. 1·022 to 1·032)
Ability to dilute	40 to 80 m.Osmol/l
	(i.e. S.G. 1·002)
Ability to excrete a water load of 1 litre	800 ml excreted in next 4 hours.

* SHOCK, N. W. (1946). "Kidney function tests in aged males." *Geriatrics*, **1**, 232.

DAILY URINARY EXCRETIONS

Twenty-four-hour output, on a mixed diet. These
figures are given only as a guide

AMMONIA	30 to 60 mEq
CALCIUM	80 to 400 mg
COPROPORPHYRIN, total . .	14 to 100 μg
CHLORIDE	80 to 200 mEq
CREATINE: .	
Children	up to 150 mg
Women	small amounts
Men	nil
CREATININE	0·8 to 1·8 g
DIASTASE	8,000 to 30,000 units
GLUCOSE	16 to 132 mg
POTASSIUM	80 to 200 mEq
pH	4·8 to 7·4
SODIUM	80 to 200 mEq
TITRATABLE ACID . . .	20 to 30 mEq
(Hydrogen ion)	
UREA	16 to 35 g
URIC ACID	0·1 to 2·0 g
UROBILINOGEN	Less than 2 mg
VOLUME	1,000 to 2,000 ml

PLASMA CONTENTS

			Useful average
ALBUMIN	4·0 to 5·7 g/100 ml		4·8 g/100 ml
ALBUMIN/GLOBULIN RATIO	1·2/1 to 4/1		2/1
BICARBONATE (see CARBON DIOXIDE)			
BILIRUBIN (total) . .	Less than 0·8 mg/100 ml		
CALCIUM	Total .	8·5 to 10·5 mg/100 ml	9·5 mg/100 ml
	Diffusible .	3·6 to 5·6 mg/100 ml	
	Non-diffusible .	2·8 to 6·1 mg/100 ml	
CARBON DIOXIDE . .	25 to 31 mEq/l		27 mEq/l
CHLORIDE . . .	99 to 108 mEq/l		103 mEq/l
CHOLESTEROL . .	Total, 120 to 240 mg/100 ml		200 mg/100 ml
	Ester, 60 to 80% of total		70% of total
CREATINE . . .	0·2 to 0·6 mg/100 ml		0·4 mg/100 ml
CREATININE . .	0·8 to 1·4 mg/100 ml		1 mg/100 ml
DIASTASE . . .	90 to 160 units/100 ml		
FIBRIN(OGEN) . .	200 to 400 mg/100 ml		300 mg/100 ml
GLOBULIN . . .	1·5 to 3·0 g/100 ml		2·4 g/100 ml.
GLUCOSE: *Capillary* .	Fasting or noon, 80 to 120 mg/100 ml		100 mg/100 ml
Venous . .	About 10 mg/100 ml lower		
OSMOLALITY. . .	275–285 m.Osmol/l		280 m.Osmol/l
pH	7·37 to 7·4		7·40
PHOSPHATASE: *Alkaline* .	King-Armstrong, 3 to 13 units/100 ml		
	Bodansky, 1·5 to 4·0 units/100 ml		
Acid .	King-Armstrong-total 1 to 5 units/100 ml		
	King-Armstrong-formaldehyde stable, 0 to 4 units/100 ml		
PHOSPHORUS. . .	Adults, 2·4 to 4·5 mg/100 ml		4·0 mg/100 ml
(inorganic) . .	Children, 4·0 to 6·5 mg/100 ml		
POTASSIUM . .	4·0 to 5·5 mEq/l		5 mEq/l
SODIUM . . .	137 to 148 mEq/l		142 mEq/l
SULPHATE . . .	0·5 to 1 mEq/l		
UREA	15 to 35 mg/100 ml (adults)		25 mg/100 ml
	10 to 25 mg/100 ml (pregnancy)		
URIC ACID . . .	3 to 5 mg/100 ml		

APPROXIMATE COMPOSITION OF VARIOUS BODY FLUIDS

Fluid	HCO_3 mEq/l	Cl mEq/l	P *mM/l	Na mEq/l	K mEq/l	Protein g/l	Water g/l
Serum . . .	25	100	2	142	4·3	70	940
Interstitial fluid .	28	111	—	145	3·3	traces	993
Spinal fluid . .	21	125	—	147	2·8	0·3	993
Gastric juice . .	—	145	—	50	12·0	mucus	993
Bile	38	108	—	150	5·0	mucus	990
Pancreatic juice . .	110	40	—	140	5·0	mucus	993
Jejunal juice . .	30	110	—	138	5·0	mucus	993
Sweat† . . .	—	40	—	42	—	—	993
Intracellular fluid:		mEq/kg	mM/kg	mEq/kg	mEq/kg	g/kg	
Skeletal muscle amounts per kg of intracellular water }	—	3	107	7	155	306	

* mM, or millimole, is the molecular weight in milligrams.
† The composition of sweat may vary considerably.

BODY CONTENTS OF SODIUM AND POTASSIUM. RED CELL MASS AND FLUID VOLUMES

	Man 70 *kg*	*Woman* 57 *kg*
Total exchangeable sodium	2,950 mEq	2,250 mEq
Total exchangeable potassium	3,200 mEq	2,300 mEq
Plasma volume	2·83 l	2·40 l
Red cell mass	2·1 l	1·8 l
Extra-cellular fluid	14 l	11 l
Intra-cellular fluid	25 l	20 l
Total body water	39 l	31 l

EQUIVALENT AND MOLECULAR WEIGHTS

Equivalent Weights:

N	14	Mg	12
K	39	P	16 (variable)
Ca	20	Cl	35·5
Na	23	O	8

Molecular Weights:

Na Citrate ($2H_2O$)	29·40
Na Cl	58·5
Na Lactate	112·0
Na HCO_3	84·0
Na_2 HPO_4 ($12H_2O$)	358·2
Na H_2PO_4 (H_2O)	156·0
K HCO_3	100·1
K Cl	74·6
K_3 Citrate (H_2O)	324·4
K Acetate	98·1
K_2 HPO_4	174·2
NH_4 Cl	53·5
Ca CO_3	50·0
Ca gluconate (H_2O)	448·4
Ca Cl_2	111·0
Ca Lactate ($5H_2O$)	308·3
Mannitol	180·0
Glucose	180·2

Index